INTERNATIONAL PERSPECTIVES IN PHYSICAL THERAPY 8

Muscle Strength

SERIES EDITORS

Ida Bromley MBE FCSP

Ida Bromley is a freelance consultant in London. From 1979–1986 she was the manager of the physiotherapy service for the Hampstead Health Authority in London. She has also worked in Australia, and for many years was in charge of physiotherapy at the Stoke Mandeville Hospital in England. She has lectured and run workshops in many countries including Turkey, U.S.A., South Africa and Australia, and written articles for several journals on subjects ranging from 'Rehabilitation of the Severely Disabled' to 'Problem Oriented Medical Recording and Audit'. She is also author of a well-known textbook, *Tetraplegia and Paraplegia.* From 1978–1982, she was Chairman of the Council of the Chartered Society of Physiotherapy. She is a past President of the Organization of District Physiotherapists and the Society for Research in Rehabilitation.

Nancy Theilgaard Watts RPT PhD

Nancy Watts is Professor Emerita at the MGH Institute of Health Professions at Massachusetts General Hospital in Boston. A physical therapy teacher for over 30 years, since 1965 most of her work has been in establishing advanced study programs for experienced therapists. Her major academic interests and publications concern methods of clinical teaching, economics of health care, and analysis of the process of judgment used by clinicians. Her clinical research has varied widely, ranging from studies of the effects of cold on spasticity to cost-effectiveness comparisons of different methods of treatment for common orthopaedic disorders. Dr Watts has served on a number of national and international commissions, and frequently teaches and consults in Britain, Scandinavia, and Latin America. She has also helped to prepare physical therapy teachers for schools in over 20 different countries.

VOLUME EDITOR

Karin Harms-Ringdahl Dr Med Sc RPT
Dr Karin Harms-Ringdahl qualified as a physiotherapist from the medical university Karolinska Institute, from where she also graduated as a Doctor in Medical Science. After a long period as clinician specializing in manual therapy, she is now an associate professor in physiotherapy at the Department of Rehabilitation Medicine, Karolinska Institute, Stockholm, Sweden. She is a senior lecturer in the postgraduate preresearch programme in physiotherapy. She was a member of the Kinesiology Research Group at the Karolinska Institute during her doctoral studies and her research is still focused particularly upon rehabilitation, occupational biomechanics, exercise biomechanics and assessments of load-elicited pain. Dr Harms-Ringdahl is the author of many scientific articles.

For Churchill Livingstone:
Publisher: Mary Law
Project Editor: Dinah Thom
Copy Editor: Andrew Gardiner
Indexer: Helen McKillop
Production Controller: Mark Sanderson
Sales Promotion Executive: Hilary Brown

INTERNATIONAL PERSPECTIVES IN PHYSICAL THERAPY 8

Muscle Strength

Edited by

Karin Harms-Ringdahl Dr Med Sc RPT
Associate Professor and Senior Lecturer in Physiotherapy, Department of Rehabilitation Medicine, Karolinska Institute, Stockholm, Sweden

CHURCHILL LIVINGSTONE
EDINBURGH LONDON MADRID MELBOURNE NEW YORK AND TOKYO 1993

CHURCHILL LIVINGSTONE
Medical Division of Longman Group UK Limited

Distributed in the United States of America by Churchill Livingstone Inc., 650 Avenue of the Americas, New York, N.Y. 10011, and by associated companies, branches and representatives throughout the world.

First published 1993

British Library of Cataloguing in Publication Data
A catalogue record for this book is available from the British Library.

Library of Congress Cataloging in Publication Data
Muscle strength/edited by Karin Harms-Ringdahl.
p. cm. — (International perspectives in physical therapy; 8)
Includes bibliographical references and index.
ISBN 0-443-04336-1
1. Muscle strength. 2. Physical therapy.
I. Harms-Ringdahl, Karin. II. Series.
[DNLM: 1. Muscles—physiology. W1 IN827JM v. 8 / WE 500 M9847]
QP321.M8945 1993
615.8'2—dc20
DNLM/DLC
for Library of Congress

92-48964

The publisher's policy is to use **paper manufactured from sustainable forests**

Produced by Longman Singapore Publishers (Pte) Ltd
Printed in Singapore

Contents

Contributors

Richard W Bohannon PT EdD NCS
Dr Richard Bohannon, a board certified specialist in neurologic physical therapy, is an associate professor at the University of Connecticut (Storrs, Connecticut) and the Coordinator for Clinical Research in the Department of Rehabilitation of Hartford Hospital (Hartford, Connecticut). He received his Bachelor and Master of Science degrees in Physical Therapy at the University of North Carolina, and his Doctor of Education degree at North Carolina State University. He is the author of more than 100 scholarly publications and serves on numerous editorial boards. His involvement in patient care, which spans more than 12 years, is primarily with patients who have suffered strokes.

Jan Ekholm MD PhD
Dr Jan Ekholm is Professor of Medical Rehabilitation, particularly Physical Medicine, at the Karolinska Institute and the Head of the Department of Rehabilitation Medicine at the Karolinska Hospital, Stockholm, Sweden. He published his first studies on joint sensory physiology in the early 1960s. Since then he has published a great number of studies about functions and biomechanics of joints and muscles, and about pain. During the 1970s he founded the Kinesiology Research Group of the Karolinska Institute, and as its director he has supervised physical therapists in their research studies and been involved in higher education of physical therapists.

Bette Ann Harris MS PT
Bette Ann Harris has been a member of the faculty at MGH Institute of Allied Health Professions, Boston, MA, USA, since 1985. As Assistant Professor and Interim Director, Graduate Program in Physical Therapy, her primary responsibilities include coordinating the orthopaedics/sports specialization, coordinating the advanced clinical practicum and teaching concepts in orthopaedics, muscle physiology and radiology for physical therapists. She also is a clinical consultant and clinical research associate in the Department of Physical Therapy at Massachusetts General Hospital, Boston. She earned a Bachelor of Science degree and Certificate of Physical Therapy in 1972 from Simmons College and a Master of Science degree in 1983 from the MGH Institute of Health Professions. She has conducted and published descriptive, methodological and experimental studies in the areas of orthopaedics, physical therapy treatment and measurement of muscle performance.

Kathleen A Hinderer MS MPT PT
Kathy Hinderer obtained her Bachelor of Science degree and Certificate in Physical Therapy from the University of Michigan in 1980. She received her advanced Master of Physical Therapy degree in 1986 and Master of Science degree in Rehabilitation Medicine in 1988 from the University of Washington in Seattle. She has had extensive clinical experience with pediatric and adult rehabilitation clients using

traditional manual muscle testing and quantitative myometry techniques for strength measurement. Additionally, Kathy has conducted five research studies examining the reliability and validity of manual muscle testing as compared to myometry. She is currently a doctoral candidate in the Division of Movement Science at the University of Michigan, Ann Arbor.

Steven R Hinderer MD MS PT

Dr Steve Hinderer obtained his Bachelor of Science degree and Certificate in Physical Therapy in 1978, and his MD degree in 1983 from the University of Michigan. He completed physical medicine and rehabilitation residency training in 1986 and a PM&R research fellowship in 1987 at the University of Washington in Seattle. He was a faculty member in the PM&R Department at the University of Michigan from 1987–1990 and has been on the faculty in the PM&R Department at Wayne State University in Detroit, Michigan from 1990 to the present. Dr Hinderer is the Medical Director of Research at the Rehabilitation Institute of Michigan, where he is helping to develop a clinical rehabilitation research unit. The primary emphasis of the research unit is quantification of human function and performance, including quantification of muscle strength. He has been a coinvestigator on several research studies assessing the reliability and validity of traditional manual muscle testing versus myometry.

Vladimir Janda MD

Dr Vladimir Janda graduated from the Charles University, Faculty of Medicine, in Prague, Czechoslovakia in 1952, and specialized in neurology and rehabilitation medicine. Currently he is a Professor of Neurology and Rehabilitation Medicine, Charles University, Director of the Department of Rehabilitation Medicine, University Hospital Prague 10, and Director, Chair of Rehabilitation Medicine, Postgraduate Medical Institute, Prague. He is responsible for the Physiotherapy School, a branch of the 3rd Medical Faculty. Dr Janda has published 14 books and around 150 scientific papers, and has lectured in almost all of the European countries, as well as the USA, Canada and Australia. He is a visiting professor at the Physiotherapy Department, University of Queensland, Brisbane, Australia. For many years he has been a consultant to the WHO in rehabilitation medicine.

Anne Elisabeth Ljunggren PhD PT

Dr Anne Elisabeth Ljunggren qualified as a physiotherapist in Norway in 1964 and received her PhD in functional anatomy in 1977. After varied clinical practice and postgraduate studies in Scandinavia, she is now a senior lecturer with an emphasis on anatomy and biomechanics, low back pain and research methodology. In 1986 she was elected as a member of the International Society for the Study of the Lumbar Spine. She is also an author of several scientific papers on pain description and clinical trials on lumbago-sciatica. At present she is Research Physiotherapist at the Clinical Research Unit, Ullevål University Hospital, Oslo, and Professor in the program of the Master of Science Degree in Physiotherapy, University of Bergen, Norway.

Esko Mälkiä PhD PT BA

Dr Esko Mälkiä is Assistant Professor in Physiotherapy, specializing in special education and adapted physical activity. He is the Director of the MSc and PhD program in PT at the Department of Health Sciences, University of Jyväskylä, Finland. His research work centres on physical performance in aging and in different occupations, especially concerning ergonomics in forest and agricultural work. His rehabilitation studies concern neuromuscular and pulmonary diseases and low back pain. His main interests lie in the abilities of different populations, exercise therapy and research strategies in PT. Clinically, he has worked within the fields of physiotherapy and rehabilitation of patients with neuromuscular diseases.

Dianne J Newham MCSP MPhil PhD

Dr Dianne J Newham trained for physiotherapy as a mature student at The Prince of Wales School of Physiotherapy in London, having worked previously as a laboratory technician in England and Nigeria. On qualification, she worked as a basic grade physiotherapist and then as a senior in neurology and human metabolism at University College Hospital, London. This was followed by a period of full time research over ten years in the departments of Medicine and then Physiology at University College, London. During this time she acquired an MPhil and a PhD. In 1989 she was appointed as a Reader in Physiotherapy and Head of the Physiotherapy Group at Kings College, London (Biomedical Sciences Division). Her research interests are human skeletal muscle — function, fatigue and control.

Mary P Watkins MS PT

Mary P Watkins has been a member of the faculty at Hanemann University, Philadelphia, PA, USA since 1980. As Associate Professor, her primary teaching responsibilities have included kinesiology, clinical evaluation of the neuromuscular system and clinical research processes. She earned a Bachelor of Science degree in 1959 and a Master of Science degree in 1974 from Boston University. She has conducted and published descriptive and experimental studies in the areas of primary muscle disease and orthopaedics. Former appointments include Assistant Professor at Northeastern University, Boston, Research Physical Therapist at Case Western Reserve University, Cleveland, Ohio and Clinical Research Associate at the Massachusetts General Hospital, Boston.

Birgitta Öberg Dr Med Sc RPT

Dr Birgitta Öberg is a Senior Lecturer in the Department of Caring Sciences, in the Faculty of Health Sciences, Linköping University, Linköping, Sweden. She is also Head of the Department for Development of care at the Linköping University Hospital. Dr Öberg is a registered physiotherapist and graduated in 1973. Her postgraduate education was at the University of Linköping, where she earned a Doctor in Medical Science degree in 1984. Her dissertation, in the field of sports medicine, was titled *Lower Extremity Muscle Strength in Soccer Players.* Her present research concerns methods for evaluation of flexibility, strength and functional performance to be used within the development of rehabilitation programs for patients with musculoskeletal and neurological disorders.

About the Series

The purpose of this series of books is to provide an international exchange of ideas and to explore different approaches in professional therapy practice. The books are written primarily for experienced clinicians. They are not intended as basic texts nor as reports on the most recent research, though elements of these aspects may be included.

Articles written by experts from a number of different countries form the core of each volume. These are supported by a commentary on the current 'state of the art' in the particular area of practice and an annotated bibliography of key references.

Each volume covers a topic which we believe to be of universal interest. Some are concerned with a troublesome symptom; others are related to problems within a broad diagnostic category, for example this volume.

I. B
N. T. W.

Preface

The intention with many therapeutic exercises is to improve muscle function and muscle strength, often of great concern to physical therapists and their patients. Sometimes strengthening exercises are also used for reducing load-induced pain or for pain prevention. However, many current textbooks describe muscle strength and exercise programs for healthy people from a *sports* perspective, and this may not always be relevant in rehabilitation programs for injured or disabled people. This book adopts a *physiotherapeutic* perspective on the function of muscular strength as it applies in rehabilitation and secondary prevention. The intention is to give basic information about muscle strength; how muscle strength can be measured; the relations between strength and functional capacity and between strength and pain; to consider biomechanical viewpoints on exercises. How strength is related to different age groups and to some patient groups where therapeutic exercises might be used is also described. Some examples of exercise protocols are given. Another aim has been to summarize research results elucidating different aspects of muscle strength, in order to provide physical therapists wishing to evaluate their treatments with a tool for their studies.

I am grateful to Professor Nancy Watts and Miss Ida Bromley, editors of the Churchill Livingstone Series *International Perspectives in Physical Therapy*, for their constructive support during the preparation of this volume, and to the authors for their cooperation and their contributions. The cooperation of the staff of Churchill Livingstone has also been much appreciated.

Stockholm 1993 K.H-R

1. Introduction

Karin Harms-Ringdahl

Twenty-five years ago, muscle strength was a rather 'easy' concept in physical therapy. It was evaluated by the physical therapist with their hands, and usually rated as *normal, reduced* or *none (paralyzed).* Sometimes a dynamometer was used, isometric strength being measured at one joint angle with the subject lying down. For strengthening exercises, manual resistance was applied in motion patterns enhancing proprioneuromuscular facilitation (PNF), or isometrically in a pain free part of the motion sector. Very often, the patient was supine or prone and the exercises were given 10–15 times in half hour sessions.

From research during the intervening years, we have learned much of importance concerning the complex relationship between muscular strength and performance and function. We have learned that muscular strength performance is specific, i.e. that muscular strength improvement will be greatest for the strength modality exercised. Thus isometric exercises give isometric strength, concentric exercises improve concentric strength, most of all for the angular speed exercised. Strength is not a valid measurement of function if isometric measurements at one joint angle are compared with measurements of dynamic performance over a range of movement angles. Analyses of performance at work and in leisure must be used to set the goal with regard to the exercise modality. Here the requirements may be sustained high load with few repetitions or endurance during continuous or repetitive contractions at rather low load levels but for more prolonged periods. Is the strength needed for isometric contractions, concentric contractions or eccentric contractions — and at what joint angles?

If strength is defined as the net muscular moment of force about a joint axis, and not as the gross force in single muscles, it is also possible to analyze how strength is influenced by pain and neurological disabilities. Besides using strengthening exercises, increased strength and function can thus be obtained by interventions aiming to reduce pain or spasticity.

Electromyography studies have shown that different muscles are very rarely activated alone. Usually there is coactivation at different levels during the motion range both in agonists and antagonists. Although the same subject tends to activate muscles similarly on different occasions during the same task, there is wide variation among subjects in muscular activation and the contribution of the various muscles to exert an induced load moment. In view of the modern theories about motor learning and movement performance, where the task being performed governs the movement performance, we have to ask ourselves whether strengthening exercises with the subject lying supine represents the optimal way to improve strength for performance in other postures, involving both stabilizing of joints and different movement speeds. However, we also have to recognize the different phases in rehabilitation. If the strength is insufficient for postural support, we might need to start increasing muscle mass or to compensate for postural stability. During the polio period, the supine position was the only way to establish safe posture; but when enough strength is available to support the body segments, we need to exercise strength and endurance in situations as similar as possible to those in which the muscular performance is going to be required.

Studies of muscular activity levels in relation to strength further show the impossibility of predicting activity levels in single muscles from strength measurements, or vice versa. Although muscle activity discharge as measured in microvolts is related to strength as measured in Newton metres, the two concepts are entirely different. This is because, e.g. EMG activity increases with speed during concentric contractions while muscular strength decreases. Further, the strength–activity relationship is sometimes linear, sometimes non-linear. Hence, relative muscle activity levels can be underestimated from induced load moment calculations and strength measurements. In addition, the EMG activity levels say nothing about how the load is shared between muscle activity and connective tissue structures.

The use of computers has developed strength measurement methods. Thus, it is now possible to measure strength in a reliable way, isometrically, concentrically and eccentrically at determined joint angles and angular speeds. Moreover, it is possible to measure fatigue and endurance in muscle groups for the same kinds of contraction. However, the necessary devices are large and expensive and can not usually be used in ordinary clinical settings. Also, many devices only allow motions in defined planes where, e.g. a rotational component during flexing-extending movements cannot be taken into consideration. Functional tests, where strength and endurance requirements are analyzed, number of repetitions measured, performance timed and perceived load and fatigue assessed offers another way of developing reliable and valid tests of muscular performance. Many of the chapters in this book deal with this issue.

In designing exercises for improving strength and endurance, the load level chosen, number of repetitions and the duration of the exercise period seem important. If the load is too low, no strength will occur; if too high, there will be a risk of overloading weak structures. If the repetitions are too few, endurance will not improve. If the exercises are not similar to the load requirements in daily life, no improvement in function will be obtained. Over the first three weeks, strength improvements are due mainly to improved neuromuscular function, and to other factors such as decreased pain or decreased spasticity. Hypertrophy of muscle cells requires exercises over 8–12 weeks. Muscle insertions and tendons weakened by trauma or disuse require longer (6–12 months) than muscle fibres for strength quality to be normalized. Another question is where therapeutic interventions end — when the patient has required adequate function for activities of daily life, for work or for continuing with different sport activities? Thus the goals and duration of the exercise period have to be carefully determined and discussed with the patient before being settled.

Many strengthening exercises focus on isometric and/or concentric contractions, whereas almost all movements in daily activities also involve eccentric contractions. Hence more emphasis is needed on exercises for improving eccentric muscular function. In addition, it seems clear that exercise dosage still needs much investigation, as recovery after fatiguing exertion takes longer than for other types of contractions.

Strength and endurance is often decreased in patients with long lasting pain conditions. Exercises are often used as one of the interventions. Theories from behavioural medicine suggest that it is very important to find out what activities the patient can do and to set realistic goals for training. Other important components of training seem to be the promotion of anti-pain behaviour, group exercise at a tempo that can be maintained for a working day, and exercise with work-related activities/movements.

This book describes different notions of muscle strength as used by physical therapists. Basic knowledge and recent research are presented as well as measurement methods used by clinicians and researchers. Training principles and biomechanical aspects of exercise are included. Some conditions in life which influence muscle strength are also described, e.g. childhood, adolescence, aging, implications for sport and work, painful conditions, and the situation after stroke.

2. Muscle performance: principles and general theory

Bette Ann Harris   Mary P. Watkins

INTRODUCTION

Muscle strength can be defined as the ability of skeletal muscle to develop force for the purpose of providing stability and mobility within the musculoskeletal system, so that functional movement can take place. This definition, however, implies not only force production in magnitude (intensity), but also the ability to maintain force for a period of time (endurance). The more general term *muscle performance* permits us to consider conceptually the role of skeletal muscle, because the requirements of 'strength', or the magnitude of force production, and 'endurance' are interrelated when analyzing human musculoskeletal function.

In order to understand the complex role of skeletal muscle in movement, we need to consider the anatomical and physiological components of muscle, and biomechanics. Furthermore, we need to understand the role of the central nervous system. The ability to generate force can be viewed as a dynamic interaction among muscle components, excitation-contraction processes, types of motor units, size of motor units, frequency and pattern of motor units discharge, neural recruitment and metabolic support (aerobic and anaerobic). If there is an abnormality affecting these interactions, then we would expect a change in the ability of a muscle to generate force. Other factors affect muscle performance such as age, training, motivation, immobilization, inactivity and pathology. Consideration of all of these elements enables us to be specific in our therapeutic approaches for enhancing functional movement. The purpose of this chapter is to review muscle structure and physiology and their relationship to normal functional movement starting from a basic level. We will also discuss current research in terms of its clinical applicability.

ANATOMICAL AND PHYSIOLOGICAL COMPONENTS OF SKELETAL MUSCLE

Types of muscle contraction

When skeletal muscle contracts, force is generated; however, the effect on the skeletal levers varies depending upon the amount of force generated in relation to externally applied forces on the lever system. Three types of skeletal muscle contractions can be observed. If the force generated by a muscle is greater than the externally applied forces, the muscle will shorten in *concentric* contraction. If the force generated by a muscle is equal to the externally applied forces, no motion will take place: an *isometric* contraction. If the force generated by the muscle is less than the externally applied force, the muscle will lengthen while maintaining its tension: *eccentric* contraction. In this latter case, the effect of this contraction is to control the moving lever from accelerating as it is being subjected to external forces. These different types of muscle contractions allow skeletal muscles to function as springs, movers, shock absorbers and stabilizers.

Each of these contractions has different properties related to metabolic requirements, force capabilities and central nervous system control. Until recently, much of our understanding of the differences among these contractions has been from research using muscle preparations from animal models. With the development of isokinetic testing devices and other objective muscle performance testing instruments, we are beginning to gain a better understanding of the differences in these types of contractions in human subjects.

Contractile elements of skeletal muscle

The contractile elements of skeletal muscle are the muscle fibres (cells). The muscle cell is cylindrically shaped, multinucleated and covered with a plasma membrane called the sarcolemma. Each muscle cell is usually innervated by a single motor neuron. The major subcellular division of the muscle fibre is the myofibril which has a longitudinal orientation and is composed of repeated sarcomeres.

The sarcomere is the basic contractile unit of the muscle cell. Heavy dense lines, called Z lines, define the boundaries of each sarcomere. Thin and thick filaments located within the sarcomere are arranged to give the muscle fibre its striated appearance. The thick myosin filaments have projections which, when activated, form crossbridges with the thin actin filaments during muscle contraction.

Voluntary contraction of skeletal muscle is the result of a series of events beginning with the excitation of cells in the motor cortex. The resultant action potentials are delivered to the anterior horn cells in fibres of the corticospinal tract. Concurrent interactions between the cortex, basal ganglia, cerebellum and less discrete areas of the reticular formation influence the impact of descending information to cause either facilitation or inhibition of those anterior horn cells. When the sum of excitatory postsynaptic potentials is adequate for depolarization of anterior horn cells, the process which creates muscular contraction has begun.

Muscle cells are surrounded by a weblike sarcoplasmic reticulum which communicates with the muscle membrane and the T tubules, which penetrate into the sarcomeres. When the nerve action potentials arrive at the myoneural junction of each muscle cell, acetylcholine (Ach) is released and diffuses across the synaptic cleft. Ach channels on the postsynaptic membrane open, permitting passage of sodium ions (Na^+) and potassium ions (K^+), which create a muscle action potential. The muscle action potential travels via the sarcoplasmic reticulum and T tubular systems, making contact with stored pockets of calcium (Ca^{2+}) along the Z lines of the sarcomeres. Ca^{2+} is then released into the sarcomere and acts as the catalyst responsible for the crossbridge formation between the actin and myosin molecules, and tension is generated. The series of events from the electrical activity of depolarization to the chemical activity creating the actin-myosin bonds is called *excitation-contraction coupling.*

The magnitude of tension developed is affected by the number of crossbridges formed in the process. In an elongated or stretched muscle, few filaments are able to make contact, and little tension can be developed. As sarcomeres are allowed to shorten more crossbridges are formed, hence greater tension is developed. If sarcomeres are in a very shortened position or compressed state, tension will be lower because actin filaments overlap, interfering with available binding sites for myosin. This phenomenon is in part responsible for the length tension curve which is discussed later in this chapter (Knuttgen 1980).

The tension created by the actin-myosin bonds will continue as long as Ca^{2+} ions are present. Relaxation depends on the return of calcium to the sarcoplasmic reticulum, which occurs by a pumping action. Within muscle, both contraction and relaxation utilize adenosine triphosphate as the fuel to support these chemical events. ATP in skeletal muscle is derived from the processes of glycolysis and oxidative phosphorylation. These biochemical processes are mentioned as a reminder that medical conditions which interfere with delivery, as in cardiorespiratory disorders, or in synthesis of required component metabolic substrates, as in diabetes mellitus, will have a negative impact on a patient's ability to improve functional muscle performance (Astrand & Rodahl 1986).

Non-contractile elements of skeletal muscle

The contractile components of muscle are connected in series with the non-contractile components, namely the matrix and sarcoplasmic reticulum. There is also a parallel elastic component of connective tissue which surrounds the actin and myosin contractile fibres. Each muscle fibre is covered by a fine connective tissue, the endomysium. Muscle fibres are grouped into bundles surrounded by the perimysium. These bundles are then encased in fibrous connective tissue, the epimysium. These structures, taken together, merge at the peripheral ends of muscles to form the myotendinous junction. The attachment of the tendon to bone completes the structural chain which allows for movements during muscular contraction.

The non-contractile components of skeletal muscle also contribute to force production. The parallel elastic component is activated when the muscle is stretched beyond its so-called resting length. When the contractile components within the muscle fibres shorten, the surrounding connective tissue actually lengthens. The elastic properties of this connective tissue matrix function to dampen the effects on the contractile unit and contribute to smooth muscle function. The passive elastic properties of non-contractile components allow for energy to be stored. The efficient use of this stored energy can increase human muscle performance. The stretch shortening cycle as described by Komi (1986) utilizes this stored energy for subsequent muscle contraction. This type of action occurs in activities such as running and jumping, when a concentric contraction is immediately preceded by an eccentric contraction.

MUSCLE FIBRE TYPES

The purpose of skeletal muscle contraction is to produce appropriate amounts of force at the appropriate speeds to accomplish functional movement. Governed by the central nervous system and modulated by sensory feedback mechanism, the entire musculoskeletal system acts by coordination and intricate cooperation among many groups of muscles for any specific functional activity. As a feature of cooperation and coordination, some muscles are enlisted more often to provide stability, while others are enlisted more often to provide dynamic mobility. For example, the soleus and back extensor muscles are required to contract isometrically with gentle shifts between concentric and eccentric contractions to maintain standing posture. They may need to be active for long periods of time but the magnitude of force and speed of contraction may be low, if the mechanical alignment of the musculoskeletal system is normal. When lifting a box from floor to a table the function of these muscles, with the addition of the gluteus maximus, quadriceps and upper extremity, is very different from their actions in maintaining a standing posture. In this case, high concentric forces must be generated dynamically in the muscles.

To meet such varied performance requirements, skeletal muscle is composed of fibre types which vary structurally, histochemically and metabolically (Astrand & Rodahl 1986, Baldwin 1983). The distributions of fibre types within any given muscle is determined by neural influences, use and perhaps in part by genetic predisposition (Komi 1986, Henneman & Olson 1965, Thorstennsen et al 1976, Johnson et al 1973, Komi et al 1977). Several classification schemes have been described over the years, refleting characteristics related to physiological or metabolic properties (Saltin et al 1977, Costill 1976, Thorstenssen 1977). Most of the data on fibre types have been derived from animal studies and, therefore, direct application to human muscle performance may be conjectural at best. However, a number of elements are worthy of consideration in relating skeletal muscle function to muscle fibre types.

Two major categories of skeletal muscle, Type I and Type II, have been extensively studied and illustrate clear distinguishing features. These categories are based on histological, biochemical and contractile characteristics. The Type II fibres are subdivided on the basis of metabolic pathways into IIA and IIB subclasses. A third type, Type IIC, has been identified in fetal muscle and in newborns. Studies have reported an incidence of 10–50% Type IIC in newborns, diminishing to 2% within the first year of life. IIC fibres have also been found in denervated and reinnervated muscle. These fibres may represent undifferentiated or dedifferentiated fibres in transition (Brooke & Kaiser 1970).

Table 2.1 Distinguishing characteristics of fibre types of skeletal muscle

Characteristic	Type I (red)	Type II (white)
Diameter	Smaller (27 μm)	Larger (44 μm)
Myoglobin content	High	Low
Mitochondria	High	Low
Sarcoplasmic reticulum	Less developed	Highly developed
Blood supply	High capillary to fibre ratio	Less extensive
Motor end plate	Smaller	Large, flat with deep regular junctions
Nerve fibre diameter	Smaller	Larger
Motor unit size	Small	Large
Major pathway for energy production	Kreb's cycle (oxidative phosphorylation)	Glycolysis
Major substrate	Mainly fats	Carbohydrate
Nerve conduction velocity	Low	High
Contraction time	Longer (85 ms)	Short (25 ms)
Tension	Low	High
Endurance	Long period of sustained contraction	Fatigues easily

Comparison of the characteristics of these two major fibre types is shown in Table 2.1. Nerve fibre diameter, and therefore nerve conduction velocity, of the two types differs. The Type I cell body is smaller and more easily activated based on the size principle of recruitment, which states that during graded muscular contraction from low to higher force, the smaller motor units will be recruited first, followed by progressively larger units. Therefore, when low tension is required, the Type I or slow twitch fibres are recruited first. When there are demands for increasing or high tension, the larger Type II or fast twitch fibres are recruited. This size principle applies during sustained, gradually rising tension development. In more twitch like contractions or during brief bursts of high tension recruitment, the order may differ. High threshold larger units theoretically could be recruited first or simultaneously (Henneman et al 1965). With the highly developed sarcoplasmic reticulum and large motor end plates, the spread of motor action potentials is fast and extensive in Type II fibres. The combination of these factors with the rapid nerve conduction velocity results in shorter contraction time of Type II fibres (25 ms versus 85 ms). These characteristics also relate to the speed of tension development.

There are also characteristics with result in differences in the magnitude of contraction. The magnitude of tension development is affected by muscle fibre diameter and motor unit size. Higher tension is developed in Type II fibres because of the larger fibre diameter and motor unit size compared to the Type I fibres (Astrand & Rodahl 1986, Gollnick et al 1973). Metabolic support systems of the two major fibre types influence fatiguability. Type I fibres depend primarily on aerobic metabolism (oxidative phosphorylation) for energy supply. The demand for oxygen is met by the high myoglobin content, high number of mitochondria and high capillary to muscle fibre ratio. Type IIB fibres primarily use the process of glycolysis. This energy supply is immediate, but limited. The process is anaerobic and cannot be sustained for long periods of time. The Type IIA fibres are capable of utilizing both anaerobic and aerobic pathways and their fatiguability falls in between the Type I and IIB fibre (Holloszy & Booth 1976).

To summarize in functional terms, Type I fibres are better suited for long sustained periods of activity at low tension levels such as walking, long distance running and most functional activities of daily living. Type II fibres fatigue easily but are better suited for rapid, high power explosive contractions such as heavy lifting activities. Physical therapists need to be aware of the specificity of these fibre types when planning therapeutic exercise programmes. Training programmes will be most effective if the types of contractions they emphasize are matched to those types of functional tasks the patient will need to perform. For example, with an older patient whose functional goal is to be ambulatory in the community and independent in performing households tasks, a program geared to low load, high repetitions may be appropriate to achieve these goals. However, a 35-year-old construction worker, whose job involves lifting heavy loads, may need a strengthening component to challenge the Type II fibres to increase force development. The addition of an aerobic conditioning programme for both types of patients will serve to increase the amount of oxygen available to the muscle to sustain activity over time.

FUNCTIONAL BIOMECHANICS

Length-tension relationships

Blix (1892-1895) described the effect of muscle length on the capacity of muscle to develop tension, showing that muscle in a very shortened or very lengthened state generates less force than in mid-ranges. The resultant length-tension curve was discussed in terms of lengthening or shortening relative to the 'resting length' of muscle. Blix's work was based on isolated muscle preparations and length changes were imposed passively. The maximum amount of force at each tested length was produced by applying electrical stimulation to tetany.

Human muscle, in situ, also displays a length-tension curve under both dynamic and static conditions. We are able to describe the curves in relation to joint angle, assuming that muscle changes length with the change in rotation of bony levers. The shape of the curve for each individual muscle varies somewhat from Blix's original description which was based on the behavior of muscle alone. The factors responsible for this variability in situ include not only sarcomere length, and the number of overlapping cross-bridges, but also the structural relationships of muscle to tendon and tendon to bone. In situ, the curves are measured by recording the force of the rotary component applied through the anatomical lever to the force recording device. Therefore, the curve only reflects that applied rotary force of the contracting muscle. Depending on the angle of muscle force application on the bony lever, there is also either a compressive or distracting force vector in addition to the rotary vector. Therefore, in situ, total muscle force is not recorded. Furthermore, in the extreme lengthened range, non-contractile (passive) musculotendinous elements contribute to the recorded force.

Length-tension curves can be demonstrated for all three types of muscle contractions. Singh and Karpovich (1966) demonstrated that at a given joint angle, human muscles (specifically elbow flexors and extensors) could develop more dynamic tension during maximal voluntary eccentric muscle action than during maximal voluntary concentric or isometric muscle actions. Bennett and Stauber (1986) reported similar results when testing the quadriceps. However, the absolute force differences among the types of contractions for the quadriceps were not as great as those found for the elbow musculature. The differences in force capability may be specific to the muscle being tested, the test instrument joint angles at which the muscles are tested.

Force velocity

The magnitude of muscle force is affected also by speed of contraction (Hill 1938, Katz, 1939). The original experiments by Hill (1938) using isolated muscle preparations, demonstrated that during concentric contractions, the magnitude of force generated declines with increasing speed of contraction. Thorstenssen et al (1976) demonstrated the same force-velocity relationship in healthy men for maximal concentric contractions of the quadriceps femoris tested at the angular velocities of 15, 30, 60, 90 and 180 degrees per second, using an isokinetic device which controls the velocity at which a limb can move.

The original laboratory studies also documented that during eccentric contraction, force production increases with increasing speed of contraction. In human subjects, preliminary data have shown that the eccentric force production will not rise with increasing speed; in fact, at higher velocities, force may decline (Hodson & Johnson 1990). This may reflect that other factors, such as soft tissue constraints and central motor control, are limiting the amount of eccentric force that human subjects will tolerate voluntarily (Stauber 1989).

Although eccentric force exceeds concentric force when tested at any given velocity, studies have shown that muscle activity recorded by integrated electromyography (IEMG) is less during eccentric contractions than during concentric activity. Consistent with these findings, energy expenditure of working muscle, measured by oxygen uptake, is less during eccentric contractions than during concentric contractions (Komi & Bosco 1978, Komi 1986). Although the physiologic explanation for this phenomenon is incomplete, it may reflect the greater contribution of passive elastic tension resulting from stretching imposed by external forces during eccentric contraction.

CLINICAL CONSIDERATIONS

The maintenance of force capabilities of skeletal muscle depends upon use through daily activity or exercise and intact neuromuscular mechanisms. The ability of skeletal muscle to develop force will diminish for a variety of reasons including disuse, immobilization and local pathology affecting the musculotendinous unit or joints. In addition, comorbidity factors such as the presence of systemic disease, medication, nutritional status, age, motivation and previous level of fitness may influence the ability to develop muscle force. When evaluating muscle status, all of these factors must be taken into account to plan an appropriate course of therapeutic intervention. This section will focus on the physiologic responses of muscle to local factors affecting performance. Other chapters in this text will discuss the effects of age related changes, specific disease processes and effects of previous conditioning.

Disease and immobilization

Skeletal muscle will atrophy when it is not used. Atrophy may be defined as a decrease in whole muscle cross-sectional area or a loss of muscle mass. Much of our understanding about the effects of disuse come from studies using the experimental model of immobilizing healthy animal limbs. In general, when there is a decreased demand for muscular contraction, as in immobilization and disuse, changes in muscle include decreases in myofibrillar proteins, phosphocreatine, glycogen, potassium and the enzymes necessary for both glycolysis and oxidative phosphorylation. Capillary density, and therefore oxygen uptake, is diminished. There is evidence of thinning of the sarcolemma and connective tissue with a resultant loss of elasticity. All of these factors reduce both the aerobic and anaerobic capacity of the inactive muscles resulting in decreased endurance and decreased force (St. Pierre & Gardiner 1987). As a result of decreased neuromuscular activity and decreased sensory stimulation, especially during immobilization, there is diminished perception, motor coordination and muscle tone. As a part of this problem, there is little or no retention of previous training effects. Therapeutic exercise that addresses the components of both force and endurance can be effective in countering the effects of disuse.

The extent of these changes is dependent upon the duration of immobilization and the position of limb fixation as it affects muscle length. Generally, the rate of atrophy is rapid during the first few weeks of immobilization and then continues more slowly (Booth 1977). The greatest amount of atrophy occurs when the muscle is held in a shortened position (Gossman et al 1982). In the shortened position, adult muscle loses sarcomeres, which contributes to the diminished ability of the muscle to develop tension (Tardieu et al, 1980, 1982; Spector et al 1982). Following immobilization in the shortened position, techniques geared to restoring length should be instituted. As the muscle stretches out, more weakness may become apparent until it structurally readapts to a more normal length for optimal use. Muscle responds with less atrophy and may even hypertrophy when immobilized in a lengthened position. It appears that muscle responds to the chronic stretch by increasing the number of sarcomeres. A maintained lengthening of muscle results in a shift of the length tension curve so that the muscle will be developing maximal force at a different point in the range of motion as compared to healthy muscle (Gossman et al 1982). When the muscle is supposed to perform optimally in biomechanical terms at a particular joint angle, and its location of maximal tension has shifted away from that range, functional efficiency of that muscle may be compromised (Kendall & McCreary 1983). In this case, the technique of shortened held resisted contractions may be appropriate to facilitate muscle contraction in a more functional range.

To date, human studies are inconclusive as to whether disuse and immobilization selectively affect one muscle fibre type more than others (Haggmark et al 1983, Sargeant et al 1977, Young et al 1982). Loss of cross-sectional area of both Type I and Type II fibres has been reported. The findings relative to the proportional loss of one or the other fibre type may have been affected by selection of muscles studied, diagnosis, length of immobilization and age. For example, studies involving older subjects report a greater loss of Type II cross-sectional area following immobilization, but this finding may simply be a reflection of the effect of age alone (Sirca & Susec-Michieli 1977).

Local pathology

Local pathology involving connective tissue or joint structures can cause muscle atrophy and decreased muscle performance. The response of the body to musculoskeletal injury is in itself a cause of muscle atrophy. Muscle function is inhibited during the inflammatory process secondary to pain and swelling. Chemical mediators have a direct effect on inhibiting muscle through their activation of nociceptors. Investigators have studied the effects of knee effusions on quadriceps muscle performance in healthy subjects and in patients with chronic arthritis (Spencer et al 1984, Fahrer et al 1988). Fahrer measured isometric quadriceps strength in 13 patients with chronic knee effusions. Following aspiration of fluid, quadriceps strength increased an average of 13.6% in these patients. When lidocaine was injected into the knee joints, a further increase in strength was documented. These findings suggest that the mechanical deformation of tissue caused by effusion and afferent firing of joint receptors can influence muscle function. In the presence of active inflammation, such as joint effusion, vigorous resistive exercise is inappropriate. Intervention should be aimed at reducing the pain and inflammation.

The formation of scar tissue is the normal end point of healing and can be a primary cause of loss of connective tissue elasticity. Disuse, microtrauma, disease and aging also contribute to this loss. Loss of elasticity can occur within the tendon, at the musculotendinous junction or in the connective tissue matrix within skeletal muscle. The affected connective tissue is less capable of storing elastic energy and becomes less able to contribute to production of dynamic forces (Akeson et al 1977, Vidik 1973, Hardy 1989, Williams & Goldspink 1984).

Muscles are at risk of injury when scar tissue is formed because the healing (new) tissue is weaker until it has a chance to mature (Kellet 1986). Vigorous, heavy resistance exercise during the healing phase could place the muscle at risk for further damage, setting up a cycle of repeated trauma. However, passive motion and carefully controlled exercise stress have been shown to be effective for promoting tensile strength of non-contractile tissue (Clarkson & Tremblay 1988).

SUMMARY

In order to have optimal muscle performance both the contractile and non-contractile components of skeletal muscle must be structurally and physiologically sound. Optimal muscle performance is dependent upon an intact central nervous system and the efficient use of cardiopulmonary support systems. The expectation that therapeutic intervention will achieve optimal performance must be tempered by careful consideration and evaluation of the patient's problems. Gaining a greater understanding of the effects of pathology, disuse, aging, training and other comorbidity factors will enable physical therapists to plan effective treatment strategies and establish realistic goals. Other chapters in this text address many of these topics in depth.

The authors gratefully acknowledge Louise Ornstein for her assistance in typing this manuscript.

REFERENCES

Astrand P, Rodahl K 1986 Textbooks of work physiology: physiological basis of exercise. McGraw Hill

Baldwin K M 1983 Structural and functional organization of skeletal muscle. In: Bove, Lowenthal (eds) Exercise medicine. Academic Press, New York, p 3–18

Bennett J G, Stauber W T 1986 Evaluation and treatment of anterior knee pain using eccentric exercise. Medicine and Science of Sports Exercise 18: 526–530

Booth F W 1977 Time course of muscular atrophy during immobilization of hindlimbs of rats. Journal of Applied Physiology 43: 656–661

Brooke H M, Kaiser K K 1970 Muscle fibre types: how many and what kind? Archives of Neurology 23: 369–379

Clarkson P M, Tremblay I 1988 Exercise induced muscle damage, repair and adaptation in humans. American Physiological Society 1–6

Fahrer H, Rentsen H V, Gerber N J et al 1988 Knee effusion and reflex inhibition of the quadriceps. Journal of Bone & Joint Surgery 70-B: 636–638

Gollnick P D, Armstrong R B, Saltin B et al 1973 Effect of training on enzyme activity and fibre composition of human skeletal muscle. Journal of Applied Physiology 34: 107–111

Gossman M E, Sahrmann S A, Rose S J 1982 Review of length associated changes in muscle: experimental evidence and clinical implications. Physical Theraphy 62: 1799–1808

Haggmark T, Jansson E, Erikson E 1981 fibre type, area, metabolic potential of the thigh muscle in man after knee surgery and immobilization. International Journal of Sports Medicine 2: 12–17

Hardy M A 1989 The biology of scar formation. Physical Therapy 69: 1014–1024

Henneman E, Somjen G, Carpenter D D 1965 Functional significance of cell size in spinal motorneurons. Journal of Neurophysiology 28: 560–580

Henneman E, Olson C B 1965 Relations between structure and function in the design in skeletal muscles. Journal of Neurophysiology 28: 581–598

Hill A V 1938 The heat of shortening and the dynamic constraints of muscle. Proceedings of the Royal Society of London Serial B 126: 136–195

Hodson L I, Johnson E B 1990 Force-velocity relationship of quadriceps femoris in vivo. Masters Thesis, MGH Institute of Health Professions, Boston, MA

Holloszy J O, Booth F W 1976 Biochemical adaptations to endurance exercise in muscle. American Review of Physiology 38: 273–291

Johnson M A, Polgor J, Weightman D et al 1973 Data on the distribution of fibre types in thirty-six human muscles: an autopsy study. Journal of Neurological Science 18: 111–129

Katz B 1939 The relation between force and speed in muscular contraction. Journal of Physiology 96: 45–64

Kellett J 1986 Acute soft tissue injuries: a review of the literature. Medicine and Science of Sports Exercise 18: 489–500

Kendall F P, McCreary E 1983 Muscus: testing and function, 3rd edn. Wiliams & Wilkins, Baltimore, MD

Knuttgen H 1980 Development of muscular strength and endurance. In: Knuttgen H (ed) Neuromuscular mechanisms for therapeutic and conditioning exercise. University Park Press, Baltimore, MD p 99–100

Komi P V, Bosco C 1978 Utilization of stored elastic energy in leg extensor muscles by men and women. Medicine and Science in Sports 10(4): 261–265

Komi P V, Vitasalo J H, Haru et al 1977 Skeletal muscle fibres and muscle enyzme activities in monozygous and dizygous twins of both sexes. Acta Physiologica Scandinavica 100: 385–392

Komi P V 1986 The stretch-shortening cycle and human power output. In: Jones N L, McCartney N, McComas A J (eds) Human muscle power, human kinetics. Champlain, Illinois ch 3: 27 p 27–39

Komi P V 1986 Training of muscle strength and power: interaction of neuromotoric, hypertrophic and mechanical factors. International Journal of Sports Medicine 7: 10–15 (suppl)

Lemkuhl L D, Smith L K 1983 Brunnstrom's clinical kinesiology, 4th edn. FA Davis, Philadelphia, p 130

Saltin B, Henriksson J, Nygaard E 1977 fibre types and metabolic potentials of skeletal muscles in sedentary man and endurance runners. Annals of the New York Academy of Sciences 301: 3–29

Sargeant A J, Davies C T, Edwards R H et al 1977 Functional and structural changes after disuse of human muscle. Clinical Science and Molecular Medicine 52: 337–342

Singh M, Karpovich P V 1966 Isotonic and isometric forces of forearm flexors and extensors. Journal of Applied Physiology 21: 1435–1437

Sirca A, Susec-Michieli M 1977 Selective type II fibre muscular atrophy in patients with osteoarthritis of the hip. Journal of Neurological Science 301: 3–29

Spector S A, Simard C P, Founier M et al 1982 Architectural alterations of the rat hind-limb skeletal muscles immobilized at different lengths. Experimental Neurology 76: 94–110

Spencer J D et al 1984 Knee joint effusion and quadriceps reflex inhibition in man. Archives of Physical Medicine & Rehabilitation 65: 171–177

St. Pierre D, Gardiner P F 1987 The effect of immobilization and exercise on muscle function: a review. Physiotherapy, Canada 39: 24–35

Stauber W 1989 Eccentric action of muscles: physiology, injury and adaptation. Exercise and Sports Science Reviews, American College of Sports Medicine, Williams and Wilkins, 7: 157–185

Tardieu C, Tabary J C, Tabary C, Tardieu G 1982 Adaptation of connective tissue length to immobilization in the lengthened and shortened positions in the cat soreus muscle. Journal of Physiology (Paris) 78: 214–220

Tardieu C, Tabary J C, Tardieu G et al 1980 Adaptation of sarcomere number to the length imposed on the muscle. Advances in Physiological Science 24: 99–114

Thorstensson A, Grimby G, Karlsson J 1976 Force-velocity relations and fibre composition in human knee extensor muscles. Journal of Applied Physiology 40: 12–16

Thorstensson A, Grumby G, Karlsson J 1976 Force-velocity relations and fibre composition in human knee extensor muscles. Journal of Applied Physiology 40: 12–16

Vidik A 1973 Collagen cross linking alterations in joint contractures: changes in periarticular connective tissue collagen after nine weeks of immobilization. Connective Tissue Research 5(1): 15–19

Williams P, Goldspink G 1984 Connective tissue changes in immobilized muscle. Journal of Anatomy 138: 343–350

3. Evaluation of skeletal muscle performance

Mary P. Watkins, Bette Ann Harris

INTRODUCTION

The assessment of skeletal muscle performance has become an integral element of physical therapy practice. Identification and documentation of the capability or inability of muscle to generate and sustain force are needed as part of the description of a patient's status whenever normal physical performance is compromised. The information derived from testing is used to plan therapeutic intervention or determine therapeutic effectiveness and may contribute to the definition of the underlying pathology.

In selecting a method for testing, the clinician must consider the specific aspects of muscle function which need to be described. Generally, the functional deficit or treatment goal is a major factor in this determination. The older patient who has had a total knee replacement may need to be able to rise from sitting and climb stairs. These activities require sufficient concentric quadriceps femoris force to lift body weight through a definable range of motion. In this case, an isometric test at 60° of knee flexion will not provide relevant information. Perhaps this test would be appropriate for the downhill skier whose flexed knee position has to be sustained during a race.

The testing protocol should also be relevant to the purpose of testing. For example, if a patient has a suspected peripheral neuropathy, the purpose of testing is to document the level and distribution of involvement by identifying the muscles which are compromised. Testing should be comprehensive, screening musculature throughout the body. A complete manual muscle test might be a reasonable choice. The approach and instrument selected will be very different for testing the young athlete who is recovering from a period of single lower extremity immobilization and who has been independent, using crutches for all activities of daily living.

The athlete's deficit is limited and the goal will be to achieve normal strength and endurance of muscles in the involved extremity so that he or she can return to competition. Testing would have to include information about force, speed of contraction, work and the ability to perform work over a period of time. The clinician might consider utilizing isokinetic instrumentation, in this situation specifically to evaluate hip, knee and ankle musculature.

In order to obtain relevant and useful information about skeletal muscle performance, we must recognize the use and limitations of the several available testing procedures. In this chapter we will review the commonly used clinical measures of muscle performance and will begin with a discussion of general considerations which should be included in the process of selecting and utilizing an appropriate testing protocol.

GENERAL CONSIDERATIONS

The validity of information obtained by testing skeletal muscle performance depends upon three essential components: the patient, the examiner and the instrument.

All assessment procedures depend on the *voluntary* effort of the patient. The first consideration, therefore, is: Is the patient willing and able to be evaluated? Since most procedures include asking patients to do their 'best', 'most', 'maximum', the potential for getting this kind of response has to be determined. The patient must be able to understand instructions, be alert and positively motivated. General anxiety or fear that testing may be painful will interfere. This problem may be alleviated by careful, thoughtful communication between the clinician and patient. But there will be times when the patient, for whatever reason, simply will not cooperate. Smith et al (1989) demonstrated that when normal subjects consciously performed submaximal grip contractions, force values were inconsistent with repeated trials compared with sincere efforts to produce maximal contractions. This demonstrates the negative impact of patient cooperation on the reliability of measuring maximum voluntary contraction.

A patient's medical condition may preclude accurate assessment as well. Patients with spasticity, rigidity or ataxia may have seriously limited voluntary motor control. Patients with poor cardiorespiratory function may have seriously limited energy. Although motor control and cardiopulmonary function are reflected in skeletal muscle performance, testing in the sense of assessing the capability of muscle is inappropriate in such circumstances. There are other things directly related to the musculoskeletal system, such as pain, swelling, joint instability and limited range of motion that may interfere with accurate muscle performance testing. These confounding variables should be isolated and defined during the evaluation, prior to testing muscle function.

The skills of the examiner related to conducting tests and interpreting the derived information will affect the usefulness of muscle performance data. The examiner is obliged to follow a standardized protocol which specifies patient position, verbal instructions or demonstration to the patient, alignment of an instrument or hand placement and direction of examiner resistance in the case of manual testing.

As clinicians, we have a tendency to overinterpret the results of muscle performance tests by assuming that the information means more than the tests can possibly indicate. For example, in assessing the isokinetic performance of the quadriceps muscle in a patient who has had a medial meniscectomy, the clinician may assume that achievement of 80% torque production on the involved limb compared to the uninvolved limb means that the patient is ready to resume full athletic activity. The potential mistake in this assumption is that the so-called uninvolved limb may not be 'normal' and we do not know that the 80% value is adequate to meet the functional demand. Comparative strength from side to side is only one factor among many, such as healing and endurance, which must be taken into account in making the judgement of return to function.

The selection of a measurement protocol should be based not only on the purpose of testing as mentioned earlier, but also in consideration of the factors of sensitivity, reliability, validity and practicality. Sensitivity refers to the ability of the test to discriminate the changes that need to be detected, e.g. the manual muscle test is not sensitive to change when the force capability of a muscle is in the 'good' or 'normal' range. Conversely, a muscle that is very weak cannot be assessed using dynamometry when that muscle cannot exert sufficient force against the instrument to obtain a reading.

A test can only be meaningful if it is reliable and valid. Reliability is the stability, reproducibility and accuracy of the measurements. There are a variety of statistical tests that may be used to determine the reliability of measures (Shrout & Fleiss 1979). Validity means that the test is measuring what it is purported to measure and that

Table 3.1 Clinical methods of measuring muscle performance

	Type of contraction			Controlled variables		
	Concentric	*Eccentric*	*Isometric*	*Gravity*	*Force*	*Velocity*
Manual muscle testing	X		X	X	X	
Hand-held dynamometer	X		X	X	X	
PRE	X	X	X		X	
Cable tensiometer			X			
Isokinetic devices*	X	X	X	X	X	X

* Variety of combinations available, depending on the manufacturer. Not all devices perform the same.

any conclusions and assumptions made from the test results reflect the actual state or condition of the characteristic being defined.

In choosing a test to measure muscle performance clinicians need to decide whether the information obtained is worth the time and effort on the basis of reliability, validity, sensitivity and practicality. Many commonly used testing procedures have been developed. Tables 3.1 and 3.2 summarize the specific aspects of muscle performance which each test is designed to assess.

MEASURES

Manual muscle testing

Manual muscle testing is a system for describing muscle 'strength' based on the ability of muscle to move its bony lever in relationship to gravity and resistance applied manually by the examiner. The role of gravity is controlled by positioning the patient so that the muscle will be working against gravity or with the effect of gravity minimized. Manual resistance is applied by the examiner either through the excursion of movement or at a specified point in the range of motion. Depending upon the testing protocol, muscles are evaluated during concentric contraction or isometric contraction or both.

Table 3.2 Advantages and disadvantages of the clinical methods of measuring muscle performance

	Advantages	Disadvantages
Manual muscle testing	• Does not require use of equipment • Relatively inexpensive • Tests individual muscles	• Requires skill and use of a well-defined protocol • Inadequate stabilization, position of examiner, consistency of examiner may influence results • Questionable reliability for muscle rated *F*+ and above
Hand-held dynamometer	• Provides quantitative data • Equipment is portable • Tests individual muscles	• Requires same attention to protocol, stabilization, skill as MMT
PRE	• Provides quantitative data	• Measures the amount of force the muscle can develop at the weakest point in the range of motion • Tests muscle groups, not individual muscles
Cable tensiometer	• Provides quantitative data	• Limited applicability • Tests muscle groups, not individual muscles • Requires relatively expensive equipment • Not portable
Isokinetic testing	• Provides quantitative data • Some devices allow for testing reciprocal contractions	• Not portable • Tests muscle groups, not individual muscles • Expensive

The grading system is based on muscle performance in relation to the magnitude of manual resistance applied by the examiner. The two most widely used grading systems in the United States are those described by Daniels & Worthingham (1980) and Kendall & McCreary (1983). Both systems of grading use the ordinal scale of measurement. Scores are ranked from no contraction to a contraction which can be performed against gravity and can accept 'maximal' resistance by the examiner. However, the implication of grades is limited to interpretation of 'better' or 'worse', 'stronger' or 'weaker' and no assumption can be made about the magnitude of difference between grades.

Table 3.3 Grading criteria (adapted from Daniels & Worthingham 1980)

Normal	=	motion through full range against gravity and maximum applied force
Good	=	motion through full available range against gravity and less than maximum applied force
Fair	=	motion through full available range against gravity
Fair minus	=	motion through at least ½ of full available range but not complete against gravity
Poor plus	=	motion is initiated against gravity, but does not reach ½ of the available ROM
Poor	=	motion through full range with gravity diminished
Poor minus	=	motion through partial range with gravity diminished
Trace	=	palpable contraction but no movement
Zero	=	no palpable contraction

The manual muscle test is the only available tool which permits description of muscle performance or deficits when muscle cannot move a part through a full range of motion against gravity or accept externally applied resistance. The scores of *zero, trace, poor* and *fair* apply to muscles with serious 'weakness'. If testing procedures are clearly described and followed and grades are specifically defined, objective assessment of severe weakness can be reliably made (Beasley 1961, Lilienfeld et al 1954, Iddings et al 1961, Frese et al 1987). The system can be refined if interim grades between *trace* and *fair* are added (Table 3.3) (Daniels & Worthingham 1980, Kendall & McCreary 1983).

We would like to emphasize two points about the application of this grading system. First, the definitions regarding range of motion should take into account the available range. Therefore, passive range of motion must be measured prior to grading performance, e.g. if passive knee extension is limited from 90° to 30°, i.e. lacking 30° of full extension, a grade of *fair* would be assigned if the quadriceps were able to extend the knee to 30°. Clinicians are often tempted to apply resistance to a part which can not be moved through the full available range of motion. Using the manual muscle test system, the application of resistance for any grade below *fair* is inappropriate based on the grading definitions.

Secondly, although there should be little doubt about the assignment of grades *fair* and below, the appropriateness of manual muscle testing and the validity of the grading system is questionable when muscles can move or hold against external resistance. The grades *good* and *normal* imply an arbitrariness, in that the amount of manual resistance is described as *minimal*, *moderate* or *maximal*, which requires a subjective judgement on the part of the examiner. Furthermore, a grade of 'normal' or '100%' suggest full recovery or normal strength, which may not be so. For example, in one study the so-called uninvolved thigh musculature in patients with hemiparesis was graded 'normal' by manual muscle testing; however, significant deficits in torque production by those muscles were recorded by isokinetic testing (Watkins et al 1984). Manual muscle test grades above *fair*, therefore, may lack acceptable reliability, validity and sensitivity. When a patient can perform in these ranges of 'strength', other more objective measures should be selected for more precise description of performance (Beasley 1961, Rothstein 1986).

Hand-held dynamometer or myometer

A hand-held dynamometer is an instrument which is designed to measure isometric force exerted between the examiner and the limb segment being tested. As the examiner holds the instrument against the limb segment to be tested, the patient is asked to push or pull maximally and then to hold for several seconds against the instrument. The force (in pounds or kilograms) exerted through the input plate or piston is recorded. The advantage of this type of instrument is that numerical values can be assigned for manual muscle test grades of *good* and *normal*, within the limit of the instrument and the ability of the examiner to oppose the patient's force.

Several studies have been conducted to examine the reliability of the hand-held dynamometer used with specific testing protocols (Stuberg & Metcalf 1988, Bohannon & Andrews 1987, Riddle et al 1989, Nicholas et al 1978, Marino et al 1982, Agre et al 1987).

In general, the reported reliability values ranging from $r = 0.84$ to $r = 0.99$ are acceptable when testing patients who have documented force deficits. However, Riddle et al (1989) reported low test-retest reliability scores for wrist extensors ($r = 0.21$) and for the quadriceps femoris ($r = 0.56$) on the uninvolved muscles in brain-damaged patients. These findings may exemplify one of the difficulties with hand-held dynamometers. At times, positioning of the instrument and examiner is awkward. The plate of the dynamometer may be uncomfortable for the patient, especially when applied over bony surfaces such as the dorsum of the hand. The examiner may not be able to match the holding contraction of large muscle groups. In this case, the measurement reflects the resistive ability of the examiner, rather than the patient.

The results of these studies indicate that this instrument, when used with a standardized testing protocol, can measure isometric force generated by muscles at specific joint angles. The limitations of this testing include the difficulties inherent in stabilization, position and examiner strength particularly when testing large muscle groups.

Cable tensiometer

The cable tensiometer is another instrument designed to record isometric tension. A calibrated cable is interposed within a fixed cable or chain system which is secured to a stable base, such as a floor or wall, at one end and applied to the patient at a pre-selected angle at the other end. The force, translated through the calibrated length of cable is recorded in pounds or kilograms using a tensiometer attached to that cable. An advantage of this system of measurement is that by altering patient position or the angle of application of the cable, a muscle or muscle group can be tested at several points in the arc of motion (Clarke et al 1952, Clarke 1954, Currier 1972, Alderman 1969, Asmussen et al 1959).

Progressive resistance exercise (PRE) testing

One of the earliest systems described by Delorme (1945) for quantitating the amount of force a muscle can develop concentrically is the determination of '10-repetition maximum' (10 RM). This procedure involves loading weights on the distal limb segment and asking the patient to lift the weight against gravity 10 times. Weight is added until the patient can not complete the 10 required repetitions. The next lower amount of weight is recorded as that patient's 10 RM.

The original purpose of establishing the 10 RM was to establish a treatment protocol for patients in which the 10 RM was designated as the maximum exercise load to be used during a treatment session (DeLorme & Watkins 1951). However, using a standardized method including positioning, stabilization, instructions to patients and supervision, this procedure can be used to provide objective information about the concentric, eccentric or isometric force capability of tested musculature.

PRE testing may be performed using free weights or on exercise devices such as the Universal Gym, Nautilus equipment, Elgin table, Eagle system and other pulley systems. Using free weights is practical, reliable, portable and inexpensive. However, when assessing patients with joint dysfunction and instability, free weights need to be used carefully in order not to apply torsion or stress on the affected structures, which can be contraindicated. The use of closed systems can be safer in these cases. The main disadvantage of using PRE testing is that the amount of weight determined to be the maximum (e.g. 10 RM) is based on the muscle's capability at its weakest point in the range of motion being tested. If the original purpose of PRE testing is kept in mind, evaluating muscle performance in this manner is appropriate because it suggests to the examiner the amount of weight a patient should use for training. A baseline can be established and amount of weight lifted may be modified as the patient progresses.

There are many variations of the 10 RM protocol; these include determining the 1 RM and testing the muscle in the eccentric as well as the concentric mode through a predetermined range of motion. All of these protocols essentially give similar information provided that the protocols are standardized and instructions are consistent. Repeated assessments must be done using the same protocol over time in order for the results to be meaningful.

Isokinetic testing

The concept of isokinetic exercise and the introduction of isokinetic dynamometers interfaced with computers have expanded the choice of instrumentation for clinical measurement of muscle performance. Isokinetic systems provide muscle loading by controlling the velocity of limb movement as opposed to loading by external weight. This allows a muscle group to be maximally loaded throughout its range of motion. Assessment of concentric, eccentric and isometric muscle contractions can be measured depending on the specific instrument used. These instruments can be used to quantitatively document torque during muscle contraction and joint motion. Work, power and fatigue can be calculated from the data.

There are many testing protocols in existence which stress two kinds of measures: 'strength' and 'endurance'. Strength in this context is defined as the ability of a muscle to develop torque.

Commonly used isokinetic measures of strength include peak torque, average peak torque and calculated values such as antagonistic muscle group ratios, power and work. Endurance in this context is defined as the ability of a muscle to sustain torque over time. Isokinetic measures of this concept actually quantify the converse of endurance, i.e. fatigability. Isokinetic fatigue measures include the percent decline of torque over time, total work over time and time to 50% decline. Several measurements using isokinetic systems have been reported and discussed in the literature. Most studies have focused on testing the knee musculature, although data on the shoulder, elbow, hip and ankle have also been presented (Clarkson et al 1980, Smith et al 1981, Knapik & Ramos 1981).

Peak torque is defined as the highest point on the generated torque curve and is recorded in foot-pounds* or Newton-metres depending on the specific instrument used. This value reported in the current literature may represent the highest single value obtained during a series of repetitions (Gilliam et al 1979, Smith et al 1981, Richards 1981) or the mean value of a series of repetitions (Murray et al 1980, Knapik & Ramos 1981). If the purpose of testing is to determine an individual's maximum capability to generate torque, then the highest value may be an appropriate indicator. When assessing the injured or deconditioned individual, however, the mean and standard deviation or range of values may be a better measure of functional capability. Studies have shown that peak torque values are affected by age, sex, height and weight of the subject (Molnar & Alexander 1974, Gilliam et al 1979). These factors, therefore, should be taken into account when making intersubject comparisons. It is likewise important to test subjects at a consistent pre-set speed in serial evaluations because, following the principles of the force-velocity relationship, torque values change inversely with changing speed during dynamic, concentric contractions (Thorstensson 1976).

In recent years eccentric muscle testing has become available and preliminary data reveal that, in general, following the force-velocity relationship, eccentric contractions generate more torque than concentric contractions at any given test speed. However, in contrast to the original data obtained on isolated muscle preparations, eccentric torque values do not significantly increase when tested at progressively higher velocities (Hodson & Johnson 1990).

*1 foot-pound = 1.356 Newton-metres, 1 Newton-metre = 0.7375 foot-pounds

A related measure is the *joint angle at which peak torque occurs.* Testing speed apparently affects this measure as well. Comparing the findings of Moffroid et al (1969), Thorstensson et al (1976), Osternig (1975) and Watkins & Harris (1983), the evidence suggests that quadriceps peak torque occurs later in the range of motion with increasing speeds.

The interrelationship between antagonistic muscles can be described in part by determining the *hamstrings to quadriceps torque ratio*. In all studies reporting both quadriceps and hamstrings torque values and using similar subject positioning, the quadriceps has been found to generate higher torque than the hamstrings (Moffroid 1969). The reported ratios obtained on normal subjects and athletes tested isometrically or at relatively slow speed (up to 60° per second) range from 0.50 to 0.60. Smith et al (1981), Wyatt & Edwards (1981) and Watkins & Harris (1983) have found that the ratio is higher (approximately 0.77) at the testing speed of 180° per second. Comparison of torque values for quadriceps and hamstrings obtained at slow speed versus fast speed indicate that the decline in quadriceps torque from slow to fast speed is greater than the decline in hamstrings torque, which may explain the change in ratio. Marked deviations from these normal ratios may serve as an indicator of pathomechanics or pathophysiology of the knee musculature, e.g. Watkins et al (1983) have reported a mean hamstrings to quadriceps ratio of 1.36 in a series of patients following patellectomy. Furthermore, deviations from this normal ratio may reflect the result of training in specific sports, e.g. Gilliam et al found that in high school football players, linemen had a significantly higher hamstrings to quadriceps ratio at slow speed than the receivers and backs (0.65 vs. 0.59) (Gilliam 1974).

The derived values of work and power are also used as measures of strength. These measures supposedly represent the ability of a muscle to sustain tension or torque through the muscle contraction. These measures may potentially be correlated with functional abilities, although this suggestion has not been validated in the literature. Briefly, work may be defined as a force moving a resistance through a distance. Work is calculated as the area under the torque curve and is expressed in units of force times distance, such as foot-pounds or Newton-metres (Laird & Rozier 1979). Power is the rate of doing work or the amount of work done over time. Power has been defined in several ways throughout the isokinetic literature and the commonly used terms are average power, peak power, rate of power production, instantaneous power and contractile power (Ivy et al 1981, Laird & Rozier 1979, Moffroid & Kusiak 1975).

Measures of *fatigability* or indicators of *endurance* using the Cybex instrumentation have been defined in several ways. All definitions, however, are based on the decline in torque occurring over some prolonged series of repeated contractions, commonly performed at a relatively high speed (180° per second). One method of determining fatigue is to have the subject perform repeated contractions until torque values drop to 50% of the initial torque value obtained at the test speed. In this case, the measure is the *time* taken to lose 50% of the initial torque production (Moffroid et al 1969). A second method is to determine the *per cent decline* after a predetermined number of repetitions (Thorstensson 1976). If a reciprocal alternating contraction test mode is used, whereby antagonistic pairs of muscles are studied simultaneously, the fatigue rates of the two muscles may be different because of differences in metabolic demands, histological make-up or training effects (Thorstensson 1977, Barnes 1981). A third method of testing fatigability, which avoids undue stress on the more easily fatigued muscle, is to measure the *per cent decline in torque within a time limit*. Using this latter method, Watkins & Harris (1983) documented that in normal untrained subjects the per cent decline in torque over a 15 second run of repeated contractions was greater for the quadriceps than for the hamstrings (means of 25% and 16% respectively).

The reliability of an isokinetic testing protocol is critical to the interpretation of test results. If the reliability of a specific protocol has not been established, differences in torque with repeated tests may represent measurement error instead of actual changes in muscle performance. Potential sources of error can be due to the instrument, the testing protocol or the subject. The equipment must be calibrated according to the specific manufacturer's instructions. Testing protocols should be standardized and specific as to patient position, stabilization, selected test velocities, alignment of the joint axis to the dynamometer, testing instructions, warm-up and rest periods.

Isokinetic systems offer several advantages over free weights. These instruments provide 'accommodating resistance', meaning that maximal muscular force can be generated throughout an arc of motion. Speed can be adjusted to tailor exercise performance to subject's need. If pain or cramping occurs at any point in the exercise and the subject stops moving, the apparatus stops, which is a safety feature of these systems.

Disadvantages of isokinetic testing include the fact that the equipment is very expensive and constant velocity is an artificial condition. Normal motion occurs at variable velocities and in multiple planes of motion. The knee and elbow, although not true hinge joints, are the easiest to stabilize and test. Although positioning techniques are improving because of modifications in the equipment, there are limitations in testing multiaxial joints. The effect of gravity may also produce distortion in the test results (Winter et al 1981, Sapega 1990). According to several investigators, this distortion is greater during high speed testing (Davies 1985). Gravity correction procedures are reported in the literature and are available on some of the newer models of isokinetic equipment.

In summary, physical therapists have adapted test protocols to suit their specific needs and goals. The selection of measures to be used in assessment of patients or clients should depend on the training or treatment goals in each situation. As the body of knowledge about the relative value of each measure grows, the choice of studying torque, angle, timing or endurance factors will become more clear.

FUNCTIONAL ASSESSMENT

The tests of muscle performance are valuable for treatment planning and recording of specific intervention strategies. However, for the patient and for understanding the role of specific muscular activity in overall musculoskeletal function, evaluation should not be limited to specific muscle tests. Since we still do not know 'how much' strength a particular muscle 'needs' to be able to perform an activity, direct assessment of the activity is an appropriate, practical element of evaluation. For example, a patient who sustained a distal femoral fracture which is healed clinically and by radiograph is referred to physical therapy for strengthening of the lower extremity and for progressive functional training. There is no limitation of range of motion of the lower extremities, no swelling and the patient reports that he is pain free. Manual muscle test results show that the lower extremity musculature is generally *normal* throughout with the exception of the quadriceps, which is graded *good.* Isokinetic testing of the quadriceps documents a 50% quadriceps deficit at low speed compared to the uninvolved side. The patient wants to know if he can discontinue the use of crutches. In this case, direct assessment of the patient's gait will give the therapist the additional information needed to make the judgement of whether he is ready to walk without assistive devices. Because functional performance of activities of daily living, work or sports is usually the goal of therapeutic intervention, the final outcome measure should be in keeping with the practical aspect of patients' lives. As with more direct methods of muscle performance testing, discrimination of functional performance must be conducted in a consistent, reproducible manner.

Functional abilities may be recorded by questionnaire, whereby the patient is asked to answer questions or to describe what activities are possible or not. This method of documentation is quite different from an observational analysis whereby an examiner actually observes the patients' performance. The Functional Status Index (FSI) described by Jette (1980) is an example of a self-report instrument which measures basic and instrumental activities of daily living. The FSI uses an ordinal scale to measure the level of difficulty and the amount of assistance required to perform activities such as transfers, toileting, walking and shopping. Advantages of using self-report measures of function include ease of administration and lower cost than direct observation. In addition, complex functional activities can be assessed. Whether the data obtained by these methods are an accurate reflection of the patient's functional disability has not been definitively established. Some investigators have compared patient self-report of disability with professional judgement in an attempt to examine the validity of self-report measures (Nelson et al 1983). Harris et al (1986) compared the results of the FSI with direct observation of the functional activities in an elderly population. The results of these studies indicates that self-report is a valid method of assessing basic level of function. When discrepancies between self-report and direct observation or professional judgement were noted, patients tended to underestimate their abilities.

Functional assessment scales have been developed to document performance of activities of daily living (ADL). The ADL scales are qualitative in nature and are used to note improvement or decline in functional status. These assessment scales have been developed to meet needs of specific patient populations, e.g. the Katz ADL Index was developed to evaluate the status of elderly patients in the nursing home environment (Katz et al 1970). Scoring is based on observation of very fundamental activities such as dressing, toileting and bathing. There are many other functional scales available for clinical use, including the Barthel Index, Waddell and Main

Disability Index and the Functional Assessment Inventory (FAI)(Mahoney & Barthel 1965, Waddell et al 1982, Rose et al 1986).

Functional performance may be quantitatively described, e.g. using a stop watch, the time it takes to rise from a chair, climb a standard flight of stairs or walk a fixed distance can be recorded to describe the efficiency of selected activities (Vignos et al 1963). The Jebsen Hand Function Evaluation is an example of a timed functional test (Jebsen et al 1969). In this evaluation, patients are asked to perform activities such as writing, turning objects, picking up and placing objects while being timed with a stop watch. In these examples, *time* is the recorded value.

In the analysis of ambulation, *distance* factors may be recorded. The Cooper Walk-Run Test measures the distance traversed over a fixed period of time (Cooper 1968). As originally described, this is a 12 minute test documenting how far a patient walks or runs 'as fast as possible' in a 12 minute period. This can be modified to shorter periods of time depending on the realistic abilities of patients in specific diagnostic groups.

Foot print analysis is another method of documenting gait performance. The basic implements of the method described by Boenig (1977) are a mat or paper strip secured to the floor, inked tapes on the shoes of the subject and a stop watch. This method permits documentation of spatial gait characteristics, such as step length, stride length, base of support and foot angle.

In summary, there are a variety of functional performance tests available for clinicians to use to evaluate the patient's ability to use the affected musculature. Selection of the appropriate test must be based on the functional goals of the patient.

SUMMARY

The development of more sophisticated testing instruments has been stimulated by an increased understanding of how muscles work under different conditions. Currently, there is much interest in developing reliable and valid methods to quantitate the more subtle changes in muscle performance as a means of documenting deficits, measuring response to treatment and correlating specific aspects of dynamic muscle performance with functional activities. However, until the validity of these measures is established, the direct clinical application of the data remains limited. Caution must be used when interpreting test results and clinicians must recognize that muscle performance tests are only one part of a physical therapy examination. At present, there is no single 'best test' for all situations. Selection of the appropriate test still depends on the specific needs of the individual patient.

REFERENCES

Agre J C, Magness J L, Hill S Z et al 1987 Strength testing with a portable dynamometer: reliability for upper and lower extremities. Arch Phip Med Rehabil 68: 454–457

Alderman R B, Banfield T J 1969 Reliability estimation in the measurement of strength. Research Quarterly 40: 448

Asmussen E, Heeboll-Neilsen K, Molbech S V 1959 Methods for evaluation of muscle strength. Comm Dan Natl Assoc Infant Paralysis 5.

Barnes W S 1981 Isokinetic fatigue curves at different contractile velocities. Archives of Physical Medicine and Rehabilitation 62: 66–69

Beasley W C 1961 Quantitative muscle testing: principles and applications to research and clinical services. Archives of Physical Medicine and Rehabilitation 42: 398–428

Boenig D 1977 Evaluation of a clinical method of gait analysis. Physical Therapy 57: 795

Bohannon R W, Andrews A W 1987 Interrater reliability of hand-held dynamometry. Physical Therapy 67: 931–933

Clarke H H 1954 Comparison of instruments for recording muscle strength. Research Quarterly 25: 398

Clarke H H, Bailey T L, Shay C T 1952 New objective strength tests of muscle groups by cable-tension methods. Research Quarterly 25: 398

Clarkson P M, Kroll W, McBride T C 1980 Plantar flexion fatigue and muscle fiber type in power and endurance athletes. Medicine and Science in Sports and Exercise 12: 262–267

Cooper K 1968 A means of assessing maximal oxygen intake. Journal of the American Medical Association 203: 201–204

Currier D P 1972 Maximal isometric tension of the elbow extensors at varied positions. Physical Therapy 52: 1043

Daniels L, Worthingham C 1980 Muscle testing: technique of manual examination, 4th edn. W B Saunders, Philadelphia

Davis G 1985 A compendium of isokinetic in clinical usage, 2nd edn. S & S Publishers, LaCrosse, Wisconsin

Delorme T L 1945 Restoration of muscle power by heavy resistance exercise. Journal of Bone and Joint Surgery 27: 645

Delorme T L, Watkins A 1951 Progressive resistance exercise: technic and medical application. Century-Crofts, New York

Frese E, Brown M, Norton B 1987 Clinical reliability of manual testing. Physical Therapy 67: 1072–1076

Gilliam T B, Sady S P, Friedson P S et al 1979 Isokinetic torque levels for high school football players. Archives of Physical Medicine and Rehabilitation 60: 110–114

Harris B A, Jette A M, Campion E W, Cleary P D 1986 Validity of self-report measures of functional disability. Topics in Geriatric Rehabilitation 1: 31–42

Hodson L I, Johnson E B 1990 Force-velocity relationship of quadriceps femoris in vivo. Masters Thesis, MGH Institute of Health Professions, Boston, MA

Iddings D M, Smith L K, Spencer W A 1961 Muscle testing part 2: reliability in clinical use. Physical Therapy Review 41: 249–256

Ivy J L, Withers R T, Brose G et al 1981 Isokinetic contractile properties of the quadriceps with relation to fiber type. European Journal of Applied Physiology 47: 247–255

Jebsen R, Taylor N, Trieschmann R, Trotter M, Howard L 1969 An objective and standardized test of hand function. Archives of Physical Medicine and Rehabilitation 63: 269

Jette A M 1986 State of the art in functional status assessment. In: Rothstein J M (ed) Measurement in Physical Therapy, Churchill Livingstone, New York, ch 5, p 137–168

Jette A M 1980 Functional status index: reliability of a chronic disease evaluation instrument. Archives of Physical Medicine and Rehabilitation 61: 395

Katz S, Downs T, Cash H, Grotz 1970 Progress in development of the index of ADL. Gerontologist 10: 20

Kendall F P, McCreary E K 1983 Muscles: testing and function, 3rd edn. Williams and Wilkins, Baltimore, MD

Knapik J J, Ramos M R 1981 Isokinetic and isometric torque relationships in the human body. Archives of Physical Medicine and Rehabilitation 61: 64–67

Laird C E, Rozier C K 1979 Toward understanding the terminology of exercise mechanics. Physical Therapy 59: 287–292

Lilienfeld A M, Jacobs M, Wiles M 1954 A study of the reproducibility of muscle testing and certain other aspects of muscle scoring. Physical Therapy Review 34: 279–289

Mahoney F, Barthel D 1965 Functional evaluation: the Barthel index. Maryland State Medical Journal 14: 61

Marino M, Nicholas J A, Gleim G W et al 1982 The efficacy of manual assessment of muscle strength using a new device. American Journal of Sports Medicine 10: 360–364

Mayhew T P, Rothstein J M 1988 Measurement of muscle performance with instruments. In: Rothstein J M (ed) Measurement in Physical Therapy. Churchill Livingstone, New York, ch 3, p 57–102

Moffroid M T, Whipple R H 1969 Specificity of speed of exercise. Physical Therapy 50: 1699–1700

Moffroid M T, Kusiak E T 1975 The power struggle: definition of power of muscular performance. Physical Therapy 55: 1098–1104

Moffroid M T, Whipple R, Hofkosh et al 1969 A study of isokinetic exercise. Physical Therapy 49: 735–747

Molnar G E, Alexander J 1974 Development of quantitative standards for muscle strength in children. Archives of Physical Medicine and Rehabilitation 55: 490–493

Murray M P, Gardner G M, Mullinger L A et al 1980 Strength of isometric and isokinetic contractions: knee muscles of men ages 20-86. Physical Therapy 60: 412–419

Nelson E, Conger B, Douglas R et al 1983 Functional health status levels of primary care patients. Journal of the American Medical Association 249: 3331–3338

Nicholas J A, Sapega A, Kraus H et al 1978 Factors influencing manual tests in physical therapy: the magnitude and duration of force applied. Journal of Bone and Joint Surgery (American) 60: 186–190

Osternig L R 1975 Optimal isokinetic loads and velocities providing muscular power in human subjects. Archives of Physical Medicine and Rehabilitation 56: 152–155

Richards C L 1981 Dynamic strength characteristics during isokinetic knee movements in healthy women. Physiotherapy Canada 33: 141–150

Riddle D L, Finucane S D, Rothstein J M, Walker M L 1989 Intrasession and intersession reliability of hand-held dynamometer measurements taken on brain-damaged patients. Physical Therapy 69: 182–192
Rose S J, Shulman A D, Strube M J 1986 Functional assessment of patients with low back syndrome. Topics in Geriatric Rehabilitation 1: 9–30
Sapega H, Nicholas J, Sokolow D, Saraniti A 1982 The nature of torque 'overshoot' in cybex isokinetic dynamometry. Medicine and Science in Sports and Exercise 14: 368–375
Shrout P E, Fleiss J L 1979 Intraclass correlations: uses in assessing rater reliability. Psychological Bulletin 86: 420–428
Smith D J, Quinney H A, Wenger H A et al 1981 Isokinetic torque outputs of professional and elite amateur ice hockey players. Journal of Sports Physical Therapy 3: 42–47
Smith G A, Nelson R C, Sadoff S J, Sadoff A M 1989 Assessing sincerity of effort in maximal grip strength tests. American Journal of Physical Medicine and Rehabilitation 2: 73
Stuberg W A, Metcalf W K 1988 Reliability of quantitative muscle testing in healthy children and in children with Duchenne muscular dystrophy using a hand-held dynamometer. Physical Therapy 68: 977–982
Thorstensson A, Grimby G, Karlsson J 1976 Force-velocity relations and fiber composition in human knee extensor muscles. Journal of Applied Physiology 40: 12–16
Thorstensson A, Karlsson J 1976 Fatigability and fiber composition of human skeletal muscle. Acta Physiologica Scandinavica 98: 318–322
Vignos P J, Spencer G E, Archibald K 1963 Management of progressive muscular dystrophy in childhood. Journal of the American Medical Association 184: 89–96
Waddell G, Main C J, Morris E W et al 1982 Normality and reliability in the clinical assessment of backache. British Medical Journal 284: 1519–1523
Watkins M P, Harris B A 1983 Evaluation of isokinetic muscle performance. Clinics of Sports Medicine 2: 27–53
Watkins M P, Harris B A, Wenders et al 1983 Effect of patellectomy on the function of the quadriceps and hamstrings. Journal of Bone and Joint Surgery 65-A: 390–395
Watkins M P, Harris B A, Kozlowski B A 1984 Isokinetic testing in patients with hemiparesis. Physical Therapy 64: 184–189
Winter D A, Wells R P, Orr G W 1981 Errors in the use of isokinetic dynamometers. European Journal of Applied Physiology 46: 397–408
Wyatt M P, Edwards A M 1989 Comparison of quadriceps and hamstrings torque values during isokinetic exercise. Journal of Sports Physical Therapy 3: 48–56

4. Biomechanical aspects of exercise

Karin Harms-Ringdahl, Jan Ekholm

INTRODUCTION

Biomechanical analyses of load on locomotor system structures are important parts of physical therapy programs for the rehabilitation of disabled people and for the prevention of musculoskeletal problems. Induced load moment, and also muscular activity levels, will influence the strain on the different structures involved in movement. In designing training exercises, one of the main problems is to achieve an appropriate level of muscular activity without creating the risk of excessive load on joint structures and/or muscle insertions, particularly if the latter are weakened by disease or injury (Moritz et al 1973, Ekholm et al 1982). Various approaches have been suggested for dealing with the problem, all with their advantages and limitations. Isokinetic devices seem to have several advantages, e.g. Grimby et al (1980) used an isokinetic device in postsurgical training for patients with knee ligament injuries. The authors suggested that good strength improvements were caused by the ability of the device to give maximal loading throughout the motion range. In an isokinetic exercise, the resistive load moment (moment (Nm) = force (N) x moment arm (m)) corresponds to the maximum muscular moment (strength, or torque) through the motion range. However, isokinetic devices are very expensive, large and impractical to use for home exercises. Another disadvantage is that the movements are not very similar to the movements carried out in daily life.

Most exercises are still performed without complicated devices and hence it is useful to analyze how the effectiveness of these simple exercises can be optimized. In certain situations, exercise in water and other forms of suspended exercise might offer ways of achieving low load and high muscular activity. However, these types of exercise might not provide the axial weightbearing load needed for, e.g. preventing osteoporosis (Sinaki 1989). Analysis of the underlying biomechanical factors is needed before an appropriate exercise program can be designed for any patient with muscle weakness.

Although much has been written on the effects of exercise on muscular function (e.g. Basmajian & Wolf 1990, Bouchard et al 1990, Grimby & Thomeé 1988, Saltin & Gollnick 1983), there is less literature available on the biomechanics of resistive exercises for developing increased strength or endurance, i.e. how loading forces and moments really influence muscles, tendons or joint structures involved in the various exercises commonly used.

Strength and joint angles

In many human actions several muscles are simultaneously activated to perform a movement or to counteract a resistive load moment. The relative activity levels of the muscles vary through the motion range, as do the moment arms of these muscle forces. The moment arm is the perpendicular distance from the line of action of the muscle force to the joint motion axis. Thus, strictly speaking, the force in a single muscle can not be estimated directly in clinical situations. However, the resistive load moment can be measured or calculated and the counteracting muscular moment (i.e. strength, sometimes denoted *torque*) can thus be estimated. Muscle fibre type, composition and cross sectional area also influence the contribution to the muscular moment.

Maximum muscular isometric strength varies over the movement sector, as described by, amongst others, Williams & Stutzman (1959), Haffajee et al (1972) and Moritz et al (1973). Strength curves have been summarized by, e.g. Kulig et al (1984) and Svensson (1987). As some muscles produce force across more than one joint, the position of a nearby joint may or may not influence the maximum strength in a muscle group as measured in another joint (Williams & Stutzman 1959, Németh et al 1983).

The resistive load moment induced by the body segment weights (and, e.g. the weight of the resistance arm of the training device) also varies through the motion range. Thus, the muscle strength capacity used to counteract the resistance during the exercise also varies. The muscular strength utilization ratio (% MUR) in each part of the motion sector can be calculated as a ratio between the resistive load moment and the maximum muscle strength in each joint angle. An important problem is that when the exercise load level is set, it is always the relatively weakest point (lowest % MUR) in relation to the load in motion range, which sets the limit for movement performance.

In Figure 4.1A, a schematic situation is illustrated where the resistive load moment and the maximum muscular moment are well adapted to each other over the motion range. The relative load level can be chosen to suit strength or endurance training purposes without risk of excessive load in certain parts of the movement sector. In Figure 4.1B, the resistive load gives a very low relative load in the beginning of the motion sector with no strength-increas-

A

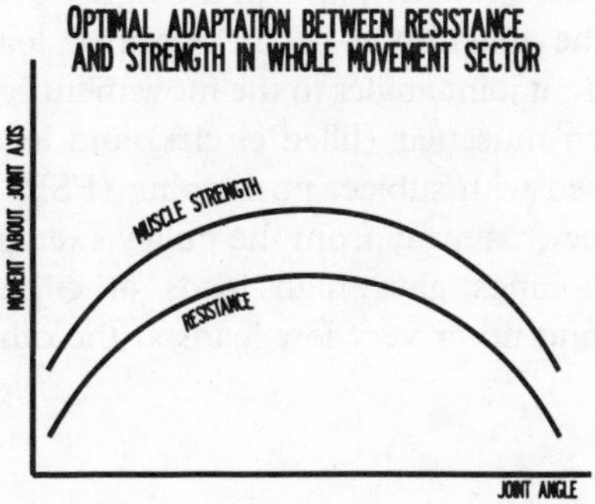

B

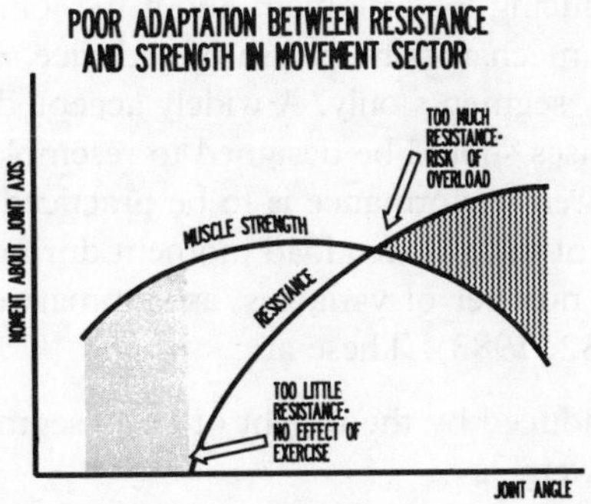

Fig. 4.1 Schematic illustration of muscular (muscle strength) and induced (resistance) load moments of force (Nm) about a joint axis in relation to joint angle over the motion sector. (A): The muscular and induced load moments are well adapted throughout the motion sector. (B): There is a mismatch between the moments, with too little resistive load for training effects in the beginning of the motion sector and too much resistance, with risk of overload, in the other part of the motion sector.

ing effect, and in combination with too high a relative load in other parts with risk of overload. If one still tries to perform such an exercise, lower resistance levels must be chosen to avoid the excessive load, giving even lower resistance, or none at all, in other parts of the motion sector. An example of this is given in Figure 4.2, where shoulder external rotation is being performed with a pulley exerciser as the resistive device (Harms-Ringdahl et al 1985). The upper curve in Figure 4.2, with filled circles, represents mean maximum isometric external rotation strength at different joint angles in five subjects. The drawings to the right show a transversal plane of the seated subject in relation to the pulley. The positioning of the subject, i.e. the angle between the frontal plane and a line from the pulley to the shoulder joint (in the figure denoted FSP), is crucial for how the magnitude of the resistive load moment is distributed at different joint angles in the movement sector. The best covariation between muscular (filled circles) and load (solid lines) moments is achieved with subject positioning (FSP) – 20°, i.e. the subject turned somewhat away from the pulley exerciser. The other two subject positionings gave high loads at either end of the movement sector and no or very low loads at the other.

BIOMECHANICAL VARIABLES INFLUENCING EXERCISE LOAD

The resistance inducing load moment about the joint axis may be applied manually, mechanically by use of a device, or by utilizing the weight of body segments only. A widely accepted standpoint is that training exercises should be designed to resemble the situation in which the acquired performance is to be practiced.

The magnitude of the induced load moment during the exercises is influenced by a number of variables, as summarized by Ekholm & co-workers (1982, 1983). These are:

- load moment induced by the weight of body segments
- magnitudes of weights
- moment arm (or lever arm) length (i.e. direction of the loading force)
- sum of different load moments
- load moment magnitude distribution over the different joint angles of the movement sector
- motion speed and acceleration.

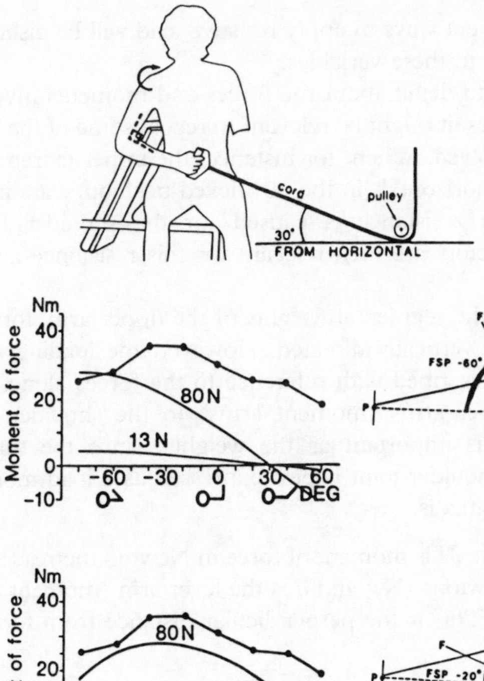

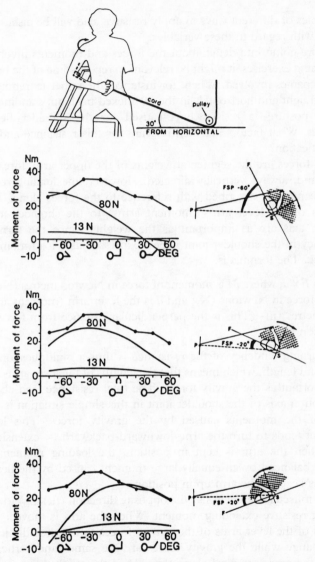

Fig. 4.2 The upper diagram shows the exercise arrangement. The three diagrams below, left, show the effects of different positioning, illustrating muscular strength (filled circles) and resistance load moment (solid lines) during external rotation of the shoulder at different joint angles. The moment of force (Nm) is shown on the *y*-axis and the joint angle (degrees) on the *x*-axis. Symbols below the *x*-axis define the shoulder joint angles. To the right, subject positioning in relation to the pulley is illustrated. Angle FSP is the angle between the frontal plane and a line from the shoulder joint to the pulley at distance 1.3 m: –20°, +20° and –60°. 80 N and 13 N indicates two different weights applied to the cord. (Modified from Harms-Ringdahl et al 1985.)

Examples of different ways to apply resistive load will be discussed below with regard to these variables.

Before going into detail about the forces and moments involved in training exercises, it might be relevant to repeat some of the basic biomechanics involved. When, for instance, the upper extremity is kept straight and horizontal (in the 90° flexed position, standing or sitting posture) a resistance is caused for the shoulder flexor muscles. What factors are then relevant for this resistance and its quantification?

The forces are the segmental weights of the upper arm, forearm and hand, always vertically directed. However, the loading resistance cannot be described with reference to the forces alone. The lengths of the lever arms (moment arms) to the shoulder joint motion axis are as important as the weights, since the turning tendency in the shoulder joint is best expressed as a load moment of force. The formula is:

> $M = F \times d$, where M is moment of force in Newton metres (Nm); F is force in Newtons (N); and d is the lever arm (moment arm) in metres (m) (This is the perpendicular distance from force to motion axis).

The turning tendency of the resistance is thus a multiplication of force and length, which means that the lengths of the lever arms are as important as the gravity forces. The total resistance load about the motion axis of the shoulder joint in this simple situation is the sum of the moments caused by the gravity forces. This load moment tends to turn the arm downward-backward (= extension) and when the arm is kept in position, the loading moment is counterbalanced by an equally large moment caused by the flexor muscles keeping the arm up in position.

The muscular moment has the opposite direction (flexing) to the loading resistive extending moment. When the arm is moved, the lengths of the lever arms of the gravity forces to the shoulder joint axis change while the gravity forces are the same (and vertical). When the arm is vertical along the side of the trunk the moment arms are zero and the moment becomes zero too. When the shoulder joint is flexed, the lengths of the moment arms increase to a maximum at 90° of flexion, then they decrease again up to 180°, where they again become zero. If an extra weight such as a dumb-bell is carried, its loading effect follows the same principle as that of the body segments weights, i.e. the length of the lever arm of the gravity force is as important as the weight per se. In principle the

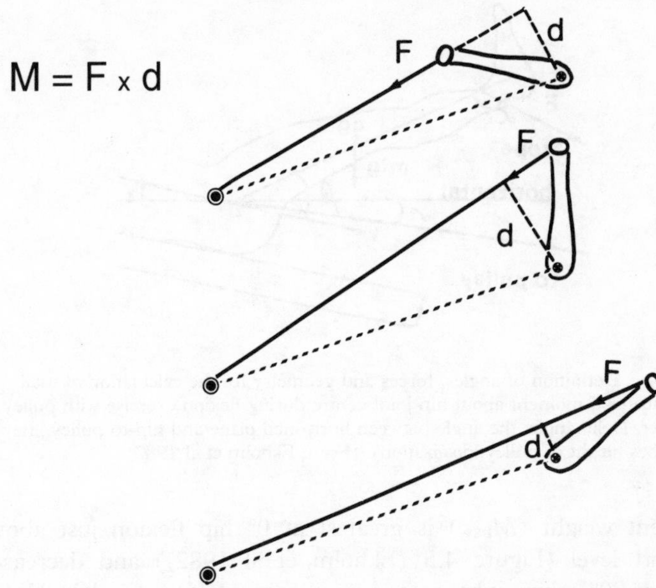

Fig. 4.3 Schematic drawings of a plane perpendicular to the humerus and with the forearm and hand to show the shoulder external rotation exercise in Fig. 4.2. Filled circle: pulley; dotted line: distance from pulley to longitudinal motion axis of humerus; *F:* cord force; *d:* lever arm of cord force (perpendicular distance from cord force vector *F,* or its line of action) to joint motion axis. Note the different lengths of *d* through the motion sector (internally rotated position: top figure; neutral position: middle; and externally rotated: bottom figure). As the cord force *F* is the same through the motion, the resistive moment $M = F \times d$ changes with the length of lever arm *d.*

length of the moment arm also varies in a similar way when the cord of a pulley exerciser is used as a resistance (Fig. 4.3).

The total resistive load moment about a given axis of motion during an exercise movement often consists of moments caused by the gravity forces of some body segments involved plus an extra force caused by the exercise device or the gravity forces of applied extra weights. As an example, Figure 4.4 (Ekholm et al 1982) shows forces and angles at the hip joint during a supine hip flexion movement with extra resistance from a pulley exerciser. The weight of the lower limb (*mg*) is one important force of the system. The cord of the pulley exerciser provides an extra force (*F*) applied at the ankle. With the trunk horizontal, the load moment of the body

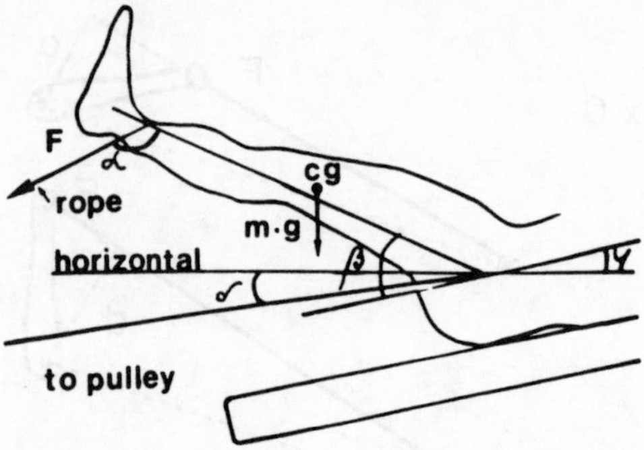

Fig. 4.4 Definition of angles, forces and geometry for the calculation of total resistance load moment about hip joint centre during flexion exercise with pulley exerciser. Delta angle: the angle between horizontal plane and hip-to-pulley line (describes height of pulley localization). (From Ekholm et al 1982)

segment weight (M_{bsw}) is greatest at 0° hip flexion just above support level (Figure 4.5 (Ekholm et al 1982)) and decreases towards 90°, where it becomes a zero moment. If the trunk had been vertical (standing on one leg, γ angle = 90° in Fig. 4.4) the induced load moment (M_{bsw}) would instead have been zero at 0° hip flexion and would have increased towards a maximum at 90° of flexion.

The effect of a change in the height of the pulley (angle δ) of the exerciser on the total resistive load moment (M_{load}: continuous curve) of the hip joint is also illustrated in Figure 4.5. In the upper diagram, the cord (connected to a 4 kg weight) comes from below (angle δ = 20°) and gives an extra moment (M_{wpc}) with a flat peak at about 45° of flexion. This moment and the moment induced by the body segment weights (M_{bsw}) are added and cause the total resistive load moment (M_{load}), which in this case runs fairly parallel to the example of maximum strength of the hip flexors indicated by the uppermost curve (filled circles).

In the lower diagram of Figure 4.5, the cord from the pulley is elevated above the horizontal plane (angle δ = –60°) and the hip-to-pulley line makes an angle of 60° to the horizontal. In this situation, the extra force of the cord supports the movement up to 60° of flexion, so the total resistive moment (continuous curve) becomes flatter, giving an undesirably low relative load in the beginning of the movement. Note that it is important to consider the moment caused by body segment weights, particularly at joints such as the hip, where such moments can be large compared with moments caused by the resistive device. The loading moment about

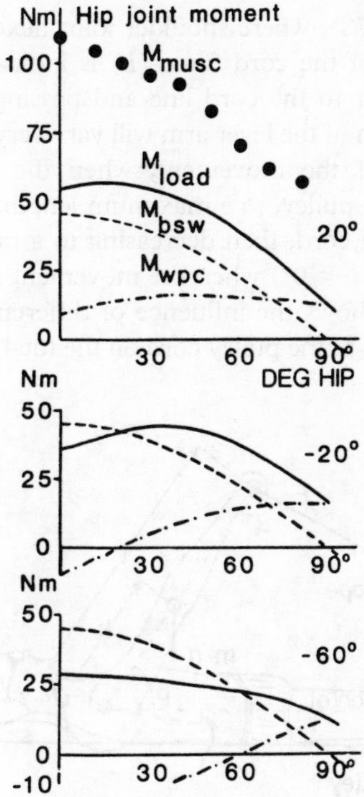

Fig. 4.5 Diagram showing effects of changes on height of pulley localization (delta in Fig. 4.4) on total hip resistance load moment. *y*-axis: moment of force (Nm). *x*-axis: joint angle (degrees). An example of maximum isometric muscular moment (strength) of hip flexors (M_{musc}) is indicated by filled circles in the top diagram. Components of total resistance load moment (M_{load}) are shown: moment due to weight of body segments (M_{bsw}) and moment due to pulley cord force (M_{wpc}) 40 N. Upper diagram: δ 20°, cord from below: middle diagram: δ = –20°, cord from above; lower diagram: δ = –60°, more from above. (From Ekholm et at 1982)

the hip joint due to the weight of the horizontal lower limb is about 30 Nm (Németh et al 1983), and in prone position, these weights of the body segments use up to 24% of the maximum hip extensor strength in young subjects.

The magnitude per se of the applied weight of the pulley exerciser, of course, also influences the induced load moment. However, the effect also depends on the length of the lever arm of this force with regard to the joint motion axis at each angle of the motion sector. An example of this is shown in Figure 4.6A and B

(Arborelius et al 1978), where shoulder joint flexors are exercised. The line of action of the cord force (*F*) is indicated and its lever arm is perpendicular to the cord line and passing to the shoulder joint axis. The length of the lever arm will vary very much from zero in the beginning of the movement, when the subject's arm is directed towards the pulley, to a maximum length, when the arm is perpendicular to the cord, then decreasing to a rather short length (or zero if the angle $\delta = 0°$) when the movement angle approaches 180°. Figure 4.6B shows the influence of different weights (1.5, 3 and 4.5 kg) attached to the pulley cord on the total resistive moment

A

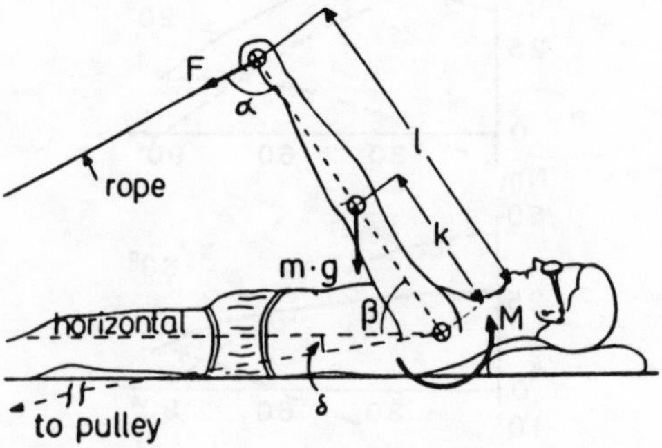

B

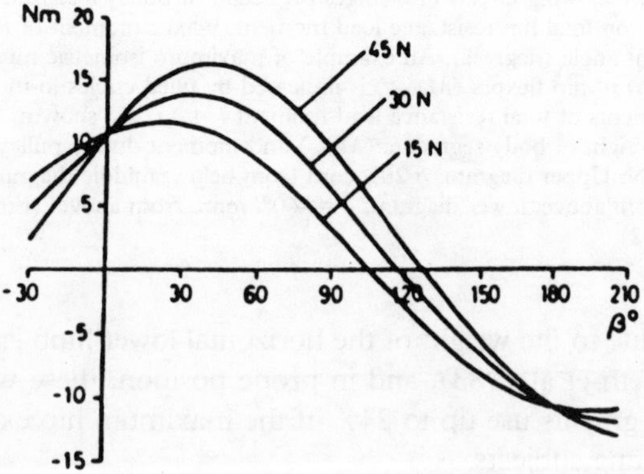

Fig. 4.6 Shoulder flexion exercise using a pulley device as resistance. (A): Biomechanical illustration of forces (*F, mg*), distances and angles (α, β, δ). (B): Diagram showing the influence of different weights (15, 30, 45 N) attached to pulley cord on total resistance moment of the shoulder joint axis. β = shoulder joint angle. Body weight: 70 kg. Shoulder-pulley distance: 2 m. (From Arborelius & Ekholm 1978.)

in the situation shown in Figure 4.6A. Compared to the 3 kg weight (30 N), the added 1.5 kg (to 45 N) increases the peak of total load moment by 3 Nm and the peak occurs later in the movement.

The total resistive moment about a joint motion axis is usually the sum of the moment caused by the weight of the body segments involved and the moment of the extra force caused by a gravity force of the weight (e.g. dumb-bell) applied to a body segment. Note that both the moment caused by weight of body segments and the moment caused by the force from a pulley cord can turn into a negative 'resistance', i.e. into a supporting moment of force. This depends on which side of the joint motion axis the line of action of the force will pass. Since these two kinds of moment are usually present concomitantly, when they are combined in a concerned and calculated way, the total resistive load moment, can to a considerable extent be adapted to the functional capacity of the muscle group under training.

Muscle capacity in this context is characterized partly by the distribution of strength over joint angles. The rationale of exercise design would be to combine the two basic kinds of load moment so that the total resistive moment gives the appropriate load throughout the range of motion, with no unexercised sector and no part with risk of overload and injury (e.g. see Fig. 4.2).

If the moment velocity is approximately constant, no resistive force is added due to acceleration. However, if there is acceleration (of some magnitude) in the exercise movement, extra moments are induced which add to the resistive moment. The magnitude of the forces depends on the acceleration. Acceleration usually adds resistive forces in the beginning of an exercise movement when body segments and applied weights are accelerated from zero velocity.

Smidt & Blanpied (1987) analyzed the sit-up, double straight-leg lowering and prone trunk extension and found that the movements had limitations as tests of maximum trunk flexor and extensor strength but also as modes of resistive exercise. One reason for the limitations was that these manoeuvres lack the range of resistance necessary to cover the spectrum of human trunk muscle strength capacity.

The relationships between levels of muscular moment and the electrical activity of the muscle (EMG) are rather complicated. The upper diagram in Figure 4.7 (Harms-Ringdahl et al 1985) shows the total load moments about the shoulder joint axis when different weights are attached to the pulley cord (5 N, 13 N, 34 N, 80 N)

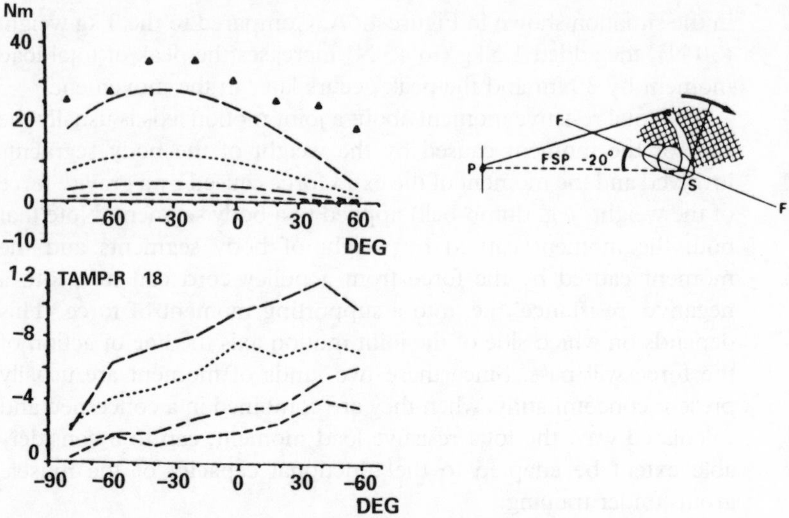

Fig. 4.7 Muscular strength (filled triangles) and resistance load moments (dashed lines) during shoulder external rotation, as in Fig. 4.2. Moments of force (Nm) on *y*-axis (top figure) and joint angle (degrees) on *x*-axis. On the right, subject positioning in relation to pulley is shown. Angle between frontal plane and line from shoulder joint to pulley (FSP): –20°, at distance 1.3 m. Different weights attached to the cord. Pulley cord forces 5, 13, 34, and 80 N are indicated by curves with interrupted lines. Bottom figure shows normalized muscle activity levels (time averaged myopotential ratio, TAMP-R) in the infraspinatus (IS) muscle for the corresponding cord forces. (From Harms-Ringdahl et at 1985.)

during shoulder external rotation movements. The lower diagram shows the corresponding EMG activity recorded from the infraspinatus muscle. Note that the EMG curves continuously increase, despite the fact that the load moments decrease after –30°. However, the curves are in the same order from lowest to highest in both load moment and level of activity in the muscle. This illustrates some of the complexity of EMG/moment relationships. It also illustrates the possibilities of finding high muscular activity levels, suitable for training, despite low mechanical load on joint structures.

Although muscles are activated to counteract induced load moments, muscle activity and muscle strength are two related but entirely different concepts. For a given load moment, muscle activity as measured by electromyography (EMG) reflects motor behaviour. Usually, several muscles are coactivated to exert a load moment, and the muscles are activated both for movements and for joint stabilization. The amplitude levels are influenced by biomechanical factors such as load moment, motion speed and joint angle. However, the electrode distance, skin impedance, fat layers and the size and number of motor units of the muscle also influence the amplitude levels. To be able to compare between different muscles, subjects and measurement occasions, the activity levels must be normalized in some way. Otherwise, it is like trying to assess how fat a person is knowing only the weight and not the height. Thus, calculations of induced and counteracting muscular load moments in relation to maximum strength offer one way of assessing muscle load. Measurements of muscle activity discharge using EMG give valuable information on how much a muscle/muscle group is activated in one situation in relation to another, but give no information as to whether the subject is strong or not.

EXAMPLES OF EXERCISES AND BIOMECHANICAL ASPECTS

Knee joint and thigh muscles

Nisell and co-workers (1989) analyzed tibiofemoral joint forces during isokinetic knee extension in a Cybex II exerciser and compared two different positions of the resistance pad (proximal and distal). At an angular velocity of 30°/s the tibiofemoral compressive force was of the same magnitude as the patellar tendon force, with a maximum of 6300 N or close to 9 times body weight (bw) (Fig. 4.8A, Nisell et al 1989). The tibiofemoral shear force (Fig. 4.8B) changed direction from initially tending to move the tibia posteriorly in relation to femur to the opposite direction with a magnitude of about 700 N or close to 1 bw. This indicates that high forces arise in the anterior cruciate ligament when the knee is straighter than 60°. The anteriorly directed shear force was considerably lowered by locating the resistance pad proximally on the leg (Fig. 4.8B). This mode may be used when the anterior cruciate stress should be minimized, e.g. in rehabilitation after ligament repairs or reconstructions.

Ericson et al (1986) analyzed knee load moment during ergometer cycling. During cycling at 120 Watts, 60 revolutions per minute with mid-saddle height and anterior pedal foot position, the mean peak flexing knee load moment was 29 Nm and the extending moment was 12 Nm (Fig. 4.9, Ericson et al 1986). For the amplitude of knee load moments, work load was the most important factor. All load moments analyzed were small compared to other

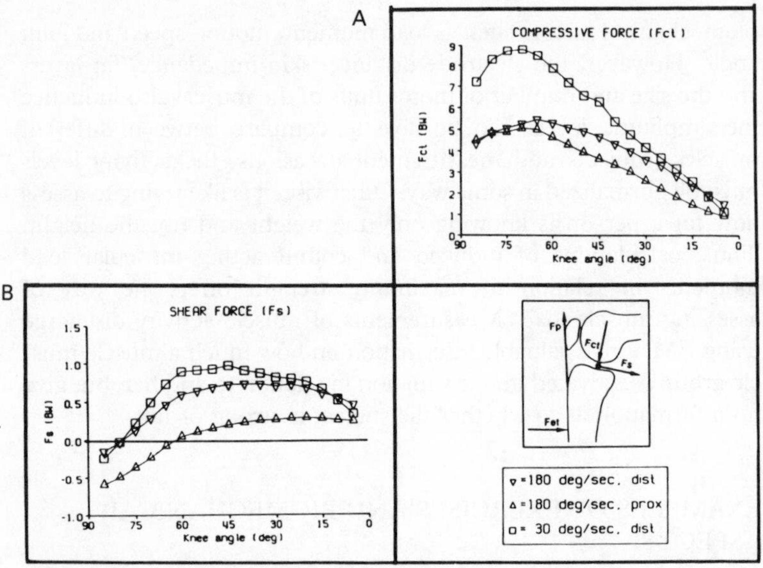

Fig. 4.8 (A) Compressive knee joint force (*Fct*) and (B) shear force (*Fs*) expressed in times body weight (BW)(*y*-axis), with distal and proximal (pyramids) resistance pad placings during maximum isokinetic knee extensions at 180°/s and at 30°/s with distal placing. Straight knee = 0° angle (*x*-axis). (From Niselly et al 1989.)

exercises or activities, such as stair climbing, etc., while the muscular activity levels in the knee extensors, medial and lateral vastus, were comparatively high (Ericson et al 1985).

Schüldt et al (1983) studied the load moment about the knee joint during exercises in rising (in an exercise device with movable trunk support). Floor-to-foot forces were recorded using a force-measuring platform. Figure 4.10 (Schüldt et al 1983) shows that the resistive load moment for one knee joint is relatively high at large knee flexion angles and that the resistance diminishes rapidly during the rising moment, giving a negative 'resistance' after 30° of flexion. The diagram also shows that the difference between extra loading by adding a 10 kg weight or unloading with a 10 kg counterbalance was small. The reason for the small difference is that a 10 kg weight is relatively small in relation to the weight of the body segments above knee level. Approximately the same biomechanical model is valid also when exercising rising from the squatting.

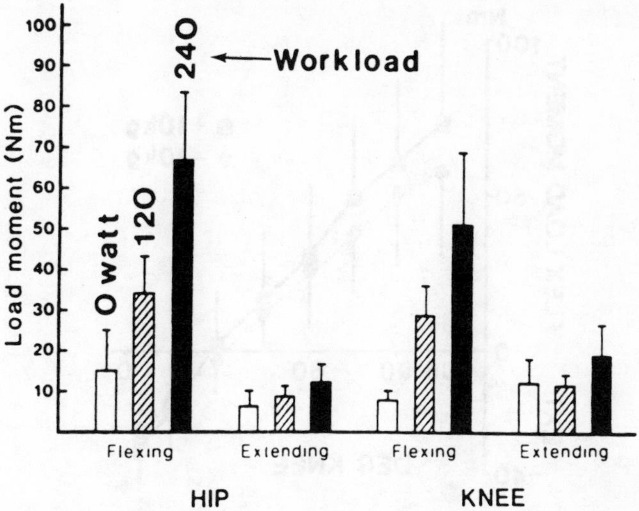

Fig. 4.9 Mean peak hip and knee joint load moments (Nm) induced during ergometer cycling with three different workloads: 0, 120 and 240 W. (From Ericson et al 1986.)

Shoulder muscles

Different ways of applying resistance against shoulder rotators, and how the resistance should be applied to fit the isometric shoulder rotator strength curves, have been analyzed (Harms-Ringdahl et al 1982, 1983, 1985). Figure 4.11 (Harms-Ringdahl et al 1982) shows dumbbell exercises in a supine position. When the subject lies inclined to 45° (feet down), the resistive load during external rotation, elbow flexed 90°, gives good covariation with the muscular strength curve through the motion range. The ideal posture is estimated to be 30° from vertical (feet down) and slightly side-lying, turned 20° backward. Lying supine and horizontal (left in figure), only gives resistance in the internally rotated joint angles (and a negative 'resistance' in the externally rotated joint angles). This position, of course, can be used if one wants to avoid load in externally rotated angles. Lying prone gives large disproportions between the resisting and the muscular moments, i.e. the resistance increases while the muscular strength output decreases. As opposed to the horizontal supine posture, there is a resistive moment only in the externally rotated positions of the shoulder joint.

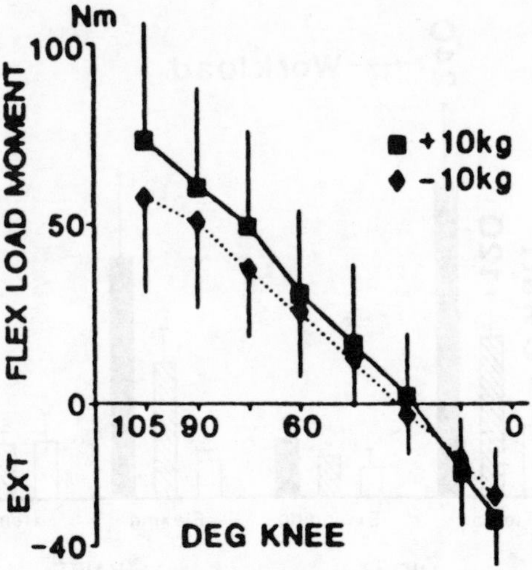

Fig. 4.10 Resistive load moment (Nm) for one knee joint in relation to joint angle (*x*-axis) during rising exercises in a device with movable trunk support. Effect of extra loading by adding 10 kg weight (= squares) and reduction of load by –10 kg (= diamonds) is shown. Trunk inclination: 10°. (Vertical bars: 95% confidence intervals; n = 6). (From Schüldt et al 1983.)

The position for exercising shoulder external rotators using a pulley exerciser is shown in Figure 4.2. Positions for internal rotators have also been studied. The position using a pulley-shoulder line to a frontal plane angle of 40° gave the best covariation between the resistance moment and the muscular strength curves, i.e. the subject was turned somewhat towards the pulley exerciser (Fig. 4.2, Harms-Ringdahl et al 1985).

Rubber exercise strips give increasing resistance with lengthening directed through the strip during the movement. The lever arm also changes. This has been studied using three qualities (elasticity modules) of strip: thin, heavy and extra heavy (Fig. 4.13, Harms-Ringdahl et al 1982). The rubber strips give a low resistance in relation to the average maximum moment (upper curves), both for internal and external rotation exercises in normal subjects. The peak of the load is, however, in an appropriate part of the movement sector for the chosen positioning of the subject. When strength is decreased, as e.g. measured in a female with tendinitis (dotted lines with triangles), the resistive load may be appropriate at least for endurance training. As when using pulley exercises, correct

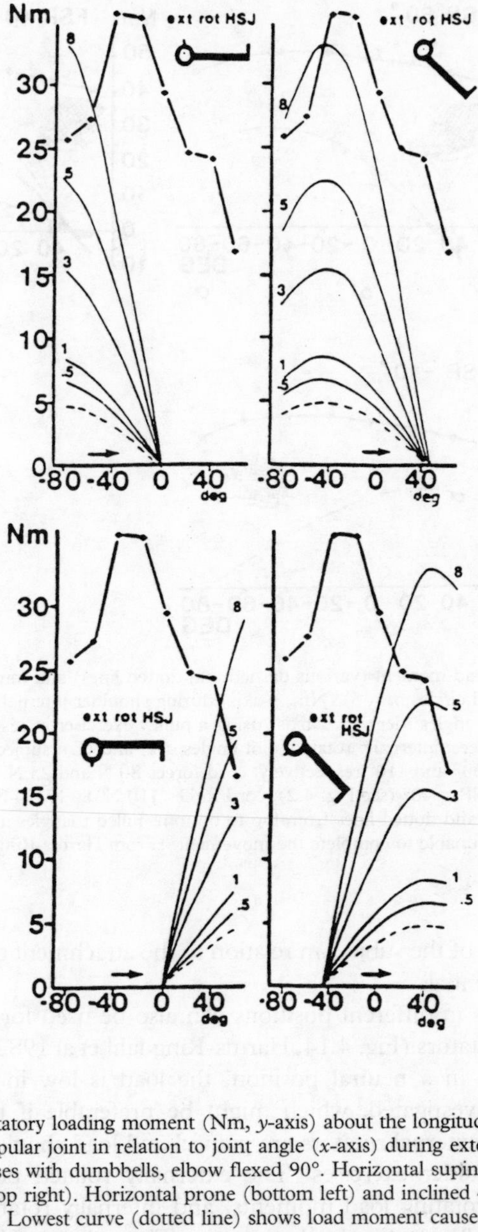

Fig. 4.11 Rotatory loading moment (Nm, *y*-axis) about the longitudinal axis of the humeroscapular joint in relation to joint angle (*x*-axis) during externally rotating exercises with dumbbells, elbow flexed 90°. Horizontal supine (top left); inclined 45° (top right). Horizontal prone (bottom left) and inclined 45° head up (bottom right). Lowest curve (dotted line) shows load moment caused by weight of forearm and hand alone. Solid line curves show total resistance moment. Dumbbell weights shown by figures alongside curves. Upper curve (diamonds) shows maximum isometric muscular moment of external rotators (n = 7). (From Harms-Ringdahl et al 1982.)

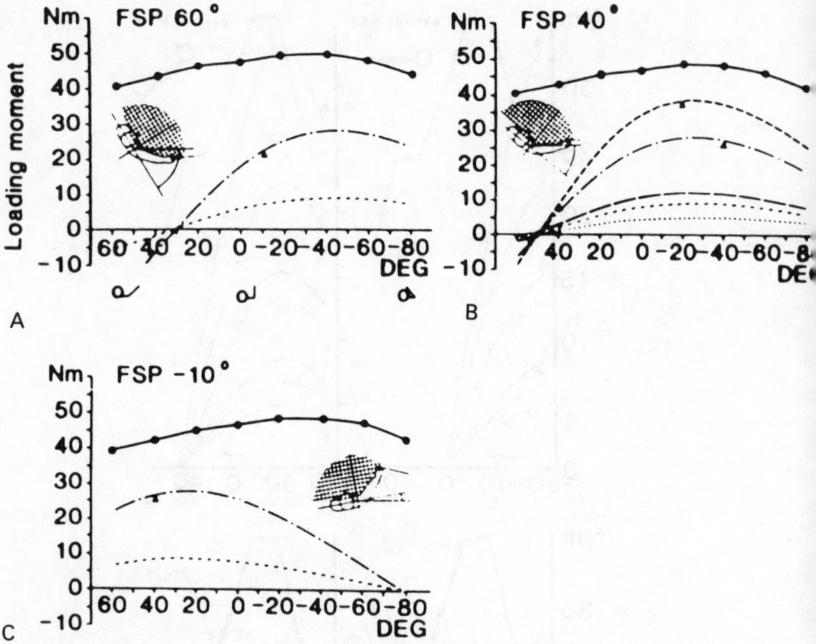

Fig. 4.12 Load moment (various dashed and dotted lines) and muscular strength (filled circles, $n = 5$) (Nm, y-axis) during shoulder internal rotation at different joint angles (degrees, x-axis) using a pulley exerciser as resistance device. Negative degrees: internally rotated joint angles. (A) and (C): subject positioning angle FSP = 60° and –10° respectively; cord forces 80 N and 25 N. (B): subject positioning FSP = 40° (see Fig. 4.2); cord forces 110 N, 80 N, 34 N, 25 N and 13 N, dashed and dotted lines from top to bottom. Filled triangles indicate where a subject was unable to complete the movement. (From Harms-Ringdahl et at 1983.)

positioning of the subject in relation to the attachment of the rubber strip is essential.

Push-ups in different positions can also be used for training the shoulder rotators (Fig. 4.14, Harms-Ringdahl et al 1982). When the shoulder is in a neutral position, the load is low in all push-up postures investigated, which might be preferable if the shoulder internal or external rotators are painful and load should be avoided during shoulder exercises. The externally rotated positions give externally rotating load moments, and internally rotated positions give internally rotating load moments. Thus, the positioning of the hands in relation to the shoulder joint is very important for the resistive load. The load is also influenced by the subject's posture. Push-ups against the floor with straight body, or kneeling with the

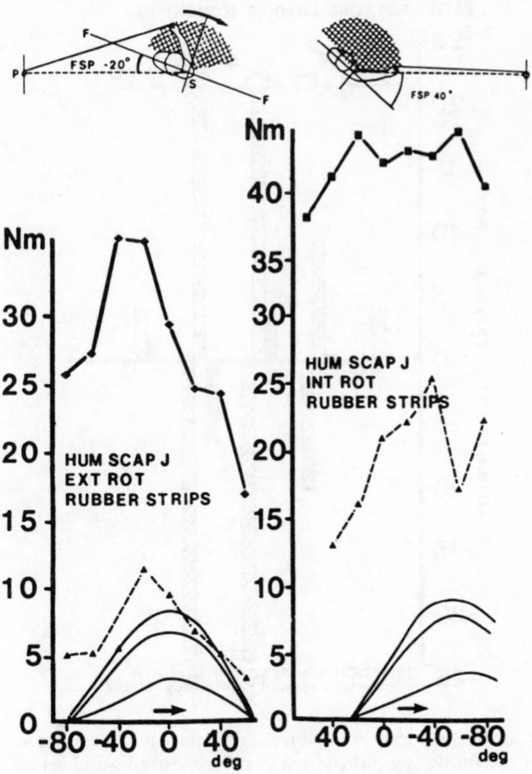

Fig. 4.13 Rotatory humeroscapular moments (Nm, *y*-axis) in relation to joint angle (*x*-axis) during rotating exercises resisted by rubber strips of three different qualities (elasticity modules). Subject positioned as indicated by drawings with an angle FSP (see Fig. 4.2) = 20° for external rotating (left) and FSP = 40° for internal rotating (right) exercises. Upper curves = maximum isometric muscular moment (strength) of the rotators in healthy subjects ($n = 7$). Dashed lines with triangles show an example of muscular strength in a patient with pain from shoulder tendinitis. The three lower continuous curves show moment caused by rubber strips. Arrows indicate direction of movement. (From Harms-Ringdahl et al 1982.)

hip flexed 45°, give high loads both in internal and external directions.

EXERCISE DOSE

Success in promoting functional increase of strength in patients is largely a matter of 'dose of exercise' and rate of increase in dose.

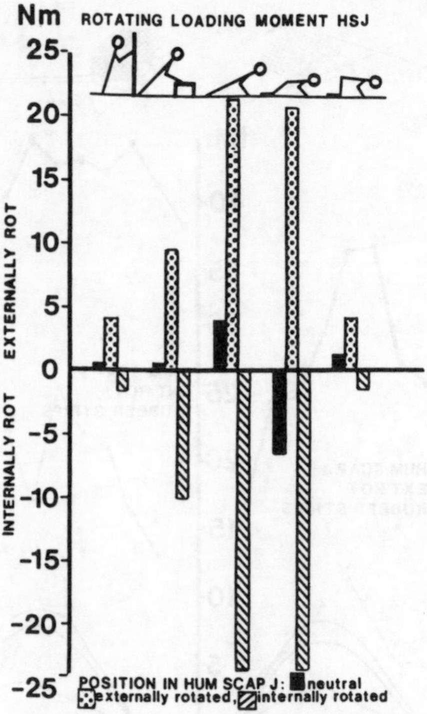

Fig. 4.14 Rotatory load moment (Nm, *y*-axis) about the longitudinal axis of the humeroscapular joint during push-ups with different hand positions leading to different shoulder rotation positions. Positive values: externally directed load moments counterbalanced by internal rotator muscles; negative values: internally rotating load moments counterbalanced by external rotator muscles. Trunk postures as indicated by drawings. (From Harms-Ringdahl et at 1982.)

Since the degree of muscular and articular impairment is individual, the optimum dose of exercise is also individual. *Thus, the functional capacity of each patient should be determined and the results used for the planning of the dose of exercise.* Motor performance, strength and endurance have to be assessed in joint angles and movements related to the situations where the functional biomechanical demands will be. As discussed in other sections of this book, isometric and isokinetic strength are correlated. For clinical purposes strength can be determined on an isometric basis, in relevant joint angles. If the functional demands require concentric muscle activity, a higher % MUR will be utilized than in the isometric test situation. Functional endurance tests can be performed and timed together with assessments of perceived exertion. When the requirements resulting from biomechanical analyses of work and leisure loads and the functional capacity of the patient have been mapped, suitable exercises can be chosen to optimize the training. For this planning an understanding of the biomechanical aspects of various exercises is necessary. The number of repetitions, load, speed and motion range can be determined from the requirements of the patient's impaired structures. For dynamic endurance training a resistance of 40% of maximal isometric strength is usually used (Hansen 1961, Petersen et al 1961). For adequate muscular strength training, resistance should be 50–70% of maximum isometric strength, as recommended by Hollman & Hettinger (1976). Depending on the physiological variation in strength through the movement sector, the applied weights are not always the most relevant factor. To find the best compromise between the curves for the resistance moment and the muscular moments, it is first necessary to find the subject's maximum muscular moment curve. For practical purposes, a fair estimate of this might be obtained by measurement at four different joint angles. With knowledge of the load moment curve caused by the resistance device, one can find the best adapted curve form and the best level of load to keep the muscle exercise at an adequate strength utilization level. For good general adaptation, the ratio between the loading moment and the maximum muscular moment (% MUR) should maintain values that are as similar as possible for as much as possible of the range of motion. However, for patients with a problem such as tendinitis or a partial tendon rupture, one might want to find exercises initially with very low, or no load, in a painful part of the motion sector.

Exercise checklist

The series of steps for designing a strengthening program is summarized in the following checklist:

1. Map the required work movements and work postures, e.g. with video.
2. Analyze the movements:
    a) biomechanically, e.g. induced forces and load moments at different joint angles for the postures and movements performed;

b) for duration of loads;
c) for type of muscle contraction (concentric, isometric, eccentric) and speed of motion.

3. Measure the patient's functional capacity for the corresponding variables, i.e. muscle strength at 3–4 joint angles (or with an isokinetic device) in the motion sector and the endurance for relevant loads and joint angles.
4. Find exercises which result in motor learning, and which lead to increases in endurance and strength in movements and postures, corresponding to no. 2 above.
5. Choose load level and duration according to the measurements in no. 3 above, aiming to improve function according to no. 2. Depending on the rehabilitation phase, the emphasis might be on different aspects of muscular performance (Grimby & Thomeé 1988), such as reduction or elimination of any reflex inhibition (Arvidsson et al 1986), recovery of muscle mass and achievement of gross motor functions by specific training for certain activities. (Note that extreme endurance and strength exercises cannot be successfully performed in the same time period.)

SUMMARY

Biomechanical methods can be applied to various therapeutic exercise situations. The effect of biomechanical factors on joint load has been mapped, such as the distribution of maximum muscular moment of force over the motion sector, the relation between resistive load and maximum muscular moments, subject positioning and the muscular strength utilization ratio. Different exercise examples are given for thigh and shoulder muscles. The load during the therapeutic exercises can be varied in many ways by adjustment of the subject's posture and position. It is concluded that guidelines based on biomechanical analyses can be found for the design and optimization of exercise movements.

REFERENCES

Arborelius U P, Ekholm J 1978 Mechanics of shoulder locomotor system during exercises resisted by weight-and-pulley circuit. Scandinavian Journal of Rehabilitation Medicine 10: 171–177

Arborelius U P, Ekholm J, Németh G, Hammarberg C 1982 Biomechanical aspects of hip joint load during exercises resisted by weight-and-pulley circuit. Europa Medico Physica 18: 245–251

Arvidsson I, Eriksson E, Knutsson E, Arnér S 1986 Reduction of pain inhibition on voluntary muscle activation by epidural analgesia. Orthopedics 9: 1415

Basmajian J V, Wolf S L (eds) 1990 Therapeutic exercise, 5th edn. Williams and Wilkins, Baltimore, USA

Bouchard C, Shepard R J, Stephens T, Sutton J R, McPersson B 1990 Exercise, fitness and health. A consensus of current knowledge. Human Kinetics Books, Champaign, Illinois, USA

Ekholm J, Arborelius U P, Németh G, Schüldt K, Harms-Ringdahl K 1982 Biomechanical research methods for analysis of factors influencing load and muscle activation during therapeutic exercise movements. Proceedings 'Man in Action', IXth International Congress of the World Confederation of Physical Therapy, Stockholm, Sweden. Part I, p 50–57

Ekholm J, Arborelius U P, Németh G, Harms-Ringdahl K, Schüldt K 1983 On the biomechanics of therapeutic exercises for strength and endurance. Proceedings 'New frontiers that influence disease and rehabilitation', 4th World Congress of the International Rehabilitation Medicine Association, San Juan, Puerto Rico, p 287–293

Ericson M O, Nisell R, Arborelius U P, Ekholm J 1985 Muscular activity during ergometer cycling. Scandinavian Journal of Rehabilitation Medicine 17: 53–61

Ericson M O, Bratt Å, Nisell R, Németh G, Ekholm J 1986 Load moment about the hip and knee joints during ergometer cycling. Scandinavian Journal of Rehabilitation Medicine 18: 165–172

Grimby G, Gustavsson E, Peterson L, Renström P 1980 Quadriceps function and training after knee ligament surgery. Medicine in Science and Sports 12: 70–75

Grimby G, Thomeé R 1988 Principles of rehabilitation after injuries. In: Dirix A, Knuttgen H G, Tittel K (eds) The Olympic Book of Sports Medicine, vol 1: 489–502

Hafajjee D, Moritz U, Svantesson G 1972 Isometric knee extension strength as a function of joint angle, muscle length and motor unit activity. Acta Orthopaedica Scandinavica 43: 138–147

Hansen J W 1961 The training effect of repeated isometric muscle contractions. Internationale Zeitschrift zur Angewante Physiologie 18: 474– 477

Harms-Ringdahl K, Arborelius U P, Németh G, Schüldt K, Ekholm J 1982 Biomechanical load and muscle activation during exercise therapy of the humeroscapular joint. In: World Confederation for Physical Therapy, Proceedings, part I, p 58–65. IXth International Congress, Stockholm

Harms-Ringdahl K, Ekholm J, Arborelius U P, Németh G, Schüldt K 1983 Load moment, muscle strength and level of muscular activity during internal rotation training of the shoulder. In: Recent Advances in Rehabilitation Medicine. Scandinavian Journal of Rehabilitation Medicine (Suppl. 9.): 125–135

Harms-Ringdahl K, Arborelius U P, Ekholm J, Németh G, Schüldt K 1985 Shoulder externally rotating exercises with pulley apparatus. Joint load and EMG. Scandinavian Journal of Rehabilitation Medicine, 17: 129–140

Hollman W, Hettinger T 1976 Sports medicine — Arbeits- und trainungsgrundlagen. F K Schattauer Verlag, Stuttgart

Kulig K, Andrews J G, Hay J G 1984 Human strength curves. Exercise in Sport and Sport Sciences Reviews 12: 417– 466

Moritz U, Svantesson G G, Haffajee D 1973 A biomechanical study of torque as affected by motor unit activity, length tension relationship and muscle force lever. In: Desmedt J E (ed) New developments in electromyography and clinical neurophysiology. Karger, Basel, 1: 675–682

Németh G, Ekholm J, Arborelius U P, Harms-Ringdahl K, Schüldt K 1983 Influence of knee flexion on isometric hip extensor strength. Scandinavian Journal of Rehabilitation Medicine 15: 97–101

Nisell R, Ericson M, Németh G, Ekholm J 1989 Tibiofemoral joint forces during isokinetic knee extension. American Journal of Sports Medicine 17: 49–54

Petersen F B H, Graudal H, Hansen J W, Hvid N 1961 The effect of varying the number of muscle contractions on dynamic muscle training. Internationale Zeitschrift zur Angewante Physiologie 18: 468

Saltin B, Gollnick P D 1983 Skeletal muscle adaptability: significance for metabolism and performance. In: Peachy L D, Adrian R, Geiger S R (eds) Handbook of physiology. Williams & Wilkins, Baltimore, USA, section 10: Skeletal muscle, p 555-631

Schüldt K, Ekholm J, Németh G, Arborelius U P, Harms-Ringdahl K 1983 Knee load and muscle activity during exercises in rising. In: Recent Advances in Rehabilitation Medicine. Scandinavian Journal of Rehabilitation Medicine, (Suppl 9): 174–188

Sinaki M 1989 Exercise and osteoporosis. Archives of Physical Medicine and Rehabilitation, 70: 220–229

Smidt G L, Blanpied P R 1987 Analysis of strength tests and resistive exercises commonly used for low-back disorders. Spine 12: 1025–1034

Svensson O K 1987 On quantification of muscular load during standing work. A biomechanical study. Thesis, Karolinska Institute, Stockholm, Sweden

Williams M, Stutzman L 1959 Strength variation through the range of joint motion. Physical Therapy Reviews 39: 145–152

5. Eccentric muscle activity in theory and practice

Dianne J. Newham

INTRODUCTION

Most of us are conditioned to think of muscle activity as falling primarily into one of two categories. The first is used to exert a stabilizing force with the muscle length remaining virtually constant, i.e. an isometric contraction. The second is a dynamic contraction, in which work is done and the muscles shorten during activity, i.e. a concentric contraction.

There is a third form of muscle activity, which is also of a dynamic nature, in which the active muscles are acted upon by external forces which lengthen them during activity. This is termed an eccentric contraction. This type of muscle activity is of great interest to both basic scientists and those concerned with physical training and rehabilitation as it has a number of characteristics which make it clearly different from both concentric and isometric muscle activity.

It would be a mistake to think that eccentric contractions are an unusual form of activity in everyday life and of little practical relevance. In general terms, a concentric contraction is followed, sooner or later, by an eccentric contraction of the same muscle. For example, we stand up by using concentric contractions of the hip and knee extensors and sit down by performing eccentric activity of the same muscle. Similarly, each time a weight is lifted by means of a concentric contractions of the elbow flexors it is lowered in a controlled manner by an eccentric contraction of these muscles. Thus eccentric contractions are commonly used by the body to exert a braking force and indeed form part of each step cycle.

The aim of this chapter is to bring attention to the known characteristics of eccentric contractions and discuss their relevance to physical training and rehabilitation. The reader should bear in mind that in addition to the term 'eccentric' contraction or activity, a number of others are used such as lengthening contractions, negative work and decelerator muscle function.

PROPERTIES OF ECCENTRIC CONTRACTIONS

i) Force generation

It has been known for a long time that the type of activity a muscle performs has a marked effect on the force it can generate. When an isolated muscle preparation is allowed to shorten, performing a concentric contraction, it generates less force than when its length is held constant in an isometric contraction (Hill 1938, Wilkie 1950). However, when the active muscle is lengthened and an eccentric contraction is performed, much greater forces are generated, up to nearly twice those of an isometric contraction (Katz 1939).

The force of a dynamic contraction is affected not only by the type of muscle activity but also by the speed of that activity. Hill (1938) showed that the force generated by a concentric contraction decreased to zero as velocity increased to the maximal. It was later shown by Katz (1939) that the force generated by an eccentric contraction increased with velocity up to a certain velocity and thereafter remained unaffected by increases in velocity. Therefore the greatest tension is generated by a fast eccentric contraction and the least by a fast concentric one. Isometric contractions generate an intermediate force which is always greater than that of a concentric contraction, but less than that of an eccentric one (Fig. 5.1).

The reason for the extra force generated by eccentric contractions is the subject of much debate and will not be discussed here in any detail. Interested readers are referred to recent reviews by Cavanagh (1988) and Stauber (1989). The different forces can be explained by the crossbridge theory of Huxley (1969) which states that the active force generated by a single crossbridge is the result of the binding between actin and myosin molecules. During a concentric contraction these bonds are broken as the myosin moves onto the next actin site. The faster the shortening velocity, a greater number of myosin molecules will be moving to the next actin site at any point in time and not generating tension. Therefore tension decreases as velocity increases. During eccentric activity the tension generated by the crossbridges is increased by the force which arises from the existing actin-myosin bonds being stretched. This is

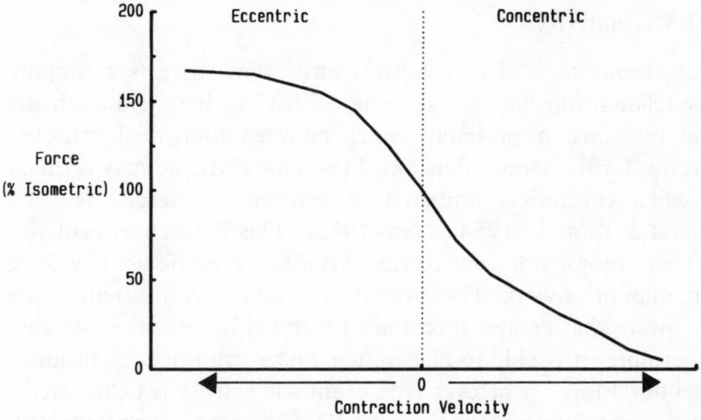

Fig. 5.1 The force–velocity relationship for skeletal muscle. The force generated by a shortening (concentric) contraction declines as velocity increases. It is always less than that generated by an isometric contraction (0 velocity). Conversely, lengthening (eccentric) activity generates greater tensions than isometric and the force increases with velocity up to a plateau value. Data derived from a number of sources.

analogous to the extra force that can be gained from an elastic band, which is already under some tension, when it is stretched further. The additional force will increase until the actin-myosin bonds are broken (without energy consumption), but the myosin can then attach to another actin and generate tension again.

Work on intact human muscle has shown that the relationship between force and speed during dynamic contractions is broadly similar to that described for isolated preparations, although there are some discrepancies. This applies to the force–velocity relationship of both concentric contractions (for review see Osternig 1986) and eccentric contractions. In the latter case it seems that the eccentric forces produced can be less than would be predicted by the isolated work, although there appear to be differences in the force–velocity relationship between individual muscles (Singh & Karpovich 1966, Komi 1973, Jorgensen 1976, Westing et al 1988). The most common explanation for this and for which there is some experimental evidence (Edman et al 1979, Triolo et al 1987), is that there is a neural mechanism which inhibits some muscles from producing their full eccentric force potential during voluntary, eccentric activity.

ii) EMG activity

During isometric and concentric contractions there is a roughly linear relationship between force and EMG activity, although the actual relationship probably varies between individual muscles. However, for the same submaximal load, the EMG activity is much less when eccentric, compared to concentric, exercise is used (Bigland & Lippold 1954, Komi 1973). This is taken as evidence that fewer motor units are recruited during eccentric activity for a given amount of work. Therefore the central nervous system seems to be aware that greater forces are generated by eccentric activity. Furthermore, it is able to alter motor unit recruitment to produce the required force, whatever type of muscle activity is being used.

During maximal contractions the EMG activity seems to remain virtually constant, while the force varies with velocity for both types of dynamic muscle activity (Komi 1973). This indicates that virtually maximal activation is possible during voluntary eccentric activity, at least in some muscles, and raises further questions about why the eccentric force–velocity relationship in some intact human muscles differs from that of isolated preparations.

iii) Metabolic factors

The metabolic cost of performing a given amount of work is less with eccentric activity than with concentric. This has been shown by measurements of oxygen uptake by human subjects (Abbott, Bigland & Ritchie 1952, Asmussen 1952, Knuttgen 1986) and also by the amount of ATP utilized by isolated preparations (Curtin & Davies 1973). The combination of high force output with a low metabolic cost means that eccentric activity is the most efficient way of doing work in mechanical terms. Due to the force–velocity relationship, the mechanical efficiency (ME) of eccentric activity increases with velocity and at the highest velocities the ME is greater than 100% (Margaria 1972, Aura & Komi 1986).

CONSEQUENCES OF ECCENTRIC ACTIVITY

The effects of performing eccentric activity depend to a large extent on whether this is an unfamiliar activity for a particular muscle, as a number of training induced adaptations have been described. Therefore the following section will deal firstly with the effects of unaccustomed eccentric activity and secondly with the effects of repeated eccentric activity.

Effects of unaccustomed eccentric activity

These fall under three main categories: pain, fatigue and damage; these will be discussed separately.

i) Muscle pain

It has been known since the beginning of this century that eccentric exercise is more likely to cause delayed onset muscle pain than other types of muscular activity. This type of pain has a very characteristic time course; it is not detectable until about 8–10 hours after exercise and reaches peak intensity one or two days after exercise (Newham 1988, Ebbeling & Clarkson 1989). Typically it is described as a dull aching sensation which is accompanied by tenderness and stiffness, the latter being subjectively alleviated by movement.

The fact that eccentric exercise is also associated with high force generation by the active fibres has led to the belief that the pain is due to some form of damage. Exactly which tissue the pain originates from has been the subject of much discussion and research, which will be discussed later. Despite this, the origin of delayed onset muscle pain is still unknown.

The main theories have included both the contractile and non-contractile, i.e. connective, tissues. The muscle spasm theory (Devries 1966) has been unsupported by experimental evidence and is now generally discounted. There is clear evidence of damage to contractile tissue, as will be described below, but there is substantial evidence that this does not cause the pain. The current evidence, albeit of an indirect nature, points in favour of connective tissue being the origin of delayed onset muscle pain. Many authors have reported that the discomfort is greatest at the promixal and distal ends of the muscles (e.g. Newham et al 1983), although this is not a universal finding. It has been suggested that such a distribution could be due to the more oblique angle of pennation in these regions, which may make the fibres more susceptible to mechanical trauma (Friden et al 1986). Alternatively, it could be an indication of damage to the connective tissue in the musculotendinous junctions (Armstrong 1984) or simply reflect the high density of nociceptors in these regions (Mense & Schmidt 1977).

People who have delayed onset muscle soreness often comment that the affected muscles feel swollen, but the experimental evidence for oedema is conflicting (Ebbeling & Clarkson 1989). Some workers have reported that there is an increase in limb volume or intramuscular pressure during the period of muscle soreness but others have failed to find any evidence of oedema. The reason for the lack of agreement may be that many different muscle groups have been studied and their anatomical compartments may vary considerably in compliance (Newham 1988). The presence of oedema in a compliant, extensible compartment would be reflected by an increase in volume which could occur in the absence of an increase in pressure. The opposite situation would be found in a relatively inextensible, low-compliance compartment.

Indirect evidence for the lack of association between delayed onset muscle soreness and oedema or swelling is provided by a number of studies which fail to show any effect of anti-inflammatory drugs, both steroidal and non-steroidal (reviewed by Ebbeling & Clarkson 1989). However there is some evidence that anti-inflammatory drugs may reduce the extent of the damage in animal experiments. There does not appear to be an increase in either neutrophils or total white blood cell counts in painful muscles after eccentric exercise, as would be expected if there were inflammation and oedema.

ii) Force fatigue

An inevitable consequence of any form of continued muscular activity is the onset of progressive fatigue. This can be measured by a decrease in either the force of isometric contractions or of dynamic ones from which power can be calculated. Historically, fatigue has usually been measured by changes in isometric force generation, largely for technical reasons. The relatively recent development of commercial dynamometers has resulted in more information becoming available about changes in dynamic force and power output, but this is still a relatively unexplored area. It is possible, but by no means certain, that fatigue as measured by a decrease in isometric force generation may underestimate the changes in dynamic force production.

Fatigue can be the result of changes within the muscle itself which decrease its ability to generate force and is thus of peripheral origin. Alternatively, there may be central changes which reduce the voluntary motor drive to the muscles, which themselves may or may

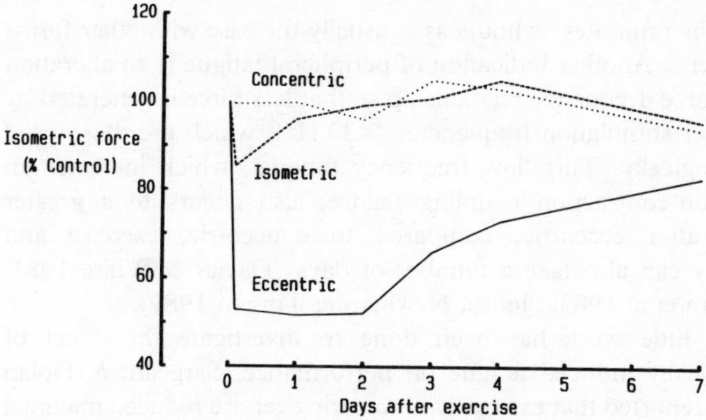

Fig. 5.2 Changes in the maximal, isometric voluntary contraction force after concentric, isometric and eccentric activity in the human elbow flexors. The subjects had performed the same number of maximal contractions of each type. Note that the eccentric activity caused the greatest force fatigue, which was also the slowest to recover (Jones, Newham & Torgan 1989)

not be showing peripheral fatigue. This is termed central fatigue and is an area in which there is an increasing amount of interest but, as yet, relatively little experimental evidence. In situations where only voluntary force generation is measured it cannot be known whether the fatigue is of peripheral or central origin. Only the use of electrical stimulation techniques provides definitive evidence about the site of fatigue (Belanger & McComas 1981, Rutherford, Jones & Newham 1986).

Eccentric activity has been shown to cause a greater reduction in isometric force than the same number of maximal isometric or concentric contractions (Fig. 5.2.) (Jones, Newham & Torgan 1989). The reduction in maximal voluntary, isometric force generation was demonstrated to be of peripheral origin by electrical stimulation techniques. Therefore it appears that during isometric contractions, muscles with delayed onset muscle pain can be fully activated during voluntary contraction and are not inhibited by pain as one might expect. However, this might not be the case during eccentric contractions as these are more painful than isometric ones. In addition to the profound loss of force after eccentric exercise (which may be up to about 50%), many workers have shown that recovery is very slow, occurring over a period of days, and on occasions more than a week (Newham, Jones & Clarkson 1987), rather than minutes or hours as is usually the case with other forms of exercise. Another indication of peripheral fatigue is an alteration in the force–frequency relationship so that less force is generated by the lower stimulation frequencies (<30 Hz), which are those used physiologically. This 'low frequency fatigue', which indicates an excitation-contraction coupling failure, also occurs to a greater extent after eccentric, compared to concentric, exercise and recovery can also take a number of days (Davies & White 1981, Newham et al 1983a, Jones, Newham & Torgan 1989).

Very little work has been done to investigate the effect of eccentrically induced fatigue on performance. Sargeant & Dolan (1987) reported that exhaustive eccentric exercise reduced maximal power output (measured during concentric cycling); the output was decreased when the muscles were showing low frequency fatigue and a reduced isometric force. The reduced power output would be expected to result in decreased performance and functional ability.

iii) Damage

Evidence of physical changes and/or structural damage to a number of tissues has repeatedly been shown to be most likely after eccentric activity. These will be described below, as will the temporal relationship between them and delayed onset muscle pain.

a) Myofibrillar damage. Direct evidence of myofibrillar damage has been obtained by both light and electron microscopy examinations of muscle biopsy samples. While it is clear that eccentric exercise is more likely to cause structural damage to the contractile machinery than other forms of muscle activity, the pattern of the changes is not clear. There appear to be two main forms of myofibrillar damage (Newham 1988, Ebbeling & Clarkson 1989, Stauber 1989).

The least severe form is only visible with electron microscopy; it is present immediately after exercise and becomes more extensive over the course of the next few days (Newham et al 1983b). The initial changes are usually restricted to individual sarcomeres which show misalignment of the contractile material and bulging Z-lines. Over a number of hours the disruption spreads and involves larger areas which include a number of adjacent sarcomeres and fibres. In these areas the normal structure of the muscle can be completely lost and there is marked streaming of the Z-lines.

The more severe form of myofibrillar damage is easily seen with light microscopy (Fig. 5.3); it also can be seen immediately after

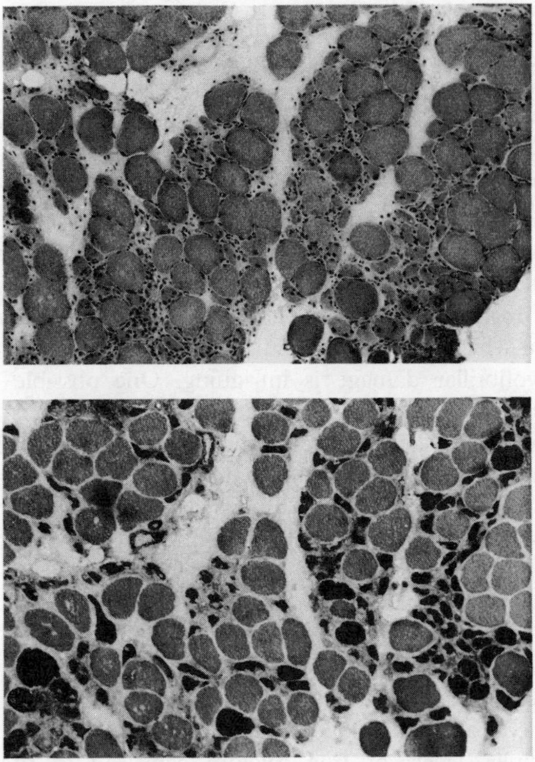

Fig. 5.3 Needle biopsy sections taken from the gastrocnemius muscle of a normal subject 12 days after performing eccentric contractions. The muscles had been very painful during the first few days after exercise, although the biopsy samples appeared normal. The pain had gone when these biopsies were taken. Twenty days after exercise the muscles appeared to have fully recovered. (A) Section stained with haematoxylin and eosin, showing many atrophied fibres and infiltration of white cells and fluid; (B) Section stained with ATPase at pH 9.4, showing the most affected fibres to be Type II, fast twitch (dark staining). Original magnification x100.

exercise and again becomes more marked over the next few hours and days. Often there is considerable atrophy of the affected fibres and also an infiltration of leucocytes and other indications of inflammation (Jones et al 1986).

Despite the progressive nature and extent of the myofibrillar damage, the repair processes are activated afer the first few days. The speed and completeness of repair and regeneration in normal, healthy subjects is remarkable and is virtually complete within three weeks of considerable disruption.

The Type II (fast twitch) fibres of human subjects are most affected by the structural changes and undergo greater atrophy (Friden et al 1984, Newham 1988). This is an interesting and surprising finding in view of the fact that the damage is thought to be due to the high tensions generated during eccentric exercise. Type II fibres are selectively recruited during high force contractions and would therefore be expected to withstand mechanical damage better than Type I (slow twitch) fibres; this finding is currently unexplained.

The major disruption is not seen until some days after the exercise which caused the damage and the progressive nature of the myofibrillar damage is intriguing. One possible explanation for this is that the high tensions generated during eccentric exercise actually break some fibres which may subsequently atrophy, especially at the break point (Stauber 1989). Another suggestion is that while some fibres are frankly damaged during the causative exercise, a greater number are less affected but are mechanically stressed. As a result of this they may be particularly susceptible to subsequent damage from the stress of normal activity (Armstrong 1984).

Mechanical disruption in a fibre could, presumably, affect the sarcoplasmic reticulum as much as any other structure. If this happened, calcium could leak out into the interior of the cell. Raised intracellular levels of free calcium can lead to tissue damage (Baracos et al 1986) and thus a chemically induced form of damage could compound that initially caused by mechanical factors (see Stauber 1989, Ebbeling & Clarkson 1989).

While it is clear that eccentric exercise is more likely to cause structural damage than other forms of muscular activity, there is no evidence that there is a causative link between this and delayed onset muscle pain. Immediately after exercise there is structural damage, although the muscles are completely pain-free. It is true that the damage is more extensive by the time the muscle become painful, but there is no reason to think that this relationship is anything other than coincidental. Consideration of the clinical situation reinforces this belief; patients with primary myopathies show abnormalities which are very similar to those after eccentric exercise, but the overwhelming majority of these patients are pain-free (Edwards & Jones 1983).

b) Membrane damage. In addition to the damage in the interior of the fibre, the fibres' membranes are affected by eccentric exercise. This results in a loss of membrane integrity and increased permeability, so that normal function is impaired and substances normally kept largely on one side of the membrane are allowed to cross in unusually large quantities. This is indicated by raised levels of muscle enzymes in venous blood and also by an increased uptake of radiolabelled substances into the fibre. This efflux of muscle enyzmes and influx of radioisotopes follow the same time course and reflect each other in magnitude (Newham 1988) and so it seems that they are manifestations of the same phenomenon.

A number of muscle specific enyzmes, such as creatine kinase (CK) and lactate dehydrogenase (LDH), are released into the circulation after many forms of exercise and also in myopathic conditions (Pennington 1981). After brief, exhaustive exercise there is a modest increase in circulating enyzmes (which approximately double the pre-exercise levels) with peak values occurring about 24 hours after exercise. In this case, energy depletion is thought to cause a small, transient change in membrane permeability (Ebbeling & Clarkson 1989).

After unaccustomed eccentric exercise there is a much more dramatic response in both the extent and time course of indications of membrane damage. In many cases the circulating levels of muscle enzymes can be similar to those found in patients with primary myopathies (Newham 1988). The circulating concentration of CK can increase by a factor of 100 and peak values do not occur until up to seven days after exercise (Newham 1988). This slow time course appears to be a true reflection of the efflux from the muscle, rather than slow clearance from either the muscle itself or the circulation (Ebbeling & Clarkson 1989). It is very unlikely that these membrane changes are caused by energy depletion, due to the low energy cost of eccentric exercise and also because of the delayed time course. In general, the magnitude of the efflux increases with the force of the contractions and it is thought that the high tensions generated during eccentric exercise cause mechanical damage to the membrane. This may also be exacerbated by subsequent metabolic disturbances such as calcium leakage from damaged sarcoplasmic reticulum.

There is a marked degree of variability in the individual response of the magnitude of the CK efflux. Eccentric training reduces this, as will be discussed later, but there is still a great variation in the response of untrained individuals. The reason for this is thought to include genetic factors (Ebbeling & Clarkson 1989).

There seems to be no causative relationship between the membrane damage and either muscle pain or myofibrillar damage. In the individuals with large enzyme effluxes, peak values occur when pain is declining and the structural damage is under repair. The magnitude of the enzyme efflux bears little or no relationship to the extent of myofibrillar damage (Jones et al 1986, Kuipers et al 1985).

c) Connective tissue damage. There is no reason to suppose that the non-contractile elements of the muscle would be spared from the damage that can be caused by eccentric exercise. However, the experimental evidence for connective tissue damage is largely either inconclusive or indirect. It has been reported that the musculotendinous junctions are particularly susceptible to injury from stretch (Garrett et al 1988). Furthermore, damage can occur in muscles which show little or no force fatigue and in which, therefore, there is no indication that the contractile elements are seriously compromised (McCully & Faulkner 1986). More indirect evidence for connective tissue damage comes from animal studies which have shown that the Type I (slow twitch) fibres have a stronger connective tissue harness than the Type II (fast twitch) fibres (Kovanan, Suominen & Heikkinen 1989) which are more affected by damage after eccentric contractions as mentioned earlier.

Muscles damaged by eccentric exercise often demonstrate an increased resistance to passive movement and the limb is held with the affected muscles at a short length. This shortening is electrically silent and therefore not due to the generation of active tension (Howell et al 1985, Jones, Newham & Clarkson 1987). It has also been shown that eccentric exercise performed by muscles at a long length causes more pain, fatigue and damage than when performed at a short length (Jones, Newham & Torgan 1989). This effect was independent of force, which was similar at both extremes of length, and is thought to be the result of additional stress imposed on the connective tissue.

Thus there is a considerable amount of data which point to injury and damage to connective tissue, although it is not known whether this affects the tendons themselves or the sheaths and fascia which surround the contractile material. It is interesting to note that pathological connective tissue disorders are usually associated with pain and tenderness. The incidence of connective tissue damage after eccentric exercise, and its association with delayed onset pain, is a topic which clearly warrants further investigation.

Effects of repeated eccentric exercise

a) Pain and damage

Most readers will be aware that delayed onset muscle pain is worse after the performance of unaccustomed exercise. Repetition of the same exercise on subsequent occasions causes a progressive reduction in pain until eventually it can be performed without any noticeable discomfort. This subjective impression of a decreased susceptibility to the undesirable consequences of unaccustomed eccentric exercise is substantiated by experimental evidence.

There are numerous studies which report that training reduces the susceptibility to delayed onset pain. Individuals who are accustomed to performing eccentric contractions in a particular muscle group are very resistant to developing delayed onset pain (Howell et al 1985, Evans et al 1986). Repeated bouts of eccentric exercise also reduce and eventually eliminate the enzyme efflux and structural changes that occur after the first bout (e.g. Friden et al 1983, Newham, Jones & Clarkson 1987, Clarkson & Tremblay 1988). It is particularly interesting that even a single bout of eccentric exercise can bring about a very significant training effect which persists for about 6 weeks (Byrnes et al 1985). Furthermore, the training adaptation can occur in the absence of changes in either muscle strength or fatigue resistance (Newham, Jones & Clarkson 1987).

In the majority of training studies, the exercise bouts have been separated by a number of weeks so that the muscles could recover between bouts, but in everyday practice training bouts are performed a number of times per week. Ebbeling & Clarkson (1988) used a protocol in which the second bout took place 5 days after the first. Recovery from the first bout did not appear to be affected by the second. However the optimal time between training bouts, which would both bring about the training effect and not delay recovery is not known.

The mechanism(s) involved in the training response are not understood at present, although the hypotheses include changes in motor-unit recruitment as well as metabolic and structural adaptation. The recruitment theory suggests that after the first bout of eccentric activity, the central nervous system learns that the generation of very high forces by relatively few fibres can cause pain and damage in the muscle. In subsequent bouts of such exercise, the tension generated by each active fibre is reduced by recruiting more motor units to generate the same total muscle tension. If this were true, then the training adaptation would only occur when submaximal contractions were being used since during a maximal contraction all, or virtually all, the motor units are recruited and there is little possibility of significant changes in the number of motor units recruited. However, it has been shown that the training adaptation does occur when maximal force contractions are used (Newham, Jones & Clarkson 1987). Furthermore, if a significantly greater number of motor units were active, the metabolic cost of the exercise would be expected to increase, but there is no evidence that this happens (Schwane, Williams & Sloan 1987). Another point is that the training effect is specific to individual muscles, rather than being a generalized phenomenon. Therefore, although the recruitment hypothesis is an attractive one, the experimental evidence does not support it.

It has been proposed that training evokes a metabolic adaptation (Nuttall & Jones 1968, Hunter & Critz 1971), but is generally thought that the adaptation takes the form of a structural change (Friden et al 1983, Knuttgen 1986, Newham, Jones & Clarkson 1987, Clarkson & Tremblay 1988, Lieber & Friden 1988). There is also debate about which tissues undergo structural change; both contractile and/or non-contractile material could be involved. Armstrong et al (1983) suggested that the initial bout of exercise caused sufficient damage to eliminate a pool of susceptible fibres, leaving only damage-resistant fibres to perform the exercise during the period of increased protection. However, the fact that subsequent bouts of exercise result in a similar amount of force fatigue, even though pain and damage are diminished, argues against this theory.

There is some direct evidence of a proliferation of connective tissue during eccentric training in both animal (Kovanen, Suominen & Heikkinen 1980) and human studies. An increased content of connective tissue is also seen in the muscles of trained individuals (MacDougall et al 1982, Siegel, Warhol & Lang 1986).

b) *Muscle strength and hypertrophy*

The fact that unaccustomed eccentric exercise causes temporary damage and a decrease in muscle force begs the question of whether this type of activity has an important role in strength training regimes — in both rehabilitation and sport.

For decades it has been accepted that a muscle will hypertrophy when it is regularly required to perform unusually high force contractions. The 'overload' principle was first brought to prominence by deLorme (1946) and has formed the basis for strength training programmes up to the present day. Despite the widely accepted belief that high force contractions are required to induce hypertrophy, neither the underlying mechanisms or the optimal regimes are known (Jones, Rutherford & Parker 1989).

Acceptance of the overload principle has led to the logical speculation that, since eccentric activity generates the highest forces, it should be the most effective type of activity to increase muscle strength. Not surprisingly, this question has been the subject of a larger number of investigations. The overwhelming majority of these have failed to show that eccentric training programmes offer any advantage in stimulating hypertrophy (for reviews see Rasch 1974, Atha 1981, Jones, Rutherford & Parker 1989). In some cases this might be due to the fact that the same training weights were used for both eccentric and either isometric or concentric contractions; this would mean that during the eccentric activity the muscles were working at a lower proportion of their maximal strength. However, this does not apply to all the studies and even in those which used the same proportion of maximal force for each type of activity, there was no additional increase in strength from training with eccentric exercise (e.g. Jones & Rutherford 1987). Numerous other studies have shown that very similar increases in strength occur whatever type of muscle activity is used.

The fact that eccentric exercise does not bring about the greatest increase in strength raises questions about the stimulus for muscle hypertrophy. If, as is commonly thought, this is simply a response to the mechanical force that is developed by the muscle, then eccentric exercise would be expected to be most effective. This is not the case, but neither is there any reason to think that metabolic depletion is the crucial factor. If this were so then the greatest increases in strength would occur when concentric contractions are used, but this is not so (Jones & Rutherford 1987). Therefore there is good reason to think that neither mechanical nor metabolic factors alone act as the stimulus for hypertrophy. It may be that some combination of the two is necessary, or that the numerous processes involved in the activation of a strong, voluntary muscle contraction act as the stimulus, perhaps in addition to hormonal factors.

The finding that eccentric exercise is not the most effective way of increasing strength also negates the hypothesis that physical damage is an important stimulus for hypertrophy. As mentioned earlier, eccentric training can produce a muscle which is resistant to pain and damage, but which is neither stronger nor less fatiguable.

Although eccentric contractions do not cause greater hypertrophy than other forms of exercise, their role in training programmes should not be ignored. The phenomenon of specificity is the subject of a growing body of literature; a frequent finding in training studies is that the greatest improvement occurs in the training exercise itself, rather than measurements of strength or size in individual muscles (e.g. Sale & MacDougall 1981, Jones, Rutherford & Parker 1989). The effects of training specificity are seen not only in a particular task or function, but also with the muscle length and velocity of contraction used during training. With respect to task specificity, it seems that there is little cross-over between the training activity and other functional activities. Thus there can be a significant improvement in a dynamic training activity with little or no change in isometric strength or power output when measured during another activity (Sargeant, Hoinville & Young 1981, Rutherford & Jones, 1986, Rutherford et al 1986). Therefore, in addition to performing weight training exercises for individual muscle groups, it is important to match the training activity to the desired functional activity.

c) Clinical applications

In general terms the discussion in the preceding section also applies to the clinical application of eccentric exercise. There are, however, some additional points which warrant consideration.

The relatively recent development of dynamometers which are capable of measuring the force of eccentric muscle activity, coupled with their high purchase costs, result in only a small amount of clinical studies investigating eccentric exercise. Nevertheless, it has become fairly common clinical practice to incorporate eccentric exercise in sports medicine and rehabilitation programmes (e.g. Standish, Rubinovich & Curwin 1986, Renstrom 1988, Grimby & Thombee 1988). It is important to remember that any particular role for eccentric exercise in rehabilitation is at present largely speculative and little evaluation has been carried out.

It has been suggested that abnormalities in the generation of eccentric force can be a contributory factor to knee pain (Hughston, Walsh & Puddu 1984) and that there is a specific deficit of eccentric force which responds to training (Bennett & Stauber 1986).

Knuttson (1987) reported an interesting finding which may have important implications for the management of neurological patients with spasticity. In these patients, eccentric training appeared to reduce the inhibition caused by activity in antagonistic muscle groups and was associated with an improvement in both muscle strength and function.

While it has been shown by a number of studies that normal, healthy subjects recover completely and rapidly from the various forms of damage that unaccustomed eccentric exercise can cause, it is not known whether this holds true for individuals who already have a primary muscle disease. In pathological conditions where muscle breakdown is increased and/or synthesis depressed, the effects of eccentrically induced muscle damage may be more profound, but this is purely speculative and there appears to be no experimental data on this issue.

CONCLUSIONS

There is a considerable amount known about the effect of eccentric muscle activity on both untrained and trained muscle. Conversely, despite the many regimes which either encourage or warn against such activity in training programmes, remarkably little is known about the role of eccentric exercise in rehabilitation and athletic training. This information can only be obtained by scientific investigations of the stimulus for muscle hypertrophy and studies of the effects of eccentric exercise in clinical practice and athletic training.

REFERENCES

Abbott B C, Bigland B, Ritchie J M 1952 The physiological cost of negative work. Journal of Physiology 117: 380–390

Armstrong R B 1984 Mechanisms of exercise-induced delayed onset muscular soreness: a brief review. Medicine & Science in Sports & Exercise 16: 529–538

Armstrong R B, Ogilvie R W, Schwane J A 1983 Eccentric exercise-induced injury to rat skeletal muscle. Journal of Applied Physiology 54: 80–93

Asmussen E 1952 Positive and negative muscular work. Acta Physiologica Scandinavica 28: 365–382

Atha J 1981 Strengthening muscle. Exercise and Sports Science Review 9: 1–73

Aura O, Komi P V 1986 Mechanical efficiency of pure positive and pure negative work with special reference to the work intensity. International Journal of Sports Medicine 7: 44 – 49

Baracos V, Greenberg R E, Goldberg A L 1986 Influence of calcium and other divalent cations on protein turnover in rat skeletal muscle. Americal Journal of Physiology 250: E702–E710

Belanger A Y, McComas A J 1981 Extent of motor unit activation during effort. Journal of Applied Physiology 51: 1131–1135
Bennett J G, Stauber W T 1986 Evaluation and treatment of anterior knee pain using eccentric exercise. Medicine and Science in Sports and Exercise 18: 526–530
Bigland B, Lippold O C J 1954 The relation between force, velocity and integrated electrical activity in human muscles. Journal of Physiology 123: 214–224
Byrnes W C, Clarkson P M, White J S, Hsieh S S, Frykman P N et al 1985 Delayed onset muscle soreness following repeated bouts of downhill running. Journal of Applied Physiology 59: 710–715
Cavanagh P R 1988 On 'muscle action' vs 'muscle contraction'. Journal of Biomechanics 21: 69–85
Clarkson P M, Tremblay I 1988 Rapid adaptation to exercise-induced muscle damage. Journal of Applied Physiology 65: 1–6
Curtin N A, Davies R E 1973 Chemical and mechanical changes during stretching of activated frog skeletal muscle. Cold Spring Harbor Symposia on Quantitative Biology 27: 619–626
Davies C T M, White M J 1981 Muscle weakness following eccentric work in man. Pflugers Archives 392: 168–171
deLorme T L 1946 Heavy resistance exercises. Archives of Physical Medicine 27: 607–630
DeVries H A 1966 Quantitative electromyographic investigation of the spasm theory of muscle pain. American Journal of Physical Medicine 45: 119–134
Ebbeling C A, Clarkson P M 1988 Exercise-induced muscle damage and adaptation. Sports Medicine 7: 207–234
Edman K A P, Elzinga G, Noble M I M 1979 The effect of stretch on contracting skeletal muscle fibres. In: Sugi H, Pollack G H (eds) Cross-bridge mechanism in muscle contraction. University Park Press, Baltimore p 297–309
Edwards R H T, Jones D A 1983 Diseases of skeletal muscle. In: Handbook of physiology: vol 10. Skeletal muscle. Williams & Wilkins, Baltimore, p 633–672
Evans W J, Meredith C N, Cannon J G, Dinarello C A, Frontera W R, Hughes V A, Jones B H, Knuttgen H G 1986 Metabolic changes following eccentric exercise in trained and untrained men. Journal of Applied Physiology 61: 1864–1868
Friden J 1984 Muscle soreness after exercise: implications of morphological changes. International Journal of Sports Medicine 5: 57–66
Friden J, Seger J, Ekblom B 1988 Sublethal muscle fibre injuries after high-tension anaerobic exercise. European Journal of Applied Physiology and Occupational Physiology 57: 360–368
Friden J, Seger J, Sjostrom M, Ekblom B 1983 Adaptive response in human skeletal muscle subjected to prolonged eccentric training. International Journal of Sports Medicine 4: 177–183
Friden J, Sfakianos P N, Hargens A R 1986 Muscle soreness and intra-muscular fluid pressure: comparison between eccentric and concentric load. Journal of Applied Physiology 61: 2175–2179
Garrett W E, Nikolaou P K, Ribbeck B M, Glisson R R, Seaber A V 1988 The effect of muscle architecture on the biomechanical failure properties of skeletal muscle under passive extension. American Journal of Sports Medicine 16: 7–12
Grimby G, Thombee R 1988 Principles of rehabilitation after injuries. In: Dirix A, Knuttgen H G, Tittel K (eds) The olympic book of sports medicine, volume I. Blackwell Scientific Publications, Oxford p 489–502
Hill A V 1938 The heat of shortening and the dynamic constants of muscle. Proceedings of The Royal Society of London (Biology) 126: 136–195
Howell J N, Chilia A G, Ford G, David D, Gates T 1985 An electromygraphic study of elbow motion during postexercise muscle soreness. Journal of Applied Physiology 58: 1713–1718

Hughston J C, Walsh W M, Puddu G 1984 Patellar subluxation and dislocation, volume 5. W B Saunders, Philadelphia, p1–191

Hunter J B, Critz J B 1971 Effect of training on plasma enzyme levels in man. Journal of Applied Physiology 31: 20–23

Huxley H E 1969 The mechanism of muscular contraction. Science 164: 1356–1366

Jones D A, Newham D J, Clarkson P M 1987 Skeletal muscle stiffness and pain following eccentric exercise of the elbow flexors. Pain 30: 233–242

Jones D A, Newham D J, Round J M, Tolfree S E J 1986 Experimental human muscle damage: morphological changes in relation to other indices of muscle damage. Journal of Physiology 375: 435–448

Jones D A, Newham D J, Torgan C 1989 Mechanical influences on long-lasting human muscle fatigue and delayed-onset pain. Journal of Physiology 412: 415–427

Jones D A, Rutherford O M 1987 Human muscle strength training: the effects of three different regimes and the nature of the resultant changes. Journal of Physiology 391: 1–11

Jones D A, Rutherford O M, Parker D F 1989 Physiological changes in skeletal muscle as a result of strength training. Quarterly Journal of Experimental Physiology 74: 233–256

Jones D A, Round J M 1990 Skeletal muscle in health and disease. Manchester University Press, Manchester

Jorgensen K 1976 Force-velocity relationship in human elbow flexors and extensors. In: Komi P V (ed) International Series on Biomechanics, vol 1A. Baltimore University Park Press, p 145–151

Katz B 1939 The relation between force and speed in muscular contraction. Journal of Physiology 96: 45–64

Knuttgen H G 1986 Human performance in high-intensity exercise with concentric and eccentric muscle contractions. International Journal of Sports Medicine (suppl) 7: 6–9

Knutsson E 1987 Analysis of spastic paresis. In: Proceedings of the Tenth International Congress of the World Confederation for Physical Therapy, Sydney, p 629–633

Komi P V 1973 Relationship between muscle tension, EMG, and velocity of contraction under concentric and eccentric work. In: Desmedt J E (ed) New developments in electromyography and clinical neurophysiology. Karger, Basel, vol 1, p 596–606

Kovanen V, Suominen H, Hiekkinen E 1984 Mechanical properties of fast and slow skeletal muscle with special reference to collagen and endurance training. Journal of Biomechanics 17: 725–735

Kuipers H, Janssen E, Keizer H, Verstappen F 1985 Serum CPK and amount of muscle damage in rats. Medicine and Science in Sports and Exercise 17: 195

Lieber R L, Friden J 1988 Selective damage of fast glycolytic fibres with eccentric contractions of the rabbit tibialis anterior. Acta Physiologica Scandinavica 133: 587–588

McCully K K, Faulkner J A 1986 Characteristics of lengthening contractions associated with injury to skeletal muscle fibres. Journal of Applied Physiology 61: 293–299

MacDougall J D, Sale D G, Elder G C B, Sutton J R 1982 Muscle ultra-structural characteristics of elite power lifters and bodybuilders. European Journal of Applied Physiology 48: 117–126

Margaria R 1972 Positive and negative work performances and their efficiencies in human locomotion. In: Cumming S R, Snidal D, Taylor A W (eds) Environmental effects on work performance. Canadian Association of Sports Sciences, Edmonton, p 215–228

Mense S, Schmidt R F 1977 Muscle pain: which receptors are responsible for the transmission of noxious stimuli? In: Rose C (ed) Physiological aspects of clinical neurology. Blackwell Scientific Publications, Oxford p 265–278
Newham D J 1988 The consequences of eccentric contractions and their relationship to delayed onset muscle pain. European Journal of Applied Physiology 57: 353–359
Newham D J, Jones D A, Clarkson P M 1987 Repeated high-force eccentric exercise: effects on muscle pain and damage. Journal of Applied Physiology 63: 1381–1386
Newham D J, Mills K R, Quigley, B M, Edwards R H T 1983a Pain and fatigue following concentric and eccentric muscle contractions. Clinical Science 64: 109–122
Newham D J, McPhail G, Mills K R, Edwards R H T 1983b Ultrastructural changes after concentric and eccentric contractions. Journal of the Neurological Sciences 61: 109–122
Newham D J 1991 Skeletal muscle pain and exercise. Physiotherapy 77: 66–70
Nuttal F Q, Jones B 1968 Creatine kinase and glutamic oxalacetic transaminase activity in serum: kinetics of change with exercise and effect of physical conditioning. Journal of Laboratory and Clinical Medicine 71: 847–854
Osternig L R 1986 Isokinetic dynamometry: implications for muscle testing and rehabilitation. Exercise and Sports Sciences Review 14: 45–80
Pennington R J T 1981 Biochemical aspects of muscle disease. In Walton J N (ed) Disorders of voluntary muscle, 4th edn. Churchill Lovingstone, Edinburgh, p 417–444
Rasch P J 1974 The present status of negative exercise — a review. American Corrective Therapy Journal 28: 77–94
Renstrom P 1988 Diagnosis and management of overuse injuries. In: Dirix A, Knuttgen H G, Tittel K (eds) The olympic book of sports medicine, volume I. Blackwell Scientific Publications, Oxford, p 446–468
Rutherford O M, Jones D A 1986 The role of learning and coordination in strength training. European Journal of Applied Physiology 55: 100–105
Rutherford O M, Jones D A, Newham D J 1986 Clinical and experimental application of the percutaneous twitch superimposition technique for the study of human muscle activation. Journal of Neurology, Neurosurgery and Psychiatry 49: 1288–1291
Rutherford, O M, Greig, C A, Sargeant A J, Jones D A 1986 Strength training and power output: transference effects in the human quadriceps. Journal of Sports Sciences 4: 101–107
Sale D G, MacDougall J D 1981 Specificity in strength training; a review for the coach and athlete. Canadian Journal of Applied Sports Science 6: 87–92
Sargeant A J, Dolan P 1987 Human muscle function following prolonged eccentric exercise. European Journal of Applied Physiology 56: 704–711
Sargeant A J, Hoinville E, Young A 1981 Maximum leg force and power output during short term dynamic exercise. Journal of Applied Physiology 51: 1175–1182
Schwane J A, Williams J S, Sloan J H 1987 Effects of training on delayed onset muscle soreness and serum creatine kinase activity after running. Medicine and Science in Sports and Exercise 19: 584–590
Siegel A J, Warhol M J, Lang G 1986 Muscle injury and repair in ultra-long distance runners. In: Sutton J R, Brock R M (eds) Sports medicine for the mature athlete. Benchmark Press, Indianapolis, p 35–43
Singh M, Karpovich P V 1966 Isotonic and isometric forces of forearm flexors and extensors. Journal of Applied Physiology 21: 1435–1437
Stanish W D, Rubinovich R M, Curwin S 1986 Eccentric exercise in chronic tendinitis. Clinical Orthopaedics 208: 65–68

Stauber W T 1989 Eccentric action of muscles: physiology, injury and adaptation. In: Pandolf K B (ed) Exercise and Sports Science Reviews, vol 17. American College of Sports Medicine Series. Williams & Wilkins, Baltimore, p 157–186

Triolo R, Robinson D, Gardner E, Betz R 1987 The eccentric strength of electrically stimulated paralysed muscle. IEEE Transactions in Biomedical Engineering 651–652

Westing S H, Seger J Y, Karslon E, Ekblom B 1988 Eccentric and concentric torque-velocity characteristics of the quadriceps femoris in man. European Journal of Physiology 58: 100–104

Wilkie D R 1950 The relation between force and velocity in human muscle. Journal of Physiology 110: 249–280

6. Muscle strength in relation to muscle length, pain and muscle imbalance

Vladimir Janda

INTRODUCTION

Muscle strength and weakness and its assessment is influenced by a broad spectrum of anatomical, physiological, mechanical and even methodological considerations (Smidt & Rogers 1982). With the exception of strength changes due to lesions of specific structures, e.g. of the second motoneuron, insufficient attention has been paid to those factors which might influence a voluntary contraction, such as the number of motor units activated, the frequency of their firing and the firing pattern. It is well known that the quality of muscle contraction together with the sequencing of activation of individual muscles during a particular movement (patterning) have a considerable influence on final muscular strength.

If there is no neurological disorder, it is — in a simplified way — presumed almost automatically that achieving a required muscle strength depends entirely or almost entirely on the quality of training and strengthening. Therefore in this chapter attention will be paid to some factors which, in a routine busy practice, may be underestimated and not appreciated as limiting in an attempt to strengthen muscles to a required level.

Myofascial trigger points, muscle tightness and tightness weakness, stretch weakness and muscle imbalance and arthrogenic weakness will be discussed.

TRIGGER POINTS AND MUSCLE STRENGTH

According to Travell & Rinzler (1952), myofascial trigger points are small hypersensitive regions within a muscle from which impulses bombard the central nervous system and give rise to referred pain. A trigger point in a skeletal muscle is identified by a localized deep tenderness in a palpably firm band of muscle. Deep palpation provokes a positive 'jump sign' as an indicator of increased irritability of the shortened muscle band.

Trigger points can develop directly, when the noxious stimulus acts upon the trigger area itself, or indirectly through the spinal cord (Travell & Simons 1983). This second type (if not both) evidently corresponds to muscle hypertonicity (spasm) due to an incoordinated muscle contraction as a result of the impaired function of the interneurons on the spinal segmental level (Janda 1991).

In a muscle that contains trigger points, three types of muscle fibres can be differentiated by electromyography, according to their excitability threshold, and clinically by deep palpation:

—a group which produces trigger points. The excitability threshold of these fibres is very low. These muscle fibres are those which are palpably firm, short and produce a local muscle hardening;

—a group in the vicinity of fibres in spasm. These fibres are hypotonic (= inhibited), which, in fact, can be palpated as a soft shallow groove along the fibres in spasm;

—a group of 'normal' muscle fibres which are remote from the trigger points.

With respect to pain, active and latent trigger points can be differentiated. Active points are those which cause episodes of referred pain and their threshold to mechanical stimulation is relatively low. The latent trigger points are clinically asymptomatic. Both types often lead to muscle weakness and impaired proprioceptive information. Thus there is not much difference between them (Travell & Simons 1983). It is understandable that when a decreased number of motor units are activated and the firing pattern is changed during active muscle contraction, the end result is muscle weakness. This muscle weakness is not associated with muscle atrophy, even if it lasts over a long period (Travell 1976). Why this is so has not been explained satisfactorily. At the present stage of our knowledge, it is difficult to say whether this decrease in muscle strength is due to a prolonged shortening of some muscle fibres (tightness weakness) or whether the muscle weakness occurs mainly due to the inhibition of muscle fibres in the neighbourhood of the trigger points. In any event, there is a decreased number of firing motor units and the recruitment of motor units is altered in terms of synchronization.

Trigger points are extremely frequent and thus, in addition to recognizing the fact that they may be a source of referred pain, they have to be taken into consideration in many, if not all, impairments of muscle function. This is particularly true in sports physiotherapy and in treatment of sports injuries. It is also important to notice that trigger points can contribute to the decrease in muscle strength in the postpolio syndrome, thus mimicking a weakness due to the progressive degeneration of the anterior horn cells.

Treatment of both active or latent trigger points, e.g. by a spray and stretch technique or postisometric relaxation, leads not only to pain relief but also to an immediate improvement in the strength of the particular muscle (Travell & Simons 1983).

MUSCLE LENGTH, MUSCLE INHIBITION AND MUSCLE IMBALANCE IN RELATION TO MUSCLE STRENGTH

An appropriate elasticity, i.e. a good flexibility (extensibility), of a muscle is an important precondition to achieving the full possible strength of the muscle. However, the terminology is vague and individual specialists dealing with the motor system quite often assign completely different meanings to the same term. In this chapter, the terms muscle tightness, reduced flexibility and extensibility are used as synonyms. Other terms used are, e.g. muscle shortening, shortness, stiffness, tautness or muscle hardening.

Muscle shortness or tightness

Muscle shortness or tightness, which develops without any evident structural neurological lesion and is apparently associated with overuse of the particular muscle, has never been properly defined. It indicates a condition in which the muscle is shorter than normal at rest and cannot be stretched either passively or actively to its normal length. Such a shortened muscle may move the joint from the normal rest position when inactive. It does not allow full range of motion. The important point is that a tight muscle — evidently in keeping with Sherrington's law* of reciprocal innervation — inhibits its antagonistic counterpart. This, then, leads not only to muscle imbalance, but — if not considered — also substantially influences the effect of therapeutic exercise (Janda 1978).

*Sherrington's Law (2): When a muscle receives a nerve impulse to contract, its antagonists recieve, simultaneously, an impulse to relax.

The result of decreased muscle flexibility is not only a lower excitability threshold, but also a changed elasticity, evidently due to hypertrophy and retraction of the retractile connective tissue in the muscle. This hypertrophy and retraction unfavourably influences the contractile ability of the muscle fibres. In addition, it may lead to impaired circulation producing ischemia and thus accelerating degeneration. Ultimately, the whole process results in a functional disability (Cailliet 1977). However, it has to be admitted that histological studies of tight muscles demonstrating these phenomena are still lacking.

The vicious circle can be described as follows: during training and/or prolonged overuse, the muscle will get shorter, stronger and readily activated (Janda 1964, 1984; Sahrmann 1987). However, the more marked the tightness, the worse the biomechanical and nutritional conditions of the muscle, and thus gradually the muscle strength decreases. Thus a tight muscle results in weakness, and we are right to speak about a *tightness weakness*. In time, adequately performed stretching may restore muscle strength.

Stretch weakness

Stretch weakness was first described by Kendall (Kendall, Kendall & Boynton 1952). It is defined as the effect on muscles of remaining in an elongated condition beyond the neutral physiological rest position, but not beyond the normal range of muscle elongation. According to Sahrmann (1987), a more accurate term is *positional weakness*. A shortened (tight) muscle may cause an altered position of a joint which in turn may lead to elongation of its antagonist.

To some extent Janda (1969, 1984, 1986) and in particular Sahrmann (1987) have developed their concepts of muscle imbalance based on Kendall's observations. Data on experimental animals reveal that a muscle shortness is associated with shorter muscle fibres (Gossman, Sahrmann & Rose 1982), whereas an elongation of the muscle is associated with elongation of muscle fibres but decrease and shortness of sarcomeres (Tardieu et al 1979). The clinical result is, however, the same — weakness.

The question is whether the final muscle weakness (due either to tightness or elongation) can be explained by this theory alone. In addition, nervous regulatory mechanisms (mainly spinal or segmental) also might participate (such as Sherrington's law considering reciprocal innervation). In such a case, a positional weakness would be rather the result of a reflex inhibition than of impaired muscle length.

Tightness-weakness and stretch-weakness may very often appear simultaneously in functionally related muscles and play an important role in the concept of *muscle imbalance*. However, even as regards the term muscle imbalance there is some confusion. Janda (1964) considers muscle imbalance as an impaired relationship between muscles which are prone to develop tightness and shortness and muscles which are prone to inhibition. Under the term muscle imbalance, therefore, a combination of at least three factors should be considered: muscle length, the irritability threshold of specific muscles and altered recruitment of these muscles. Sahrmann (1987) and, similarly, Cailliet (1977) define muscle imbalance as a failure of the agonist-antagonists relationship. Sahrmann (1987) considers muscle imbalance as active when one of a synergistic pair of muscles predominates during a movement. The result is either a diminished participation of the other muscle that leads to disuse atrophy, or excessive motion in the direction of another action produced by the dominant muscle.

Regardless of the explanation of a possible mechanism, some muscles typically develop inhibition, expressed by their hypotonia, decreased strength and (and this is particularly important) delayed activation during important movement patterns. If such a situation lasts long (several months) a mild atrophy may develop.

All these changes are not limited only to interplay between two antagonists, but have a striking tendency to generalize. In the end, a generalized muscle imbalance develops. As far as body mechanics and joint protection are concerned, muscle imbalance probably presents a much greater danger for the joint system than the muscle weakness alone.

ARTHROGENIC MUSCLE INHIBITION AND DECREASE OF MUSCLE STRENGTH

Altered proprioceptive input from an injured joint is a common situation. However, it is often not recognized as frequently as would be desirable in physiotherapy.

In principle, two types of arthrogenic atrophy associated with muscle weakness can be distinguished:

a) muscle inhibition and atrophy due to directly impaired proprioceptive information from the joint, and

b) indirect inhibition due to an impaired afferentation influencing many muscles which are often very remote from the injured area. This type is closely associated with reprogramming of motor control.

A direct, reflex muscle atrophy and weakness is well known. Probably the best known examples are atrophy of the vastus medialis in knee injuries (Morrissey 1989) and weakness of the gluteals in the dysfunction of the sacroiliac joint (Janda 1964).

Indirect inhibition is more complex and usually influences more muscles. In clinical work, it has been described mainly for injuries of the ankle region and, to a lesser degree, the knee joint. Probably the first mention of inhibition and incoordination together with some kind of muscle weakness was by Kurtz (1939). However, it was Freeman (Freeman, Dean & Hanham 1965) who described 'functional instability' in the ankle joint due to its injury and decrease in muscle strength of the lower leg muscles. Recent studies have demonstrated a decrease of strength in muscles of the thigh and buttocks as a result of ankle sprain (Bullock-Saxton, Janda & Bullock 1992).

Direct weakness may be explained in many ways, such as from pain irritation, or altered proprioceptive flow due to mechanical reasons (swelling). Freeman and collaborators explained muscle incoordination and weakness as being due to a partial denervation of the injured joint. Of course, all causes may be combined; however, they do not explain all the signs, e.g. they do not enlighten us on the question of remote muscle reaction as observed in the study by Bullock-Saxton, Janda & Bullock (1992).

Nevertheless, direct as well as indirect inhibition, if not properly treated, eventually results in muscle imbalance and tightness and/or stretch weakness. Many signs and symptoms of impaired function of the musculoskeletal system may have a hidden cause in an unrecognized arthrogenic muscle dysfunction.

THERAPEUTIC SUGGESTIONS

Rational and adequate treatment clearly depends on exact evaluation and diagnosis. This must be individualized, and the therapist has to bear in mind that one clinical picture may be the result of combination of several factors. So, for example, trigger points are probably the most frequent cause of muscle pain syndromes associated with muscle shortening. Muscle imbalance associated with muscle tightness is common even in school children, although at this age it is usually not associated with tightness weakness.

Treatment of taut and short muscle bundles associated with any type of trigger points is simple and effective. Spray and stretch techniques, as described by Travell & Simons (1983), can be considered as the treatment of choice, although the postisometric relaxation (Lewit 1986) or a modification of the muscle energy technique (Mitchell 1979) are effective as well. Simple icing, in acute cases, may be of some help. It is, however, usually ineffective in chronic stages in which degenerative changes already are assumed. It must be stressed that the 'stretch' has to be gentle and slow, and, in fact, probably works more by promoting relaxation than by a direct effect on the elastic properties of the muscle.

To improve muscle imbalance, the first step is to achieve a reasonably good length of the tight muscles. Numerous stretching techniques have been developed. However, bouncing stretches, which use the momentum of a swinging body segment to produce stretch, are not appropriate, as they usually cannot be specific. On the contrary, they might lead to an unwanted hypermobility. Slow stretches, which are perhaps best called slow stretching movements, are not very effective and the effect is usually of a short duration. Slowly applied stretch torque to the muscle followed by maintaining the muscle in a lengthened position is an appropriate technique for muscles with altered adaptability, such as in progressive muscle dystrophy. In tight muscles without any evident neurological defect, however, this technique is too time consuming. Thus the stretches of choice are techniques based on the theory of postfacilitation inhibition, as introduced in PNF technique. However, to achieve the best stretching result, the stretch should preferably be fast and in the full range of motion. Some underlying theoretical presumptions seem to be controversial, e.g. when the muscle activity is monitored by EMG recordings, stretching through the whole range of motion, and not only in a limited part, does not seem to influence the activity level and the stretching effect (Moore & Hutton 1980). Nor can EMG recordings confirm that, immediately after a static contraction, a muscle initially seems to be more resistant to change in length (Smith, Hutton & Eldred 1974). On the other hand, recent experiments support the idea of an immediate and fast stretch (Etnyre & Abraham 1985). Our clinical experience supports the technique which uses the maximum isometric contraction followed immediately by the fastest possible stretch.

Stretch weakness in many cases recovers spontaneously after the stretching of the antagonistic counterpart. This fact supports the concept of a neurological explanation for this weakness as a reflex inhibition. If the muscle does not recover spontaneously, any kind of facilitatory technique may be useful. In particular, for muscles involved in maintaining erect posture and gait, we found sensory motor stimulation to be particularly useful (Janda & Vávrová 1990, Bullock-Saxton, Janda & Bullock 1992).

Arthrogenic weakness requires facilitatory techniques. Sensory motor stimulation, PNF or stimulation as in the Kenny approach (1969) are particularly useful. Stokes & Young (1984) recommend, in addition, transcutaneous sensory nerve stimulation. However, no strengthening programme should be limited to the weakened muscle only; overall muscle coordination should be emphasized.

SUMMARY

Muscle weakness associated with muscle length changes is discussed. Special attention has been paid to trigger points, tightness weakness and stretch weakness, in particular in relation to muscle imbalance. Arthrogenic inhibition has been suggested as one of the possible hidden causes of muscle imbalance and impaired function of the musculosketetal system. Therapeutic possibilities are briefly mentioned.

REFERENCES

Bullock-Saxton J E, Janda V, Bullock M I 1992 The influence of ankle sprain injury on muscle recruitment during hip extension. *In press*

Cailliet R 1977 Soft tissue pain and disability, FA Davis, Philadelphia

Etnyre B, Abraham L D 1986 H reflex changes during static stretching and two variations of PNF techniques, Electroencephalography and Clinical Neurophysiology 63: 174–179

Freeman M A R, Dean M R E, Hanham I W F 1965 The etiology and prevention of functional instability of the foot. Journal of Bone and Joint Surgery 47B: 687–685

Gossman M R, Sahrmann S A, Rose S J 1982 Review of length associated changes in muscle. Physical Therapy 62(12): 1799–1808

Janda V 1964 Movement patterns in the pelvic and hip region with special reference to pathogenesis of vertebrogenic disturbances. Thesis, Charles University, Prague

Janda V 1978 Muscle, central nervous mechanism and back problems. In: Korr I M (ed) Neurobiologic mechanisms in manipulative therapy. Plenum Press, New York, p 27–41

Janda V 1984 Pain in the locomotor system — a broad approach. In: Glasgow E F, Twomey L T, Scull E R (eds) Aspects of manipulative therapy. Churchill Livingstone, Melbourne, p 148–151

Janda V 1986 Muscle weakness and inhibition (pseudoparesis) in low back pain. In: Grieve G P (ed) Modern manual therapy of the vertebral column. Churchill Livingstone, Edinburgh

Janda V 1991 Muscle spasm — a contribution to differential diagnosis. Manual Medicine 6: 136–139

Janda V, Vávrová M 1990 Sensory motor stimulation. Body Control Videos, Brisbane, Australia

Kendall H O, Kendall F P, Boynton D A 1952 Posture and pain. Williams and Wilkins, Baltimore

Kurtz A D 1939 Chronic sprained ankle. American Journal of Surgery 44: 158–160

Lewit K 1986 Postisometric relaxation in combination with other methods of muscular facilitation and inhibition. Manual Medicine 2: 101–104

Mitchell F, Moran P S, Pruzzo N A 1979 An evaluation of osteopathic muscle energy procedures. Pruzzo, Valley Parc

Moore M A, Hutton R S 1980 Electromyographic investigation of muscle stretching techniques. Medicine and Science in Sports 12: 322–329

Morrissey M C 1989 Reflex inhibition of thigh muscles in knee injury. Sports Medicine 7: 263–276

Pohl J F, Kenny E 1949 The Kenny concept of infantile paralysis. Bruce, Minneapolis

Sahrmann S A 1983 A program for correction of posture. Clinical Management, 3(4): 23–28

Sahrmann S A 1987 Posture and muscle imbalance. Faulty lumbar pelvic alignments. Physical Therapy 67: 1840–1844

Smidt Y L, Rogers M W 1982 Factors contributing to the regulation and clinical assessment of muscular strength. Physical Therapy 62(9): 1283–1290

Smith J L, Hutton R S, Eldred E 1974 Postcontraction changes in sensitivity of muscle afferents to static and dynamic stretch. Research Brain 78: 193–202

Stokes M, Young A 1984 The contribution of reflex inhibition to arthrogenous muscle weakness. Clinical Science 67: 7–14

Tardieu G, Thuilleux G, Tardieu C 1979 Long term effects of surgical elongation of the tendocalcaneus in the normal cat. Developmental Medicine & Child Neurology 21: 83–94

Travell J 1976 Myofascial trigger points, a clinical view. In: Bonica J J, Albe-Fessard D (eds) Advances in pain and therapy. Raven Press, New York

Travell J G, Rinzler S H 1952 The myofascial genesis of pain. Postgraduate Medicine 11(5): 425–434

Travell J G, Simons D G 1983 Myofascial pain and dysfunction, Williams and Wilkins, Baltimore

7. Muscle strength development and assessment in children and adolescents

Kathleen A. Hinderer, Steven R. Hinderer

INTRODUCTION

The measurement of muscle strength is an essential component of the evaluation of children and adolescents with neuromuscular and musculoskeletal conditions. Many of these conditions characteristically produce muscle weakness. Careful and reliable measurement of muscle strength can aid with early detection of disease processes, such as primary muscle diseases or spinal muscular atrophy syndromes. The collection of serial muscle strength data aids with detecting decreases in function resulting from disease progression or related complications, and assists with determining prognosis. Serial strength measurements are essential for monitoring individuals with muscular dystrophy or myelodysplasia, who are at risk for progressive loss of strength.

Muscle strength test results are used in neuromuscular and musculoskeletal conditions such as myelodysplasia, muscular dystrophy, hemophilia, dermatomyositis and juvenile rheumatoid arthritis to determine present and future functional capabilities in the course of planning orthopedic, surgical and therapeutic management. By determining the strength of individual muscles or muscle groups, the level of motor function can be determined according to the innervation patterns defined by Sharrard (1964) and McDonald et al (1987) for conditions such as myelodysplasia and other spinal cord lesions. Baseline measurement of muscle strength is critical for planning and monitoring the outcome of therapeutic exercise programmes. Examination of the balance of muscle strength around skeletal joints is important for orthopedic management of these individuals. Strength assessment is also important in the management of individuals with traumatic brain injury and cerebral palsy, following selective posterior rhizotomy surgery for reduction of spasticity, to determine residual strength levels.

There are several methods of testing muscle strength. Of these, manual muscle testing (MMT) is the most common method used to evaluate strength because of its adaptability in the clinic setting. Manual muscle test grades are determined by the examiner, who judges the ability of a muscle to move a limb in relation to gravity and against manual resistance. The advantages of this method are that the strength of specific muscles or muscle groups can be evaluated, and no special equipment is required. Despite the adaptability of this method, it has several disadvantages including: the subjectivity of criteria for determining grades above *fair* (grade 3/5), unequal strength increments between grades, and a limited number of strength grades (a scale of 0 to 5). As a result, the clinical relevance and sensitivity of the results of standard muscle testing are limited (Bohannon 1987). The usefulness of MMT scores in infants and children below the age of five or six is even more limited because testing and grading procedures often have to be modified (Kendall & McCreary 1983). Consequently, functional strength assessment methods are often advocated when testing children (Pact et al 1984). Functional strength grades, however, have limitations similar to MMT scores.

The need to develop objective methods for quantifying muscle strength has long been realized. As early as 1916, Lovett and Martin discussed the limitations of testing manually and proposed using a spring balance instrument. Beasley (1956, 1961) demonstrated that strength deficits of up to 50% may remain undetected by MMT. More recently, Bohannon (1986a), Griffin et al (1986), Agre, Findley et al (1987), Miller et al (1988) and Aitkens et al (1989) have confirmed these findings. Several instruments have been developed over the years to attempt to increase the objectivity of muscle testing. These instruments include the cable tensiometer and isokinetic testing devices which were described by Hunsicker and Donnelly (1955), Clarke (1966), Mayhew and Rothstein (1985), Amundsen (1990), and Wilk (1990). While these methods have been found to be reliable indicators of strength, they require the use of special equipment and are often not feasible in the typical clinic setting. Consequently, standard MMT continues to be the primary method used to assess strength.

Recently, several portable, handheld instruments have become commercially available for use in conjunction with MMT. The advantages of these instruments over the previously mentioned instruments are that they are easily applied in a clinical assessment and can be used in the standard MMT positions to obtain objective force

force readings from all muscle groups (Fig. 7.1). Testing with handheld instruments provides a more objective and sensitive measure of change than standard MMT (Bohannon 1987). Several studies have demonstrated that reliable strength readings can be obtained when testing children and adolescents with handheld instruments. The reliability of each of the various testing methods will be discussed later in this chapter. Muscle strength should be monitored using objective, reliable, valid and sensitive testing techniques in order to detect true changes in strength as early as possible in the course of disease progression or treatment intervention.

The use of handheld dynamometers and myometers, in conjunction with MMT techniques, has been shown to be an efficient, cost-effective method of obtaining meaningful strength measurements (Hinderer 1988). Consequently, this chapter will focus on issues pertinent to objective strength testing, in addition to traditional manual strength assessment methods. The issues that will be addressed include: the developmental foundations of muscle function, factors that account for fluctuations in strength, principles of strength testing, methods used to determine strength and suggestions for testing children and adolescents.

DEVELOPMENTAL FOUNDATIONS OF MUSCLE FUNCTION

When muscle testing children and adolescents, one must consider several factors. Knowledge of developmental changes in strength

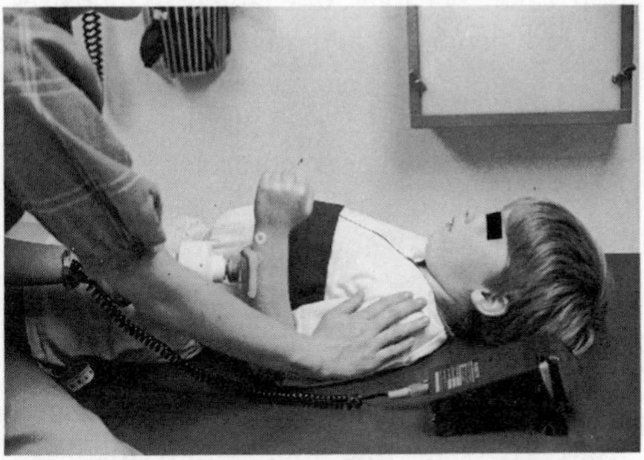

Fig. 7.1 Myometry muscle test position — elbow extensors.

due to neurological maturation, muscle tissue changes and changes in body proportions enables one to interpret muscle test results in light of the age of the individual. Sex differences across the life span must also be considered. Finally, factors that account for day-to-day variation in performance must be identified. By taking these factors into account when interpreting serial muscle test results, health care professionals can better distinguish between a true change and normal variations in strength.

Changes in muscle strength due to neurological maturation

Predictable changes in muscle strength occur across the life span as a result of neurological maturation and changes in body proportions. The pattern of these changes is genetically predetermined, but there are individual variations in the timing of these changes. According to Espenschade and Eckert (1980), development of the neuromuscular system begins during the 5th embryonic week when pre-muscle masses are being formed. A spiralling pattern of innervation of the musculature is well established by the 8th week, due to rotation that has occurred in the developing limb buds. By 16 weeks, muscular movements can be detected in utero. At birth, the neonate is capable of reflexive movement and spontanous mass activity patterns, but does not have volitional antigravity control of the musculature due to the immature state of the nervous system (Thelen 1985). Although neural conduction can occur in the unmyelinated fibres of the neonate, the movements produced are inefficient and stereotypic.

According to Hay (1984), during the first year of life the weight of the brain approximately triples, due largely to increases in the size of the neurons and dendrites and myelination of the axons. As myelination of the nervous system occurs, antigravity control develops in a cephalad to caudal, and proximal to distal direction. Consequently, the infant achieves control over antigravity neck movements before trunk control develops, and shoulder girdle musculature control occurs before distal hand function develops. The development of control of upper and lower extremity movements is phylogenetically dependent upon the maturation of the more proximal trunk musculature.

Another developmental trend seen in the human neonate is the progression from gross to fine motor movements. Antigravity control of large, more powerful extremity movements develops prior to the control of fine finger and toe movements. Increasing control of antigravity movements enables the infant to assume and maintain erect postures. This development of erect positions occurs in a predictable sequence, progressing from lower, more stable positions of the centre of gravity (supine and prone) to higher positions (sitting, four-point, kneeling and standing). During the first two years of postnatal life, the infant gains increasing control over movements within each of these positions. As a result of the infant's immature motor development, standard muscle testing procedures are not appropriate. Consequently, strength is assessed by observing spontaneous movements, functional activities and palpating the muscles. According to Schafer and Dias (1983), it is often difficult to distinguish between voluntary and reflex movements in the infant.

In addition to the increased neural control of antigravity muscle activity, muscle strength improves due to changes in muscle fibre composition. Muscles increase in length and diameter as a result of increases in the number and length of myofibril contractile units (Hay 1984). Muscle strength increases symmetrically on both sides of the body, with the dominant side of the body having slightly greater strength (Espenschade & Eckert 1980).

Changes in strength due to motor learning

Muscle strength can also increase due to motor learning. Asmussen (1973) found that strength increases more rapidly than muscle size during childhood. He attributed the greater increase in strength to the increasing skill and coordination of motor performance that occurs at this stage. Motor learning has also been found to produce increased strength in adults. Moritani and deVries (1979) reported that at the end of 2 weeks of strength training, an increase in force production occurred as a result of improved efficiency of motor unit recruitment. Increases in strength due to muscle hypertrophy were evident only after 3 to 4 weeks of training. The authors concluded that the early improvements seen in training resulted from motor learning. Edwards et al (1977) concluded that learning can occur within a given test session, because first trial readings were consistently lower than the following trial scores in their study. Based upon these findings, these investigators advocated taking three to four trials and discarding the first trial score.

Hinderer (1988), Hinderer and Gutierrez (1988), and Hinderer et al (1988) tested the strength of adults, normal children and children and adolescents with myelodysplasia, respectively. These investigators found no increasing trends across trials when a MMT trial preceded the three instrument trials. These results suggest that if a MMT trial is used to instruct the individual and warm-up the muscle, no learning effects are evident across multiple trials. Mathiowetz (1990) also reported no motor learning or practice effects across three trials of grip and pinch strength readings.

The process of measurement itself may have a training effect due to learning factors. Schenk and Forward (1965) reported that significant strength gains can result from repeated testing in the absence of any intervening strengthening programs. Tornvall (1963) found that learning effects were only observed with complex motions involving multiple joints (e.g. spinal movements and leg extension). He further suggested that the potential influence of learning factors may be reduced if frequent testing schedules are avoided. The findings of several studies support Tornvall's contention. Obtaining strength measurements at least once a week results in increased strength, while testing once every 2 weeks has not been shown to affect strength levels (Matthews & Kruse 1957, Muller 1959, Hislop 1963, Mawdsley & Knapik 1982). The results of these studies suggest that serial strength testing should not be conducted more frequently than biweekly, to minimize potential learning effects.

Changes in muscle strength due to changes in body proportions

In addition to considering nervous system maturation and motor learning factors, one must examine the effect of changes in body composition and body proportions on muscle strength during the growing years. At birth, the trunk is large in relation to the limbs, and the transverse plane of the centre of gravity is approximately 20 cm above the greater trochanter (Palmer 1944). During the first 6 months of postnatal life, the limbs and trunk increase in size proportionally. From 6 months through adolescence, however, the legs are the fastest growing part of the body. This results in a lowering of the transverse plane of the centre of gravity to 0.1 m above the greater trochanter by adulthood (Palmer 1944). The change in limb length affects the torque produced by muscles, due to increased length of the muscle and resistance force moment arms.

Changes in body proportions are accompanied by changes in body composition (Espenschade & Eckert 1980). During the first

9 to 12 months, the percentage of body fat increases due to the increased metabolism of brown fat. From 1 to 6 years of age, there is a gradual decline in the proportion of body fat, followed by a slight increase during later childhood. Following this decline in body fat, muscle atrophy is generally more apparent in disease states. During adolescence, the relative proportion of fat in females increases, while it decreases in males. The changes in the percentage of fat across the developmental years is accompanied by steady increases in muscle and bone tissue, with the exception of the rapid increase of muscle tissue in males following the onset of puberty. These changes in the relative percentage of force-generating muscle tissue to fat and bone tissue has an impact on the biomechanics of movement, due to changes in the ratio of the force producing tissue to the load of the limbs.

Age and sex differences in muscle strength

Both age and sex differences in strength are evident as children mature, with the rates of change varying throughout development (Espenschade & Eckert 1980). Metheny (1941) found that the greatest variations in strength occur during periods of rapid developmental change, with change in strength being less variable in the childhood years than the period following the onset of puberty. He further reported rapid gains in the strength of children between the ages of 3 and 6 years. Espenschade and Eckert (1980) concluded, based upon a study of 115 boys and 101 girls, that increases in isometric strength occur in a fairly linear fashion between the ages of 7 and 9. Between the ages of 9 and 11, the girls in this study demonstrated the greatest gains in strength, while the boys made much greater gains than girls between 11 and 12 years of age. Montoye and Lamphiear (1977), based upon a study of upper extremity strength of males and females between the ages of 10 and 69, found that boys continued to make steady gains in strength following puberty while gains in strength for girls tended to level off. In addition, these authors concluded that both sexes reached their peak strength values between 25 and 29 years of age.

Sex differences are evident during the childhood years with the mean strength measures for boys being consistently higher than for girls. Following the onset of puberty, the sex differences are amplified due to the much greater gains in strength that occur in males as a result of increased androgen production (Gallahue

1982). Prior to the onset of puberty, there is no known biological basis for the sex differences in strength, and these differences are thought to be culturally based (Espenschade & Eckert 1980).

FACTORS THAT ACCOUNT FOR FLUCTUATIONS IN STRENGTH

Several factors may account for day-to-day variations in performance on tests of muscle strength and must be considered in addition to the factors that occur as a result of physical growth and development discussed above. First, recent illness, injury, surgery, or immobilization may negatively affect strength levels. Secondly, physical or psychological fatigue can also result in a reduction of strength. Thirdly, neurogenic muscle weakness can result in a higher degree of variability in force production. Fourthly, the prior state of activity can affect force generation. Fifthly, seasonal variations in strength have been reported. Sixthly, temporal factors have been found to influence force production. Finally, motivation, cooperation and comprehension levels affect performance on strength tests. The potential contribution of each of these factors to random fluctuations in strength levels will be discussed below.

Illness, injury, surgery, immobilization

Fluctuations in performance may occur as a result of illness, injury, or recent surgery, particularly when coupled with a period of prolonged bedrest or immobilization in a cast. Acute infectious diseases may result in isometric strength reduction. Friman (1977) reported that significant decrements in force production were evident in individuals with acute infectious diseases, compared to no significant change for control subjects who had been confined to bedrest for a comparable period of time.

Muscle atrophy and loss of strength also occur in response to prolonged bedrest, with the greatest percentage reduction in the lower limbs and the least reduction in the upper limbs (Greenleaf & Kozlowski 1982). White and Davies (1984) indicated that atrophy results in altered muscle contractile properties, decrements in force production and reduced exercise tolerance. The magnitude of force reduction reported in the literature is variable. Taylor et al (1949) estimated that approximately a 10 to 15 pound reduction of strength occurs per week of muscle disuse. Muller (1970) estimated that strength decreases by about 5% per day in the absence of muscle contraction. Immobilization in a cast for 5 to 6 weeks has been shown to result in a 41% reduction in strength (MacDougall et al 1980). Itoh and Lee (1990) state that the rate of recovery of strength is much slower than the rate of loss.

Muscle fatigue

Muscle fatigue, defined as the reduction in the force-generating capacity of the neuromuscular system, can also produce decrements in force production. Consequently, pre-test activity levels should be consistent. Mundale (1970) demonstrated that fatigue has a short-term decremental effect upon hand grip performance. Following a 10-minute exercise period, subjects were unable to generate as much force when asked to perform a maximal voluntary contraction as they had generated prior to exercising. They were able to produce a contraction equal to pre-exercise levels, however, after a 4-minute rest period.

Neurogenic muscle weakness

Closely related to fatigue is the higher degree of variability in force production by weak muscles than strong muscles, due to the lower threshold of fatigue and slower rate of recovery of weak musculature (Steindler 1955). Local muscle endurance appears to be deficient in some neuromuscular diseases such as spastic cerebral palsy and the muscular dystrophies (Bar-or 1986). This is evidenced by a lower ratio of peak anaerobic power in these individuals compared to able-bodied control subjects. Milner-Brown and Miller (1989) examined this issue more recently by comparing EMG and fatigue indices (percent decrement in MVC) of individuals with neurogenic muscle weakness with data from control subjects for the dorsiflexors and quadriceps muscles. They found that the mean decline in rectified integrated EMG and the fatigue index was significantly greater ($p<0.001$ and $p<0.01$, respectively) for individuals with neurogenic muscle weakness.

Prior state of activity

Force production during successive trials may be potentiated by previous contractions due to the state of prior muscle activation and motor learning, thus counteracting possible fatigue effects. Preparatory warm-up activities which are similar to the strength test motions are often recommended to warm-up the muscle and enhance motor learning (Smidt & Rogers 1982, Westers 1982, Hinderer 1988). Evidence for this warm-up phenomenon is presented by Gooch et al (1990). These authors demonstrated that fewer motor spikes per second are required to sustain a 50% effort following a fatiguing 100% MVC of 1 minute duration. This effect has been noted to persist for up to an hour. The reduction was not accounted for by compensation of synergistic muscles. These results suggest that force can be maintained with a lower level of excitation following a MVC. In addition to prior activation of muscles, mental practice has been found to enhance force production (Cornwall et al 1991).

Seasonal variations

Seasonal variations in strength have been described. Espenschade and Eckert (1980) reported that seasonal variations in strength can occur in children and adolescents. The greatest gains in strength occurred in April for both males and females, with the magnitude of strength gain being greater for males. Males demonstrated the smallest gains in strength during October. Loss of strength was noted for females during the autumn season, the greatest decline occurring in October. Jones (1949) found that the seasonal difference in strength were more pronounced in females. It is important to keep seasonal variation of strength in mind when comparing measurements taken at different times of the year.

Diurnal variations

Diurnal variations in strength have also been reported. McGarvey et al (1984) found statistically significant differences in strength readings obtained in the morning, at noontime and in the late afternoon. The variations were small (ranging from 4% to 7%) and did not follow a consistent trend across different muscle groups. The investigators concluded that temporal variations in strength appeared to be clinically insignificant. Tornvall (1963) also examined temporal strength changes. Strength measurements were obtained over a 24 hour period at 2 hour intervals during the day and once during the night. The observed differences also were small and did not follow any uniform pattern in relation to time. The differences in strength reported in these two studies, therefore, could be attributed to random variations in human performance since there is no consistent relationship to temporal factors.

Motivation, attention, cooperation and comprehension

In addition to the above factors, when interpreting the results of muscle testing, one must consider the individual's level of motivation, attention, cooperation and ability to comprehend and follow directions. Consideration of these factors is especially crucial when testing children. It is also important to document the child's level of motivation and cooperation so that test results can be interpreted appropriately if optimal performance was not attained. The level of motivation can have a significant effect upon the consistency of strength measurements both between trials and between test sessions. One must also consider a child's short attention span, so play techniques should be incorporated into the testing of younger children.

According to Molnar and Alexander (1974), children may not cooperate with standard MMT procedures. Two to 5-year-olds can initiate a test position, but they often cannot sustain it because they do not understand the concept of exerting a counter-force against the examiner's resistance (Pact et al 1984). McDonald et al (1986) examined serial MMT evaluation results of 825 children with myelomeningocele between the ages of birth to 21 years and found that therapists are markedly more confident regarding test results obtained from children 5 years of age and older. Standard muscle testing and grading procedures often need to be modified for children younger than 4 to 6 years old (Kendall & McCreary 1983, Pact et al 1984, Schneider 1985). If a child is cognitively impaired or has a learning disability, the ability to follow directions or to exert resistance upon request might not be achieved until a much later age than normal. Kendall and McCreary (1983) state that it is usually not difficult to grade muscle strength up to *fair* (grade 3/5), but grading above *fair* depends upon the cooperation of the child to hold against resistance with maximal effort. Consequently, strength grades for young children should be preceded with a qualifying term such as 'apparently', since one cannot be confident that optimal performance has been obtained. In summary, when strength testing young children at least up until the age of 5, one cannot be sure if a child is exerting maximal effort.

When obtaining quantitative strength measurements, these issues are also of concern and should be documented. Mendell and

Florence (1990) and Burnett et al (1991) reported difficulty obtaining optimal performance in children aged 5 to 15 years old with Duchenne muscular dystrophy due to a lack of cooperation and motivation. In contrast, Hinderer (1988) and Hinderer and Gutierrez (1988) reported no problems with motivation, attention or compliance when testing normal children and children with myelodysplasia, respectively.

PRINCIPLES OF MUSCLE TESTING

In addition to developmental and patient factors that may account for variations in muscle strength, the type of muscle contraction, as well as mechanical, physiologic and examiner variables must be considered. The force generated varies, depending upon the type and velocity of muscle contraction. Mechanical factors affecting strength production include the moment arm, line of action of the resistance force, joint angle, stabilization of body parts proximal to the moving segment, friction and visco-elastic properties. Physiologic variables include the size and number of motor units activated, speed of tension development, influence of proprioceptive input, pre-test activity level of the muscle and synergist recruitment. The knowledge, level of experience, inherent strength and standardized testing techniques of the examiner can also affect strength test results. Consideration of these factors has led to the formulation of the basic underlying principles of strength assessment applicable to strength testing of both children and adults. These principles are outlined in Table 7.1. Detailed discussion is beyond the scope of this chapter.

MANUAL MUSCLE TESTING

Manual muscle testing is the most common method used to measure strength in a clinical setting. Dr Robert Lovett is considered to be the founder of MMT techniques. His manual methods of testing strength were first described by Wright (1912). Dr Lovett's original testing techniques have been revised over the years. Currently, the most popular methods of MMT in the United States are described by Kendall and McCreary (1983) and Daniels and Worthingham (1986). Zimny and Kirk (1987) described the similarities and differences between these two testing methods,

Table 7.1 Factors to consider when strength testing

1. *Muscle contractile properties*
   a. Muscle length
   b. Contraction rate
   c. Contraction type (concentric, eccentric, isometric, vs. isokinetic)
2. *Mechanical properties*
   a. Joint angle
   b. Stabilization
   c. Viscoelasticity
   d. Force moment arm
   e. Orientation to gravity
   f. Resistance line of action
3. *Physiological properties*
   a. Afferent input
   b. Motor unit size
   c. Activation patterns
   d. Synergist recruitment
   e. Prior muscle activation
   f. Electromechanical delay
4. *Examiner characteristics*
   a. Knowledge
   b. Verbal input
   c. Teaching skills
   d. Palpation skills
   e. Body mechanics
   f. Observation skills
   g. Testing techniques
   h. Clarity of commands
   i. Tactile & body position cues
   j. Feedback & motivation techniques

emphasizing the inherent subjectivity and limitations of MMT techniques. No studies have been conducted to assess the efficacy of one manual testing method versus another (Lamb 1985).

Manual muscle testing methods assess the ability of muscles to move body segments through normal joint excursions in relation to gravity and applied resistance. The six point rating scale (grades 0–5) is well established, but often plus and minus grades are added to provide further gradations in strength. In addition to the numerical scale, Kendall and McCreary (1983) advocate the use of percentages to denote the amount of strength deficit. These are theoretical percentages and have not been determined objectively. On the numerical scale, a grade of *fair*, or 3/5, is defined as the ability for the muscle to move the limb through its full range of motion against gravity, without any other external resistance. On the theoretical percentage scale, this is assumed to represent a 50% strength deficit. Grades at or below 3/5 have relatively specific definition criteria. Grades 4/5 and 5/5 refer to the ability of the muscle to move through the full range of motion against gravity with moderate and maximal resistance, respectively. Assigning MMT grades above *fair* involves a great deal of subjectivity on the part of the examiner. The level of force production must be judged in relation to the individual's age, sex, body habitus and lifestyle (Lamb 1985). Consequently, it is difficult to assess reliably the strength of individuals using standard MMT techniques, particularly when testing children.

The questionable reliability of MMT techniques limits the clinical usefulness of MMT measurements, since relatively large changes in strength must occur for the examiner to be confident that a true change in strength is present. Additionally, MMT methods have been shown to have poor predictive and concurrent validity. Issues of reliability and validity are essential considerations when evaluating the usefulness of any measurement technique (Hinderer & Hinderer 1993). These issues are discussed below. Studies which pertain to testing children and adolescents are highlighted.

Reliability

Only a limited number of reliability studies have been published on MMT. Considering the widespread use of this assessment technique, it is surprising that such a small number of studies have been conducted. Very few studies have been conducted on children and adolescents. Interrater reliability has been examined by Lilienfeld et al (1954), Blair (1955), Iddings et al (1961), Silver et al (1970), Florence et al (1984), Frese et al (1987) and Barr et al (1991). Test-retest reliability has been examined by Iddings et al (1961), Florence et al (1984), Wadsworth et al (1987), Florence et al (1988), Mendell and Florence (1990), Barr et al (1991), and Florence et al (1992). Percent agreement statistics are reported in all but the latter four studies. The levels of agreement attained, based upon +/– one grade were high, ranging from 89% to 97% agreement for interrater reliability and from 96% to 98% for test-retest reliability, but precise agreement levels were poor (45% to 74%) for interrater reliability and 54% to 65% for test-retest reliability). The results of these studies indicate that in order to be confident that a true change in strength has occurred, MMT scores must change more than one full grade. Consequently, the use of the limited ordinal MMT scale, which lacks sensitivity, can result in a substantial, irreversible loss of strength before any change is detected. In the latter six studies, correlation coefficients are reported. These coefficients ranged from 0.63 to 0.98 for individual muscle groups, and from 0.57 to 1.0 for a total MMT score (comprised of the sum of individual muscle grades). Significant improvement in the degree of consistency of a given examiner's scores was noted over a year period of time by Florence et al (1984). Mendell and Florence (1990) discuss the importance of considering the examiner's training effect when assessing strength via MMT. Mendell and Florence (1990) also reported improvement in the reliability of MMT scores with increasing age in a sample of 84 boys, 5 to 16 years old, with Duchenne muscular dystrophy.

Different patient populations, methods, statistical analyses and levels of examiner experience were used in the above studies, making comparisons between studies difficult. In addition, these studies inconsistently reported levels of either reliability or agreement. High reliability does not necessarily indicate absolute agreement between raters. It is important to report both reliability and agreement on the target population(s) that a clinical measure will be applied to, using typical examiners (Hinderer & Hinderer 1993). Additional reliability studies are needed, particularly for assessment of pediatric populations.

Validity

Lamb (1985) states that MMT has content validity because the test construction is based on known physiologic, anatomic and kinesiologic principles. In addition, this method of testing directly measures the torque-generating capacity of muscles. Lamb (1985) also comments, however, that there are limitations in the content domain of MMT. Not all types of muscle contraction are measured and variables such as the rate of tension development are not assessed. These inherent limitations of strength testing raise questions regarding the predictive validity of MMT, particularly with regard to functional activities.

The predictive validity of MMT has been examined in two studies on children. Murdoch (1980) examined the predictive validity of neonatal manual muscle strength assessments. The MMT grades and levels of mobility of 95 children with myelodysplasia at age 3 to 8 years were retrospectively compared with the MMT scores recorded at birth. Strength was graded on a three point scale (full muscle power, weak movement and absent function). Each child's mobility level at 3 to 8 years of age was graded on a four point independence scale. The correlation between muscle power of the newborn and subsequent mobility of the child was 'very poor'. The results of this study suggest that the predictive value to MMT during the neonatal period for children with myelodysplasia is limited using the testing methods and grading procedures suggested by these authors.

McDonald et al (1986) also examined the predictive validity of MMT scores for individuals with myelodysplasia to determine how the predictive validity of examinations varies with age and with the particular muscle group tested. Serial MMT scores were analyzed from the results of 3084 examinations performed on 825 children with myelodysplasia, according to criteria specified by Kendall and McCreary (1983) and by Daniels and Worthingham (1986). The examinations were conducted on children from birth to 21.8 years of age over a 12 year period of time by six physical and occupational therapists. These authors found that predictive validity of MMT generally increased from birth to age five. Peak asymptotic levels were obtained at age five. The probability that a given muscle test score will precisely predict future test scores varied with age and the particular muscle group tested. These probabilities ranged from 23% to 68% during the newborn period to a range of 54% to 87% in later life. The probability that a single test score will predict future strength to +/– one MMT grade ranged from 70% to 86% in the newborn period. In later life the range was from 87% to 97%. Thus, prediction to +/– one muscle grade is not as strongly influenced by age or the particular muscle tested and the probability that a given test score will predict future performance is high.

The concurrent validity of MMT has also been examined in several studies by comparing strength scores obtained manually with strength readings obtained on quantitative objective instruments. Beasley (1956) evaluated the knee extensor strength of 303 children with poliomyelitis, 9 to 12 years old. Their MMT scores were compared with their cable tensiometer readings. Manual muscle testing failed to identify muscle weakness 50% or more below the established normative values for the knee extensor muscle group measured on the tensiometer. In a later study, Beasley (1961) demonstrated that the theoretical percentages assigned to the MMT scale (where the grade of *fair* is considered to be 50% below the norm) greatly underestimated the percent strength loss for hip extensors, knee extensors and plantarflexors. More recent studies have concurred with Beasley's findings regarding the lack of concurrent validity of MMT (Bohannon 1986a, Griffin et al 1986, Agre, Findley et al 1987, Miller et al 1988, Aitkens et al 1989). The latter three studies have important implications regarding the validity of monitoring strength via MMT methods in children and adolescents and the results of these studies are described below.

Agre, Findley et al (1987) measured the hip and knee extensor strength levels of 33 adolescents with myelodysplasia. The same isometric cable tensiometer method described by Beasley (1956, 1961) was used to assess strength. The strength levels obtained on the individuals with myelodysplasia were then compared to the normative data reported by Beasley (1961). These authors found that individuals who had been classified as having 'no motor deficits' via previous MMT, actually had strength deficits for the hip and knee extensors of 40% and 60%, respectively.

Quantitative strength readings and MMT scores were obtained by Miller et al (1988) on the plantarflexors of 16 children with dermatomyositis using the Beasley (1956) cable tensiometer method. Quantitative grip strength measurements were also obtained by these investigators using the method described by Mundale (1970). Levels of strength were monitored for these two muscle groups, via the quantitative and MMT methods longitudinally over a 10 year period. Muscle strength was rated normal on the MMT scale significantly sooner, following steroid therapy, than when normal quantitative strength readings were obtained ($p<0.001$). In addition, normal MMT scores were obtained significantly prior to obtaining normal serum muscle enzyme levels ($p<0.05$). In contrast, quantitative strength changes were useful in monitoring enzyme levels. The authors concluded that quantitative strength measurements provide a more precise method of assessing clinical improvement in childhood dermatomyositis.

Aitkens et al (1989) found that MMT and quantitative isometric strength measurements were significantly correlated in 21 adolescents and adults with slowly progressive neuromuscular diseases. It was not possible, however, to reliably predict quantitative strength values from MMT scores. In addition, these authors found that more subjects were required to achieve the same level of statistical significance in a research study which monitored strength using MMT than if quantitative methods were used. Consequently, these authors advocate the use of quantitative assessment techniques over traditional MMT when monitoring the effectiveness of therapeutic regimes.

In contrast, Mendell et al (1989) demonstrated that MMT was an effective method for monitoring improvements in strength when a *total* MMT score was used (summed over 34 muscle groups). A double-blind randomized controlled study of prednisone was conducted on 103 boys with Duchenne muscular dystrophy. Monitoring total MMT scores over a 6 month period clearly demonstrated improvement in both experimental groups, whereas the placebo group followed the natural history rate of decline. Mendell and Florence (1990) point out, however, that monitoring MMT grades of *individual* muscle groups is not sensitive over time. These authors emphasize that MMT should *not* be used to monitor the strength of *individual* muscle groups and instead, they also advocate the use of quantitative methods for individual muscle assessment.

Summary

The preceding discussion has highlighted the lack of reliability and validity of MMT. Acceptable levels of agreement have been attained only when +/– one grade scores are compared, or with extensive examiner training. Precise interrater and test-retest agreement levels are poor. In order to be confident that a true change in strength has occurred, MMT scores must change more than one grade. The use of the limited ordinal MMT scale, which lacks sensitivity, to monitor strength can result in a substantial, irreversible loss of strength before any change is detected. The lack of concurrent validity of MMT compared to quantitative measurements demonstrates that MMT is severely limited in its clinical usefulness.

Despite these concerns, MMT continues to be the standard method for assessing strength in the typical clinic setting. This is most likely because it is a convenient, inexpensive method of documenting strength. No alternative method of strength measurement has emerged which is as convenient or efficient. Convenience does not justify the use of invalid and insensitive measurement techniques, however, particularly when objective, reliable methods of strength testing exist. We advocate using MMT assessments primarily as a screening tool to determine if obvious weakness exists. If weakness is suspected, objective strength readings should be obtained to establish a baseline level and to monitor changes in strength over time. Methods of objectively assessing strength are discussed below. When determining the most appropriate objective measurement tool for a given practice setting, several factors must be considered, including practicality, reliability and validity (Hinderer & Hinderer 1993).

QUANTITATIVE MUSCLE TESTING: NON-PORTABLE DEVICES

Numerous instruments have been developed since the 18th century for research and/or clinical use, to attempt to increase the objectivity of strength testing (Hunsicker & Donnelly 1955, Clarke 1966, Mayhew & Rothstein 1985, Amundsen 1990, Wilk 1990). These instruments can be classified into two categories: portable, handheld units and stationary devices. Non-portable dynamometers which have been developed primarily for clinical assessment and treatment have been described by several authors, including four studies which have been conducted on children. Molnar and Alexander (1973, 1974), and Molnar et al (1979) examined the reliability of the Cybex isokinetic exercise dynamometer and found it to be a reliable indicator of strength. Burnett et al (1991) discussed numerous problems encountered when testing the strength of children with Duchenne muscular dystrophy using the Cybex isokinetic dynamometer. These problems included limited attention span, a lack of motivation, difficulty positioning the children and instrument related problems.

Brussock et al (1992) examined the interrater and test-retest reliability of isometric force production in children with and without disabilities using a stationary electronic strain gauge. Intraclass correlation coefficients were calculated on 10 children with Duchenne muscular dystropy and their age-matched controls. The children were 4 to 14 years old. Test-retest and interrater reliability coefficients ranged from 0.85 to 0.99 and from 0.71 to 0.98, respectively. Coefficients were similar for both groups of children.

The usefulness of non-portable dynamometers in many clinic settings is limited because of the extended period of time required for testing, difficulties encountered when positioning children in equipment which was designed for adult-sized body proportions and the expense and bulkiness of the equipment required. Consequently, the use of handheld quantitative testing devices for testing children and adolescents will be emphasized below.

QUANTITATIVE MUSCLE TESTING: HANDHELD DEVICES

Due to the need for a portable, convenient, objective measure of strength, various handheld instruments have been developed over the years for use in conjunction with standard MMT (Newman 1949, Clarke 1954, Beasley 1956, Borden & Colachis 1968, Edwards & McDonnel 1974, Nicholas et al 1978, Saraniti et al 1980, Hack et al 1981, Helewa et al 1981, Marino et al 1982, Hyde et al 1983, Wiles & Karni 1983, Smidt & Rogers 1982, van der Ploeg et al 1984, Bohannon 1986a, Bohannon & Andrews 1987, Agre & Magness et al 1987, Allsop & VanWagoner 1987, Finucane et al 1988, Fischer 1988, Patterson & Baxter 1988, Surburg et al 1992).

The maximum force registered by most of these instruments is 30 kg-force (kg-f), which is approximately the equivalent of 300 N. Forces above this magnitude are difficult for examiners to stabilize and resist. Although numerous reports document the clinical applications of handheld dynamometers and myometers, there are only a few studies documenting the reliability and validity of these test instruments. Reliability, validity and clinical application of handheld dynamometers is summarized by Andrews (1991), Bohannon (1990) and Hinderer (1988). The results of reliability studies conducted on children and adolescents, using instruments which are commercially available, are summarized below. Other commercially available instruments are not discussed below, because there are currently no published data on children and adolescents. These instruments are the Dynatronics Dynatron II Strength Analysis System, Hoggan Force Evaluation and Testing System (Allsop & VanWagoner 1987), Nicholas Manual Muscle Tester (Surburg et al 1992), Minnesota System for Isometric Muscle Strength (Agre, Magness et al 1987, Patterson & Baxter 1988, Marino et al 1982) and the Universal Handheld Dynamometer (Fisher 1988). These instruments also have applications for pediatric and adolescent populations.

Reliability and validity studies

Many of the studies which have been conducted have limited clinical relevance because only a few muscle groups were evaluated, the types of muscle contraction used were not identified, the test procedures were not adequately specified, the range of strength of the subjects and examiners was not specified, few disabled populations have been studied and estimates of measurement error have not been reported. Due to the variations in the test protocol, muscle groups tested, subject populations, and experience level of the examiners, comparisons between the reported reliability of the various test instruments cannot be made. In addition, Tornvall (1963) states that comparisons between absolute values obtained using two different methods of testing should be avoided. Despite research design limitations, the results of these studies indicate that MMT, combined with the use of handheld quantitative devices, is a reliable and valid method of strength assessment in children and adolescents.

Modified sphygmomanometer

Modified sphygmomanometers have been used to assess isometric strength (Helewa et al 1981, Giles 1984, Wright & Goldsmith 1988). Strength levels up to 300 mmHg can be measured with these devices. Limited reliability data are available for this method of strength assessment. Wright and Goldsmith (1988) reported interrater and test-retest intraclass correlation coefficients of 0.79 and 0.69, respectively, when four examiners tested the hip abductor strength of four normal children.

Sparks handheld dynamometer

The clinical applications of this dynamometer have been documented in several accounts (Smidt & Rogers 1982, Bohannon & Dubuc 1984, Smidt 1984, Bohannon 1986c, Bohannon 1987, Riddle et al 1989). Five studies have examined the reliability of this instrument when testing adults (Bohannon 1986b, Byl et al 1988, Hinderer et al 1988, Rheault et al 1989) but only one study has examined these issues when testing children and adolescents. Test-retest reliability levels were assessed using the dynamometer by Stuberg and Metcalf (1988) on 14 normal children and 14 children with Duchenne muscular dystrophy, 6 to 14 years old. The isometric strength levels of four muscle groups (knee and hip extensors, elbow flexors, and shoulder abductors) were assessed bilaterally by one examiner. The test-retest Pearson product-moment correlation coefficients ranged from 0.74 to 0.99 for the normal children with all but the left hip extensor comparisons being above 0.95. Knee and hip extensor levels were not determined for most of the normal children because they exceeded the dynamometer's upper limit of 27.2 kg-f (≅270 N). For the children with muscular dystrophy, test-retest coefficients ranged from 0.83 to 0.99 and none of the children exceeded the upper limit of the dynamometer. The results of this study indicate that strength testing with the handheld dynamometer is highly reliable when the same evaluator tests normal children and children with muscular dystrophy on two different days.

Penny and Giles myometer

The clinical applications and reliability of the myometer have been documented during the various stages of its development (Hosking et al 1976, Edwards et al 1977, Edwards & Hyde 1977, Hyde 1980, Scott et al 1982, and Hyde et al 1983). In addition, normative data have been collected by Hosking et al (1976), Sykanda et al (1988), and van der Ploeg et al (1991). Acceptable reliability has been established for adults in five studies (Wiles & Karni 1983, Olds et al 1984, Hinderer et al 1988, Hinderer & Hinderer 1990, van der Ploeg et al 1991). Hosking et al (1976) asessed test-retest reliability of the Hammersmith myometer (an early version of the myometer) over a one month interval on 18 normal children between the ages of 10–13 years. For the six muscle groups tested, the authors reported that the variation did not often exceed +/– 15% of the initial values.

Hyde et al (1983) examined test-retest and interrater reliability on a disabled and normal population, respectively. Test-retest reliability was established on 12 males with muscular dystrophy, with a test-retest interval of 1.5 hours. Reliability coefficients ranged from 0.75 to 0.97 for six muscle groups. These authors also assessed interrater reliability on 14 normal children. Three physical therapists measured knee extensor and shoulder abductor strength on the same day. The experience level of the therapists varied from minimal to considerable previous experience with the myometer. The authors concluded that no significant differences existed between the readings obained by the three therapists.

Florence et al (1988) examined test-retest reliability of the myometer, testing 48 males with Duchenne muscular dystrophy, 5 to 16 years old. Five muscle groups were tested bilaterally, with a 2 week test-retest interval. The Pearson product-moment correlation coefficients ranged from 0.79 to 0.98 for the entire group. Lower correlations were noted for the 5 to 9-year-old group. This may have been due to the reduced spread of strength scores, rather than an actual difference in how young children perform on strength tests. Lower correlation coefficients are expected when testing a relatively homogeneous population (Hinderer & Hinderer 1993).

Hinderer and Gutierrez (1988) determined intertrial, interrater, and test-retest reliability levels when testing normal children. Two different methods of testing were compared in this study, the eccentric 'break' test and the isometric 'hold' test. Peak strength measurements using the myometer were obtained for the elbow extensors, hip abductors and knee flexors using both test techniques. Twenty children, 5 to 10 years old, were tested by two physical therapists who were blind to the instrument readings. The test-retest interval was 6 to 7 days. Intertrial Pearson reliability coefficients ranged from 0.91 to 0.97 for the isometric hold technique and from 0.82 to 0.94 for the eccentric 'break' test technique. Interrater coefficients ranged from 0.82 to 0.95 for the isometric hold technique and from 0.82 to 0.91 for the eccentric 'break' test technique. Test-retest coefficients ranged from 0.84 to 0.89 for the isometric hold technique and from 0.75 to 0.93 for the eccentric 'break' test technique. For the elbow extensors, interrater and test-retest 95% confidence intervals ranged from 1.6 to 2.0 kg-f (⊜ 16 to 20 N), with no significant differences between the methods. For the hip abductors, 95% confidence intervals ranged from 1.3 to 2.6 kg-f (⊜ 13 to 26 N), with the isometric confidence interval being significantly lower for the interrater comparison but not for the test-retest comparison. For knee extensors, the 95% confidence intervals ranged from 1.8 to 2.6 kg-f (⊜ 18 to 26 N), with the isometric confidence intervals being significantly lower for both interrater and test-retest comparisons. Based upon the 95% confidence intervals and t-test comparisons, the isometric hold technique was found to be significantly better regarding interrater reliability when testing hip abductors and knee flexors. The isometric technique was also found to be significantly better in terms of test-retest reliability when testing knee flexors. The methods were comparable for testing elbow extensors. Strength testing with the myometer was found to be a highly reliable method of assessing strength in normal children when the isometric test technique was used.

Hinderer (1988) determined intertrial, interrater and test-retest reliability levels when testing 66 children and adolescents with myelodysplasia. Subjects were 5 to 21 years old, with motor levels at or below L2-4 and IQ levels greater than or equal to 60. The sample was stratified according to age, motor function and gender.

Peak isometric strength readings were obtained by physical therapists who were blind to the myometer readings. One upper extremity and seven lower extremity muscle groups were tested. Intertrial coefficients ranged from 0.98 to 0.99. Interrater Pearson product-moment correlations ranged from 0.87 to 0.97 and intraclass coefficients from 0.73 to 0.96. Test-retest Pearson coefficients ranged from 0.92 to 0.96 and intraclass correlations from 0.96 to 0.98. Standard errors of measurement (based upon 95% confidence intervals) ranged from 1.5 to 5.6 kg-f (≈15 to 56 N) and from 1.8 to 3.8 kg-f (≈18 to 38 N) for the interrater and test-retest comparisons, respectively. For both comparisons, the knee flexors had the lowest measurement error and the plantarflexors had the highest. A lower standard error of measurement for the plantarflexor interrater comparison was obtained if high readings, exceeding 15 kg-f (≈150 N) were excluded. This trend was not evident for the other muscle groups, however. Variance components were negligible for the rater, trial and session effects for six of the eight muscle groups. The percentages of the variance due to raters were highest for the dorsiflexors and plantarflexors (12.5% and 4.6% respectively). The results of this study indicate that the myometer is a reliable method of assessing muscle strength in children with myelodysplasia and it provides a more sensitive and objective method of testing strength than traditional MMT.

Mendell and Florence (1990) examined test-retest reliability when testing 30 boys with Duchenne muscular dystrophy, ages 5 to 15 years. Intraclass correlation coefficients ranged from 0.50 to 0.97. In a further test-retest reliability study, these authors tested 84 boys with Duchenne muscular dystrophy. Pearson product-moment correlation coefficients for the myometer ranged from 0.71 to 1.0. Of the 84 boys in the study, only 62 cooperated with the testing procedure. The authors also noted difficulty testing some individuals due to joint contractures, especially at the ankle joint. As discussed in the earlier study by Florence et al (1988), lower correlations were obtained for the younger age group (5–9 years old). This finding could also be attributed to the relative homogeneity of scores obtained from subjects who are close in age. In a final study, Mendell and Florence (1990) evaluated the concurrent validity of the myometer for detecting changes in strength in a double-blind, randomized controlled trial of prednisone in Duchenne muscular dystrophy. Myometry strength scores were found to be an effective means of demonstrating improvement. Greater than 80% of the treated group demonstrated strength gains over a 6 month period of time, compared to 33% of the placebo group. The authors express concern regarding the improvement in the placebo group, but some gains in strength would be expected over a 6 month period of time due to maturation, as well as a result of the placebo effect.

Grip and pinch strength measurement

Grip strength measurements are predictive of overall strength and function. Serial grip strength measurements on individuals with no known disabilities have been shown to produce consistent trends over time. Aber et al (1984) reported that when using two different types of grip strength measurement tools, normal children demonstrated increases in strength with increased chronological age. Serial grip strength measurements have been suggested to be a predictor of progressive neurological dysfunction in children with Arnold Chiari II malformation (Kilburn et al 1985).

A variety of devices are available for measuring grip and pinch strength including modified sphymomanometers, squeeze bulbs and spring dynamometers. Bohannon (1991) and Mathiowetz (1990) describe various types of grip strength instrumentation. The reliability and validity, testing procedures and standardized test positions are essential factors that must be considered when measuring grip strength since grip strength has been found to vary with elbow position and the sitting versus standing position (Balogun et al 1991). Unsworth et al (1990) caution against the use of modified sphygmomanometers because the strength registered varies with the diameter, volume and initial pressure of the bag, and also with hand size, technique of squeezing and the applied load.

The linearity of three instruments which measure grip strength was compared to a universal testing machine by Solgaard et al (1984). These investigators found that the Martin Vigorimeter and the My-Gripper were both very precise instruments and recommended their use over a steel spring dynamometer, which was found to be less precise. Level (1984) advocates the use of the Martin vigorimeter and collected normative grip strength readings for 6 to 9 year olds. This device is a squeeze bulb pressure gauge instrument. It is ideal for testing children because they can readily grasp the concept of squeezing the balls and they enjoy the challenge of obtaining their highest possible score. Normative data are also available for children and adolescents using the Jamar dynamometer (Kjerland 1953, Ager et al 1984, Fullwood 1986,

Mathiowetz et al 1986) and the Harpenden dynamometer (Balogun et al 1991).

Summary

The reliability information provided in the majority of the aforementioned studies is encouraging. These studies indicate that strength can be measured reliably using handheld instruments. Different procedures were used, however, making it difficult to compare the results across studies. Many of the studies discussed have limited application in the clinic setting because issues of measurement error have not been uniformly addressed. In addition, few disabled populations have been studied. Reliability data cannot be extrapolated from one population to another.

SUGGESTIONS FOR STRENGTH TESTING INFANTS AND YOUNG CHILDREN

Manual muscle test techniques must be modified when assessing infants and children younger than 4 to 6 years of age (Kendall & McCreary 1983, Pact et al 1984, Schneider 1985). For infants and toddlers, muscle function is determined by observing and palpating muscle activity in age-appropriate developmental positions (Murdoch 1980, Schneider 1985). Observation of muscle contours is also helpful for signs of atrophy. Specific suggestions for testing infants and young children will be discussed below.

Assigning strength grades

It is often suggested that specific strength grades should not be recorded for infants and young children (Murdoch 1980, Pact et al 1984, Schneider 1985). Instead, muscle activity is often noted to be present or absent; or terms such as full strength, weak or absent may be used. The developmental level of the child should be considered when assigning strength grades. It is normal for infants to exhibit weak neck and trunk musculature, due to their low muscle tone (Kendall & McCreary 1983). These muscle groups should be graded 'normal for age' if the infant is able to perform developmentally appropriate activities.

We have found that specific strength scores do provide useful information for infants and young children with myelodysplasia. As was mentioned earlier in the section on validity of MMT,

McDonald et al (1986) found that MMT scores determined in the newborn period are predictive of future muscle function. Many of the testing techniques discussed below were utilized by the therapists who tested the infants, children and adolescents in that study.

Assessing newborns and infants

When testing newborns or infants, the state of alertness must be considered (Schneider 1985). Optimal performance cannot be elicited if the infant is sleepy or drowsy. The greatest muscle activity can be observed if the infant is alert, hungry or crying. Repeated evaluations at different times of day may need to be conducted, particularly for newborns, in order to observe the infant's muscle activity in various behavioural states. The infant's current behavioural state should be documented. If the infant is in a sleepy or drowsy state at the beginning of the evaluation, we have found that it is best to start assessing more passive parameters first, such as range of motion. The stimulus of extremity movement often arouses the infant so that muscle activity can then be observed. Additional techniques can be incorporated if the infant still is not aroused. Rocking the infant vertically stimulates the vestibular system and increases alertness (Schneider 1985). Tactile and auditory stimulation may also be effective. If, on the other hand, the infant is alert at the beginning of the evaluation, it is best to prioritize the assessment of muscle activity first, and evaluate more passive parameters later in the evaluation.

Generally, the infant's spontaneous activity should be observed first in supine, prone and sidelying positions, before the examiner starts handling the infant. Spontaneous activity is often suppressed once an infant is handled. The infant can be stimulated to move by using sounds (e.g. rattles, bells or the examiner's voice), by having the infant visually track objects or reach for toys. After spontaneous movements have been observed, begin palpating muscle activity while the infant is moving. Additional movements can be stimulated via tactile stimulation or tickling, placing extremities in antigravity positions to elicit holding responses, or by moving extremities to end range positions (e.g. fully flexed, extended, abducted or adducted) to see if the infant will perform the opposite movement to move out of the position. The opposing movements can be resisted to judge the infant's level of strength. For older babies, muscle activity can be observed and palpated in developmental positions. Resistance can be provided during activities such as crawling.

Reflexive versus voluntary movements

It is important to distinguish between voluntary and reflexive movements. This is especially challenging in infants and young children. Children with congenital or acquired spinal cord injuries may exhibit distal sparing due to preservation of spinal reflex arcs. Consequently, reflex responses may be elicited in response to stretch. Reflexive movements should be documented but they should not be considered when determining motor lesion levels.

The issue of whether the strength of individuals with upper motor neuron lesions should be assessed is often a subject of debate. Test-retest reliability of strength measurements obtained in adults with hemiparesis has been demonstrated by Bohannon (1986b), Bohannon and Andrews (1987), Riddle et al (1989) and Tripp and Harris (1991). This issue has not been examined in children, however.

Functional assessments

Functional assessments are advocated for young children, 2 to 5 years old, since they may not cooperate with traditional test procedures (Pact et al 1984). Muscle groups, rather than specific muscles, are assessed with functional tests. Muscle activity can be observed and palpated in various play activities. Activities of daily living, such as dressing and undressing, can also be used to elicit muscle activity. For example, ankle musculature will often contract to stabilize the ankle when putting on socks and shoes. Functional activities which are helpful in determining the strength of key muscle groups are outlined in Table 7.2.

Lefkof (1986) examined test-retest reliability and performance levels of 160 children, 3 to 7 years old, on three tests which functionally assessed abdominal strength. The isometric supine flexion posture and isotonic hooklying sit-up tests were more reliable than the isometric hooklying hold test. The antigravity isometric trunk flexion test could be performed by 95% of the 3 year olds. Younger children had more difficulty performing the isotonic antigravity test, but all 6 year olds could perform this test. Older children performed significantly better on all three tests, suggesting that trunk flexion strength increases with age.

Table 7.2 Functional assessment of strength in children

Position	Observations
Standing	
1. Posture (posterior and lateral views)	Symmetry and alignment, postural curves, scapular position
2. Walking	Gait deviations indicative of muscle weakness
3. Heel walking	Bilateral dorsiflexor strength
4. Toe walking	Bilateral plantarflexor strength
5. Stepping up and down a step	Leg lifted onto step via hip flexors and hamstrings (concentric contraction). Body elevated via quadriceps and hip extensors (concentric contraction). Leg and body lowered down onto step via eccentric contraction of the same muscle groups
6. One-legged stand	Strength of hip abductors (gluteus medius and minimus). Pelvis should remain level. If the pelvis drops on the non-weight bearing side, or if the trunk leans toward the weight bearing side, hip abductor weakness may exist
7. One-legged stand on tiptoes	Unilateral plantarflexor strength
8. Toe touching — rising and lowering	Eccentric and concentric contractions of back extensors and gluteus maximus
9. Squat to stand — rising and lowering	Eccentric and concentric contraction of gluteus maximus and quadriceps femoris (watch for Gower's sign, where child pushes on thighs to assist)
10. Scapular stability — arms extended against wall	Ability of serratus anterior to stabilize scapula against thoracic wall
Prone	
1. Wheelbarrow position	Triceps, latissimus dorsi, serratus anterior and neck extensors
2. Flying position (head, trunk, arms and legs extended)	Back and neck extensors, middle trapezius and posterior deltoid
3. Prone kicking (hips alternately extending)	Gluteus maximus and hamstrings
Supine	
1. Sit-up	Neck flexors and abdominals
2. Pull to sit	Neck flexors, finger flexors, biceps
3. Bridging	Gluteus maximus, hamstrings
4. Bicycle in supine	Hip and knee flexors and extensors
Sitting	
1. Sitting push-up	Upper and lower trapezius, lattissimus dorsi, triceps, hip flexors

SUGGESTIONS FOR STRENGTH TESTING SCHOOL-AGE CHILDREN AND ADOLESCENTS

Children above 4 to 6 years of age are usually able to participate in standard strength testing procedures. The key to obtaining reliable and valid results is making sure the client understands each test motion and gives a maximal effort for each test trial. The authors have found the testing techniques discussed below to optimize test performance, so that consistent test results can be obtained for children as young as 4 years old. These testing techniques are applicable to both traditional MMT and testing with handheld instruments. Recommendations regarding testing frequencies and documentation methods for stength test results will also be discussed.

Assessment intervals and recording methods

Strength should be assessed at regular intervals for individuals who are at risk from loss of function. More frequent evaluations may be indicated during periods of rapid growth. Pre- and post-intervention measurements should be obtained for individuals undergoing surgery or other therapeutic procedures which might affect muscle strength. To avoid potential biases, it is important that examiners remain blind to previous strength readings or MMT grades until after completing their assessments.

Shurtleff (1986) advocates using the Patient Data Management System (PDMS) strength testing procedures and recording format to serially monitor individuals with myelodysplasia. According to the PDMS protocol, strength levels for children with myelodysplasia below the age of two should be monitored twice per year. Strength should be monitored on a yearly basis thereafter. If progressive loss is suspected, however, more frequent evaluations should be conducted. We have found the PDMS computerized recording format to be beneficial for monitoring many patient populations because serial test results from birth to present can be efficiently scanned for each individual muscle group, to detect any evidence of changes in muscle function. Refer to Shurtleff (1991) for a detailed description of the PDMS computer program.

To permit comparison of objective strength measurements between individuals, torque values should be reported (force x lever arm lengths). An alternate, but less precise, method of normalizing strength scores between individuals is to divide by height, since overall height is closely correlated to individual limb lengths. Torque values also must be reported when monitoring strength over time in children and adolescents, until they reach skeletal maturity. The lever arm length of muscles will increase with growth, thus affecting the force generating capacity of muscles. Torque values take into account changes in both force and limb length.

It is best to obtain three trials and report the mean of the three trials. The mean score is more stable over time and between raters than any given trial score (Hack et al 1981, Hinderer 1988). In addition to recording specific strength scores, the child's level of cooperation and motivation during the evaluation should be documented.

Positioning

The use of standardized positions is essential when obtaining strength measurements, because the force produced varies with the joint angles and the stability of proximal body segments. It is also important to ensure that children are comfortable and posturally secure during the evaluation. If clients have joint contractures which interfere with positioning them in standard test positions, they should be positioned in as neutral alignment as possible, and the altered joint position(s) should be recorded. By incorporating these procedures for altering test positions, even significant joint contractures did not interfere with the reliability of testing individuals with myelodysplasia (Hinderer 1988). This is in contrast to the results reported by Mendell and Florence (1990) and Burnett et al (1991), where these procedures for altering joint positions were not employed.

Beasley (1956) found that traditional muscle test positions were not appropriate for testing with a handheld instrument. Maximum force readings could not be obtained in these positions. In addition, external stabilization, using belts, was determined by Beasley (1956) to be essential for valid testing of strong individuals. Hack et al (1981) concur with these findings. Hinderer and Hinderer (1990) compared manual fixation versus the use of external stabilization belts. They found that stabilization belts did not significantly improve the test-retest or interrater reliability of testing the strength of shoulder flexors, elbow extensors, hip abductors or knee flexors in normal adults. These issues have not been examined in children or individuals with disabilities, however. If stabilization belts are used when testing young children, an explanation should be

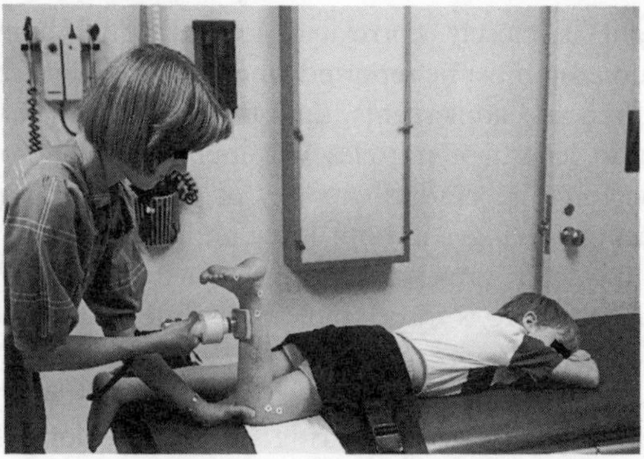

Fig. 7.2 Myometry muscle test position—knee extensors.

provided in order to avoid eliciting apprehension (e.g. 'This is a seat belt which will be used to hold you still on the table'). Descriptions of test positions which have been found to provide efficient and reproducible results in the aformentioned studies by Hinderer et al (1988), Hinderer and Gutierez (1988), Hinderer (1988), and Hinderer and Hinderer (1990) are provided in Table 7.3. An example test position is shown in Figure 7.2.

The influence of tonic neck reflexes and vision on strength has not been well established in individuals with neurologic impairments. No studies have been published examining these issues in children. Deutsch et al (1987) reported a greater influence of horizontal rotation of the neck on elbow flexor force production than sagittal plane motion in normal adult subjects. In contrast, Anderson and Bohannon (1991) reported no influence of horizontal neck rotation on elbow extensor force in normal adults. The only study which has examined the effect of neck position on neurologically involved individuals found no effect on elbow flexion force of the paretic side in hemiparetic patients (Bohannon & Andrews 1989). Since the influences of neck reflexes and vision have not been studied in children or adolescents, we recommend maintaining the head in a consistent position when testing the strength of all musculature. When testing in supine, the head should be positioned in midline without a pillow. For muscle groups tested in the prone position, the head should be turned toward the side being tested. It is important to consistently keep the head turned

Table 7.3 Handheld myometry strength testing positions

Muscle group	Body position	Starting position	End position	Application point	Fixation
Ankle dorsiflexors	Supine	Supine in anatomical position. Hips and knees extended and lower legs off the end of the plinth distal to the lateral malleoli. Feet in a relaxed plantarflexed position	Same as start position except ankle dorsiflexed to 90°	Dorsal aspects of foot at metatarsal heads	Pelvis stabilized by a belt. Anterior tibia fixed by examiner's hand
Ankle evertors	Supine	Same as above	Same as start position except ankle is everted to neutral and dorsiflexed to 90°	Lateral aspect of foot at metatarsal heads	Pelvis stabilized by a belt. Anterior tibia fixated by examiner's hand
Ankle plantarflexors	Prone	Prone in anatomical position. Knee flexed to 90° and ankle relaxed to a dorsiflexed position. Contralateral leg extended with lower leg off edge of plinth distal to lateral malleolus	Same as start position except ankle is plantarflexed to 90°	Plantar aspect of foot over metatarsal heads	Pelvis and distal thigh stabilized with belts

Table 7.3 *cont.*

Muscle group	Body position	Starting position	End position	Application point	Fixation
Elbow extensors	Supine	Supine in anatomical position. The upper extremities positioned next to the trunk. The arm to be tested fully flexed at the elbow with the forearm in neutral rotation	Same as start position except the elbow is extended to a 90° angle with the forearm in neutral rotation	The ulnar border of the forearm with the distal edge of the force pad just proximal to the ulnar styloid process	Examiner fixates shoulder and humerus with hand
Elbow flexors	Supine	Same as above except arm to be tested is fully extended at the elbow with the forearm in a position of neutral rotation	Same as start position except the elbow is flexed to a 90° angle with the forearm in neutral rotation	The radial border of the forearm with the distal edge of the force pad just proximal to the radial styloid process	Examiner fixates shoulder and proximal humerus with hand
Hip abductors	Prone	Prone in anatomical position with lower legs off the plinth distal to lateral malleoli. Hips and knees extended and in neutral rotation	Same as start position, with hips in neutral position; attempts to abduct hip by pushing into myometer force pad	Lateral aspect of distal thigh with the distal edge of the force pad just proximal to lateral epicondyle of the femur	Pelvis stabilized by a belt

Table 7.3 *cont.*

Muscle group	Body position	Starting position	End position	Application point	Fixation
Hip extensors	Supine	Supine with the hips extended and knees flexed over end of the plinth. The hips should be in a position of neutral rotation	Same as start position except tested lower extremity flexed to 90° with lower leg resting on examiner's shoulder	Posterior aspect of distal thigh, with the distal edge of the force pad just proximal to lateral epicondyle of the femur	Pelvis stabilized by a belt
Knee extensors	Prone	Prone in anatomical position with the knee fully flexed. Contralateral leg extended with lower leg off edge of plinth distal to the lateral malleolus	Same as start position except knee is extended to a 90° angle	Anterior aspect of distal leg with the distal edge of the force pad just proximal to the lateral malleolus	Pelvis and distal thigh stabilized with belts
Knee flexors	Prone	Prone in anatomical position. Towel roll placed under the distal aspect of the tibia, proximal to the lateral malleolus. Contralateral leg is extended. The towel roll diameter should be 5 cm less than 1/2 the lever arm length of the lower leg so that the end test position will be at 30°, based upon the sine of 30° •	Same as start position except texted knee is flexed 30° so that the dorsal aspect of the distal tibia is lifted 5 cm above the towel roll	Posterior aspect of the distal leg with the distal edge of the force pad just proximal to the lateral malleolus	Pelvis and distal thigh stabilized with belts

toward the ipsilateral side, to avoid any subtle influences of the asymmetrical tonic neck reflex.

Instructions

Clear, consistent instructions need to be provided when strength testing. Verbal directions are enhanced by tactile and visual cues. Passively moving the appropriate body part in the direction of movement provides tactile and kinesthetic feedback. When teaching muscle test motions, examiners should shift their body in the direction of the motion while passively moving the tested extremity through the desired motion. This visual cue of the examiner's movement also provides cues regarding the correct direction of motion. If confusion regarding the test movement is detected, the test trial should be aborted before maximum resistance is obtained, and further instructions should be provided. It is important that clients be instructed to build resistance gradually, avoiding a ballistic motion. We have found it helpful to explain that each time the 'Push!' command is given, the client should push a little harder. By the third time 'Push!' is said, the client should be pushing as hard as possible. A steady, continuous contraction should be sustained until the examiner says 'Relax'. Test instructions may be modified and repeated if needed to enhance client understanding.

It is often advantageous to refer to the names of the muscles and their function during testing, so that the procedures make sense to clients. When passively taking the extremity through the motion, it is helpful to say: 'I am going to test the strength of your *(muscle name)* muscle,' while providing tactile input to the muscle. Then say: 'Its function is to *(specify motion)*', while passively moving the extremity through the motion. 'I am going to test its strength by having you push into my hand like this' (demonstrate the motion by pushing the extremity in the correct direction while giving a light counterforce with your opposite hand). Incorporating this technique of identifying muscles and their function into the strength testing protocol seems to motivate individuals to focus on the specific test motions.

For younger children, we have found it useful to call strength testing the 'Silly Muscle Game' and to describe each muscle's function in terms of the muscle's 'job'. Children generally enjoy hearing the 'silly' scientific names of the muscles (e.g. 'Mr. Gluteus Maximus'). The child's responsibility is to make the muscle do its 'job'. It may also be helpful, when testing young children, to use a hand puppet when performing MMT or when holding a handheld myometer. Instructions can then be stated in terms of 'push the puppet over'. It is important to use a sock-style puppet made of a non-slip fabric. Use of a puppet will enhance the understanding of young children by making the testing more concrete.

Verbal commands

It is important to use short, simple, consistent commands so that the client concentrates on force production, rather than on what the examiner is saying during the contraction. Short, concise commands have been found to be beneficial in producing maximal effort during strengthening exercises (Sullivan et al 1982). This same principle can be applied to strength testing. We recommend that the examiner say 'Push!' three times during the five second contraction interval. In our experience, the 'push' command works best, regardless of the direction of motion. Varying the command with alternate choices such as 'Pull!' or 'Bend!', or by adding in additional comments, often confuses the client. Voice volume needs to be adequate to heighten the arousal state and to motivate clients to give their best effort. Examiners should increase their voice volume with each successive 'Push!' command for an individual test trial. In this way, the client will be encouraged to build resistance to a maximal level. The commands should be spaced so that the individual holds for five seconds and then relaxes. Examiners need to learn to say 'Push!' three times, with the correct timing, so that five seconds elapse between the first 'Push!' command and the 'Relax' command. The command we use is 'Ready? Hold! Push! PUSH! *PUSH*! Relax'. A variation of the Push! command that is acceptable to use to encourage clients to push harder is: 'Push! HARDER! *PUSH*!'

Reinforcement and feedback

Reinforcement should be provided following each trial using a phrase such as: 'Good!', 'Good job!', or 'Great!'. Reinforcement and feedback can influence performance levels (Schmidt 1988). Bohannon (1987) recommends that consistent verbal encouragement and feedback be given. The frequency and type of feedback provided should be documented. Verbal encouragement has been found to increase strength only slightly (2% to 4%) in normal clients or individuals with organic weakness (Peacock et al 1981, van der

Ploeg & Oosterhuis 1991). Auditory feedback has not been found to significantly influence grip strength readings (Weiss-Lambrou & Dutil 1986). In contrast, van der Ploeg and Oosterhuis (1991) found a 20% increase in strength in patients with functional weakness.

Increased strength readings were obtained by Figoni and Morris (1984) and Baltzopoulos et al (1991) when they provided subjects with visual feedback during slow speed isokinetic strength testing. Similar results have been reported by Pierson and Rasch (1964) and Berger (1967) when visual feedback was provided via the dynamometer force gauge. Electromyographic feedback and a combination of auditory and visual feedback have also been found to enhance force production (Peacock et al 1981, Middaugh et al 1982). In contrast, Buchanan (1980) and Weiss-Lambrou and Dutil (1986) reported that visual, auditory and combined visual and auditory feedback had no significant effect on elbow extensor or grip strength respectively. Schenk and Forward (1965) reported that post-test feedback does not appear to influence subsequent test performance.

The effect of various forms of feedback has not been established on children and adolescents. Permitting the client to view the force gauge during testing may bias test performance. In addition, it may distract younger clients. Therefore, until these issues are studied further, we recommend that neither the client or examiner view the force gauge during test trials, to avoid potential biases.

Resistance

Resistance should be increased gradually to match the force exerted by the client. It is very important that the contraction be maintained for 5 seconds so that adequate time is provided to build resistance. Following the third 'Push!' command, the client should be told to relax. The testing instrument should not be moved until the individual relaxes so that a rebound effect does not occur. The examiner must be careful to match the force and not overcome the client's resistance when the isometric hold test technique is used.

Type of contraction

The force generated when assessing strength varies, depending upon the type and velocity of muscle contraction. Both the eccentric 'break' resistance and the isometric hold test techniques have been advocated for use when strength testing with handheld dynamometers. We have found that it is often difficult for children to consistently sustain a contraction at the point the examiner overcomes their resistance when using the 'break' resistance technique. Consequently, optimal performance may not be elicited using this method. It is generally easier for children to grasp the concept of holding a contraction when tested using the isometric 'hold' technique. As discussed earlier in the section entitled 'Quantitative muscle testing: handheld devices' (p. 115), Hinderer & Gutierrez (1988) demonstrated that the isometric 'hold' test technique is more reliable and has less measurement error than the eccentric 'break' test technique when testing normal children, 5 to 10 years of age. Consequently, we recommend the use of the isometric 'hold' technique when testing children.

Determining the difference between force produced via the eccentric 'break' versus the isometric 'hold' technique may be useful for identifying individuals with functional weakness. This was demonstrated in a study on adults by van der Ploeg and Oosterhuis (1991). These authors also reported that forces produced by individuals with functional weakness via the eccentric 'break' method were more likely to be 'within normal limits' than forces produced via the isometric 'hold' technique. These results suggest, therefore, that the isometric 'hold' technique is more sensitive in detecting and monitoring strength deficits.

Body mechanics

The examiner should stand in the plane of motion to cue the client regarding the appropriate direction of movement (e.g. when testing shoulder flexors in the supine position, the examiner should stand at the head of the examination table, in line with the subject's arm, to cue the subject to push upwards toward the examiner). In addition, this enhances the examiner's ability to control the motion and to provide a perpendicular counter-force. The examiner's body should be positioned to have a mechanical advantage over the client. Force should be resisted by leaning in with body weight, rather than just using the upper extremities. It is much easier to appropriately grade and sustain resistance by weight shifting with one's body. Effective use of body weight also helps minimize fatigue of arm muscles. If a testing instrument is used, it should be stabilized against the examiner's body when testing so that a forward weight shift can be used to resist the client's motion. If the subject is strong or has long extremities, it may be helpful to stand on a footstool to gain more leverage when testing muscle groups such as hip flexors and extensors, knee flexors and ankle plantarflexors.

The instrument design also affects the mechanics of testing. Hinderer et al (1988) found the handle design of the Penny and Giles myometer preferable to the handle of the Sparks dynamometer, since the examiner's hand is closer to the tested extremity, allowing better directional control of resistance force applied during strength testing.

By incorporating the above principles of body mechanics, we have found no significant effect of examiner strength on test results. In contrast, Kramer et al (1991) and Wikholm & Bohannon (1991) have reported examiner effects. The procedures described in these two studies, however, did not incorporate the aforementioned principles of body mechanics.

CONCLUSIONS

Muscle strength measurement is an important evaluation tool that is useful for numerous neuromuscular and musculoskeletal conditions that occur during infancy, childhood and adolescence. When testing the strength of children, examiners need to have knowledge of normal muscle development to be able to differentiate when changes in strength have occurred due to a disease process or therapeutic intervention, versus normal variations or developmental changes in strength. Examiners should also be aware of factors that can cause fluctuation in muscle strength, particularly those factors which can be controlled for by employing proper testing techniques. Adherence to basic principles of muscle strength testing are essential to obtain reliable and valid measurements in children and adolescents, regardless of the method or device utilized.

Manual muscle testing is the most common method currently implemented for testing muscle strength. This method is convenient and inexpensive, but lacks reliability when testing children. Additionally, MMT lacks objectivity and sensitivity for detecting changes in strength.

Large fixed devices, like the isokinetic dynamometers, have been advocated by some individuals as a better method of testing. These devices are expensive, require a large amount space, and consume extended periods of time to test multiple muscle groups. Despite providing objective measurements, these devices are often not practical for broad clinical applications.

The authors recommend the use of portable, handheld, quantitative muscle strength testing devices. The current literature indicates that these devices provide reliable measurements in normal and disabled children and adolescents. The quantitative values obtained from handheld instruments provide sufficient sensitivity to detect small changes in muscle strength that a traditional MMT would miss. Because of their portability, these devices are practical for use in a typical clinic setting. Proper testing techniques and protocols must be implemented to ensure the consistency of measurements.

Testing the strength of children under the age of five requires special consideration. Young children are sometimes unable to adequately participate in standard strength testing procedures. Examiners must utilize observation and palpation skills, in addition to functional tests, to assess the strength of infants and toddlers. Manual muscle test scores have been shown to have good predictive validity, even for young infants. The results of these tests, and prognostication from them, must be interpreted with caution, however, because optimal motor performance may not have been elicited.

In summary, this chapter has discussed the clinical applications of strength assessment methods in children and adolescents, maturational changes that effect strength measurements, factors that influence strength variation and basic principles of strength testing. Testing techniques for obtaining reliable and valid strength measurements in infants, children and adolescents were specifically discussed.

REFERENCES

Ager C L, Olivett B L, Johnson C L 1984 Grasp and pinch strength in children 5 to 12 years old. American Journal of Occupational Therapy 38: 107–113

Agre J C, Findley T W, McNally M C, Habeck R, Leon A S, Stradel L, Birkebak R, Schmalz R 1987 Physical activity capacity in children with myelomeningocele. Archives of Physical Medicine and Rehabilitation 68: 372–377

Agre J C, Magness J L, Hull S Z, Wright K C, Baxter T L, Patterson R, Stradel L 1987 Strength testing with a portable dynamometer: reliability for upper and lower extremities. Archives of Physical Medicine and Rehabilitation 68: 454–458

Aitkens S, Lord J, Bernauer E, Fowler W, Lieberman J, Berck P 1989 Relationship of manual muscle testing to objective strength measurements. Muscle and Nerve 12: 173–177

Allsop K G, VanWagoner E 1987 Application of a device for the quantitative testing of muscle strength. Paper presented at 10th Annual Resna Conference, San Jose, CA., 1987

Amundsen L R 1990 Isometric muscle strength testing with fixed-load cells. In: Amundsen L R (ed) Muscle strength testing: instrumented and non-instrumented systems. Churchill Livingstone, New York, p 89–121

Anderson L R, Bohannon R W 1991 Head and neck position does not influence maximum static elbow extension force measured in healthy individuals tested while prone. The Occupational Therapy Journal of Research 11: 121–126

Andrews A W 1991 Hand-held dynamometry for measuring muscle strength. Journal of Human Muscle Performance 1(1): 35–50

Asmussen E 1973 Growth in muscular strength and power. In: Rarick G L (ed) Physical activity: human growth and development. Academic Press, New York, p 60–79

Balogun J A, Adenlola S A, Akinlove A A 1991 Grip strength normative data for the harpenden dynamometer. Journal of Orthopedics & Sports Physical Therapy 14(4): 155–160

Balogun J A, Akomolafe C T, Amusa L O 1991 Grip strength: effects of testing posture and elbow position. Archives of Physical Medicine and Rehabilitation 72: 280–283

Balzopoulos V, Williams J G, Brodie D A 1991 Sources of error in isokinetic dynamometry: effects of visual feedback on maximum torque measurements. Journal of Orthopedics & Sports Physical Therapy 13(3): 138–142

Bar-or O 1986 Pathophysiological factors which limit the exercise capacity of the sick child. Medicine and Science in Sports and Exercise 18: 276–282

Barr A E, Diamond B E, Wade C K, Harashima T, Pecorella W A, Potts C C, Rosenthal H, Fleiss J L, McMahon D J 1991 Reliability of testing measures in Duchenne or Becker muscular dystrophy. Archives of Physical Medicine and Rehabilitation 72: 315–319

Beasley W C 1956 Influence of method on estimates of normal knee extensor force among normal and postpolio children. Physical Therapy Review 36: 21–41

Beasley W C 1961 Quantitative muscle testing: principles and applications to research and clinical services. Archives of Physical Medicine and Rehabilitation 42: 398–425

Berger R A 1967 Effects of knowledge of isometric strength during performance on recorded strength. Research Quarterly 38: 507–509

Blair L 1955 The role of the physical therapist in the evaluation studies of the poliomyelitis vaccine field trials. Physical Therapy Review 37: 437–447

Bohannon R W 1986a Manual muscle test scores and dynamometer test scores of knee extension strength. Archives of Physical Medicine and Rehabilitation 67: 390–392

Bohannon R W 1986b Test-retest reliability of hand-held dynamometry during a single session of strength assessment. Physical Therapy 66: 206–209

Bohannon R W 1986c Upper extremity strength and strength relationships among young women. Journal of Orthopedics & Sports Physical Therapy 7: 128–133

Bohannon R W 1987 The clinical measurement of strength. Clinical Rehabilitation 1: 5–16

Bohannon R W 1990 Muscle strength testing with hand-held dynamometers. In: Amundsen L R (ed) Muscle strength testing: instrumented and non-instrumented systems. Churchill Livingstone, New York, p 69–88

Bohannon R W 1991 Hand grip dynamometers: issues relevant to application. Journal of Human Muscle Performance 1(2): 16–36

Bohannon R W, Andrews A W 1989 Influence of head-neck rotation on static elbow flexion force of paretic side in patients with hemiparesis. Physical Therapy 69(2): 135–137

Bohannon R W, Andrews B 1987 Interrater reliability of hand-held dynamometry. Physical Therapy 67: 931–933

Bohannon R W, Dubuc W E 1984 Documentation of the resolution of weakness in a patient with Guillain-Barre syndrome. Physical Therapy 64: 1388–1389

Borden R, Colachis S C 1968 Quantitative measurement of the good and normal ranges in muscle testing. Physical Therapy 48: 839–843

Brussock C M, Haley S M, Munsat T L, Bernhardt D B 1992 Measurement of isometric force in children with and without Duchenne's muscular dystrophy. Physical Therapy 72(2): 105–114

Buchanan C I 1980 The effect of three different types of feedback on the amount of force generated during isometric contraction of the triceps brachii muscle. Unpublished master's thesis, School of Allied Health Professions, Medical College of Virginia, Virginia Commonwealth University, Richmond

Burnett C N, Betts E F, Colby L A 1991 Muscle testing for DMD. Clinical Management 11(2): 31–34

Byl N, Richards S, Asturias J 1988 Intrarater and interrater reliability of strength measurements of the biceps and deltoid using a hand-held dynamometer. Journal of Orthopedics & Sports Physical Therapy 9: 399–405

Clarke H H 1954 Comparison of instrumentation for recording muscle strength. Research Quarterly 25: 398–411

Clarke H H 1966 Muscular strength and endurance in man. Prentice Hall, Englewood Cliffs, NJ

Cornwall M W, Bruscato M P, Barry S 1991 Effect of mental practice on isometric muscular strength. Journal of Orthopedics & Sports Physical Therapy 13(5): 231–234

Daniels L, Worthingham C 1986 Muscle testing: techniques of manual examination (5th edn) W B Saunders, Philadelphia, PA

Deutsch H, Kilani H, Moustafa E, Hamilton N, Hebert J P 1987 Effect of head-neck position on elbow flexor muscle torque production. Physical Therapy 67(4): 517–521

Edwards R H T, Hyde S 1977 Methods of measuring muscle strength and fatigue. Physiotherapy 63(2): 51–55

Edwards R H T, McDonnel M 1974 Hand-held dynamometer for evaluating voluntary muscle function. Lancet 2: 757–758

Edwards R H T, Young A, Hosking G P, Jones D A 1977 Human skeletal muscle function: description of tests and normal values. Clinical Science and Molecular Medicine 52: 283–290

Espenschade A S, Eckert H M 1980 Motor development (2nd edn) Charles E Merrill, Columbus, OH

Figoni S F, Morris A F 1984 Effects of knowledge of results on reciprocal isokinetic strength and fatigue. Journal of Orthopedics & Sports Physical Therapy 6: 190–197

Finucane S D, Walker M L, Rothstein J M, Lamb R L 1988 Reliability of isometric muscle testing of knee flexor and extensor muscles in patients with connective tissue disease. Physical Therapy 68: 338–343

Fischer A A 1988 Handheld dynamometer for clinical measurement of muscle strength. Paper presented at the meeting of the Xth Congress of the International Federation of Physical Medicine and Rehabilitation, Toronto, Ontario

Florence J M, Pandya S, King W, Schierbecker J, Robison J D, Signore L C, Mandel S, Arfken C 1988 Strength assessment: comparison of methods in children with Duchenne muscular dystrophy [Abstract]. Physical Therapy 68: 866

Florence J M, Pandya S, King W M, Robison J D, Baty J, Miller J P, Schlerbecker J, Signore L C 1992 Intrarater reliability of manual muscle test (Medical Research Council scale) grades in Duchenne's muscular dystrophy. Physical Therapy 72(2): 115–122

Florence J M, Pandya S, King W M, Robison J D, Signore L C, Wentzell M, Province M A 1984 Clinical trials in Duchenne dystrophy. Physical Therapy 64(1): 41–45

Frese E, Brown M, Norton B J 1987 Clinical reliability of manual muscle testing. Middle trapezius and gluteus medius muscles. Physical Therapy 67: 1072–1076
Friman G 1977 Effect of acute infectious disease on isometric muscle strength. Scandinavian Journal of Clinical and Laboratory Investment 37: 303–308
Fullwood D 1986 Australian norms for hand and finger strength of boys and girls ages 5–12 years. Australian Occupational Therapy Journal 33: 26–36
Gallahue D L 1982 Understanding motor development in children. John Wiley & Sons, New York
Giles C 1984 The modified sphygmomanometer: an instrument to objectively assess muscle strength. Physiotherapy Canada 36(1): 36–37
Gooch J L, Newton B Y, Petajan J H 1990 Motor unit spike counts before and after maximal voluntary contraction. Muscle and Nerve 13: 1146–1151
Greenleaf J E, Kozlowski S 1982 Physiological consequences of reduced physical activity during bed rest. Exercise and Sport Sciences Reviews 10: 84–119
Griffin J W, McClure M H, Bertorini T E 1986 Sequential isokinetic and manual muscle testing in patients with neuromuscular disease. Pilot study. Physical Therapy 66: 32–35
Hack S N, Norton B J, Zahalak G I 1981 A quantitative muscle tester for clinical use [Abstract]. Physcial Therapy 61: 673
Hay L 1984 The development of movement control. In: Smyth M M, Wing A M (eds) The psychology of human movement. Academic Press, New York, p 241–267
Helewa A, Goldsmith C H, Smythe H A 1981 The modified sphygmomanometer: an instrument to measure muscle strength. A validation study. Journal of Chronic Disease 34: 353–361
Hinderer K A 1988 Reliability of the myometer in muscle testing children and adolescents with myelodysplasia. Unpublished master's thesis, University of Washington, Seattle
Hinderer K A, Gutierrez T 1988 Myometer measurements of children using isometric and eccentric methods of muscle testing [Abstract]. Physical Therapy 68: 817
Hinderer S R, Hinderer K A 1993 Objective measurement in rehabilitation medicine: theory and application. In: Delisa J, Gans B, Currie D (eds) Rehabilitation medicine: principles and practice p 96–121
Hinderer K A, Hinderer S R 1990 Stabilized vs. unstabilized myometry strength test positions: a reliability comparison [Abstract]. Archives of Physical Medicine and Rehabilitation 71: 771
Hinderer K A, Hinderer S R, Deitz J L 1988 Reliability of manual muscle testing using the hand-held dynamometer and the myometer: a comparison study. Paper presented at American Physical Therapy Association Midwinter Sections Meeting, Washington, D C
Hislop H J 1963 Quantitative changes in human muscular strength during isometric exercise. Journal of the American Physical Therapy Association 43: 21–38
Hosking G P, Bhat U S, Dubowitz V, Edwards R H T 1976 Measurements of muscle strength and performance in children with normal and diseased muscle. Archives of Disease in Childhood 51: 957–963
Hunsicker P A, Donnelly R J 1955 Instruments to measure strength. Research Quarterly 26(4): 408–420
Hyde S A 1980 Physiotherapy in rheumatology. Blackwell, Oxford
Hyde S, Goddard C, Scott O 1983 The myometer: the development of a clinical tool. Physiotherapy 69: 424–427
Iddings D M, Smith L K, Spencer W A 1961 Muscle testing: part 2. Reliability in clinical use. The Physical Therapy Review 41: 249–256
Itoh M, Lee M H M 1990 The epidemiology of disability as related to rehabilitation medicine. In: Kottke F J, Stillwell G K, Lehmann J F (eds),

Krusen's handbook of physical medicine and rehabilitation (4th edn). W B Saunders, Philadelphia, PA, p 215–233

Jones H E 1949 Motor performance and growth. University of California Press, Berkeley, Ca

Kendall F P, McCreary E K 1983 Muscle testing and function (3rd edn). Williams & Wilkins, Baltimore, MD

Kilburn J, Saffer A, Barnes L, Kling T, Venes J 1985 The vigorimeter as an early predictor of central neurologic malformation in myelodyplastic children. Paper presented at the meeting of the American Academy for Cerebral Palsy and Developmental Medicine, Seattle, WA

Kjerland RN 1953 Age and sex differences in performance in motility and strength test. Proceedings of the Iowa Academy of Sciences 60: 519–523

Kramer J F, Vaz M D, Vandervoort A A 1991 Reliability of isometric hip abductor torques during examiner- and belt-resisted tests. Journal of Gerontology 46(2): M47–M51

Lamb R L 1985 Manual muscle testing. In: Rothstein J M (ed) Measurement in physical therapy. Churchill Livingstone, New York, p 47–55

Lefkof M B 1986 Trunk flexion in healthy children aged 3 to 7 years. Physical Therapy 66(1): 39–44

Level M B 1984 Spherical grip strength of children. Unpublished master's thesis, University of Washington, Seattle

Lilienfeld A M, Jacobs M, Willis M 1954 A study of the reproducibility of muscle testing and certain other aspects of muscle scoring. Physical Therapy Review 34: 279–289

Lovett R V, Martin E G 1916 Certain aspects of infantile paralysis with a description of a method of muscle testing. Journal of the American Medical Association 66: 729–733

MacDougall J D, Elder G C B, Sale D G, Moroz J R, Sutton J R 1980 Effects of strength training and immobilization on human muscle fibers. European Journal of Applied Physiology 43: 25–34

Marino M, Nicholas J, Gleim G, Rosenthal P, Nicholas S 1982 The efficacy of manual assessment of muscle strength using a new device. American Journal of Sports Medicine 10: 360–364

Mathiowetz V 1990 Grip and pinch strength measurements. In: Amundsen L R (ed) Muscle strength testing: instrumented and non-instrumented systems. Churchill Livingstone, New York, p 163–177

Mathiowetz V 1990 Effects of three trials on grip and pinch strength measurements. Journal of Hand Therapy 4: 195–198

Mathiowetz V, Wiemer D M, Federman S M 1986 Grip and pinch strength: norms for 6–19 year olds. American Journal of Occupational Therapy 40: 705–709

Matthews D K, Kruse R 1957 Effects of isometric and isotonic exercise on elbow flexor muscle group. Research Quarterly 28: 26–37

Mawdsley R H, Knapik J J 1982 Comparison of isokinetic measurements with test repetitions. Physical Therapy 62: 169–172

Mayhew T P, Rothstein J M 1985 Measurement of muscle performance with instruments. In: Rothstein J M (ed) Measurement in physical therapy. Churchill Livingstone, New York, p 57–102

McDonald C M, Jaffe K, Shurtleff D B 1986 Assessment of muscle strength in children with meningomyelocele: accuracy and stability of measurements over time. Archives of Physical Medicine and Rehabilitation 67: 855–861

McDonald C M, Jaffe K, Shurtleff D B 1987 Functional patterns of innervation in the lower limb musculature of children with myelomeningocele: implications for ambulation. Paper presented at International Society for Research into Hydrocephalus and Spina Bifida. Newcastle, Northern Ireland

McGarvey S R, Morrey B F, Askew L J, Kai Nan An 1984 Reliability of isometric strength testing. Temporal factor and strength variation. Clinical Orthopaedics and Related Research 185: 301–305

Mendell et al 1989 Randomized double-blind six-month trial of prednisone in Duchenne's muscular dystrophy. New England Journal of Medicine 320: 1592–1597

Mendell J R, Florence J 1990 Manual muscle testing. Muscle and Nerve 13(Suppl.): 16–20

Metheny E 1941 Breathing capacity and grip strength of preschool children. Child Welfare 18(2): 1–207

Middaugh S, Miller C, Ferdon M B 1982 Electromyographic feedback: effects on voluntary muscle contractions in normal subjects. Archives of Physical Medicine and Rehabilitation 63: 254–260

Miller L C, Michael A F, Baxter T L, Kim Y 1988 Quantitative muscle testing in childhood dermatomyositis. Archives of Physical Medicine and Rehabilitation 69: 610–613

Milner-Brown H S, Miller R G 1989 Increased muscular fatigue in patients with neurogenic muscle weakness: quantification and pathophysiology. Archives of Physical Medicine and Rehabilitation 70: 361–366

Molnar G E, Alexander J 1973 Objective, quantitative muscle testing in children: a pilot study. Archives of Physical Medicine and Rehabilitation 54: 224–228

Molnar G E, Alexander J 1974 Development of quantitative standards for muscle strength in children. Archives of Physical Medicine and Rehabilitation 55: 490–493

Molnar G E, Alexander J, Gutfeld N 1979 Reliability of quantitative strength measurements in children. Archives of Physical Medicine and Rehabilitation 60: 218–221

Montoye H J, Lamphiear D E 1977 Grip and arm strength in males and females, age 10 to 69. Research Quarterly 48: 109–120

Moritani T, deVries H A 1979 Neural factors versus hypertrophy in the time course of muscle strength gain. American Journal of Physical Medicine and Rehabilitation 58: 115–130

Muller E A 1959 Training muscle strength. Ergonomics 2: 216–222

Muller E A 1970 Influence of training and of inactivity on muscle strength. Archives of Physical Medicine and Rehabilitation 51: 449–462

Mundale M O 1970 The relationship of intermittent isometric exercise to fatigue of hand grip. Archives of Physical Medicine and Rehabilitation 51: 532–539

Murdoch A 1980 How valuable is muscle charting? A study of the relationship between neonatal assessment of muscle power and later mobility in children with spina bifida defects. Physiotherapy 66: 221–223

Newman L B 1949 A new device for measuring muscle strength. Archives of Physical Medicine and Rehabilitation 30: 234–237

Nicholas J, Sapega A, Kraus H, Webb J 1978 Factors influencing manual muscle tests in physical therapy. Journal of Bone and Joint Surgery 60: 186–190

Olds K, Colthrust A J B, Godfrey C M 1984 New technology in patient assessment: the reliability and validity of the myometer in manual muscle testing. Unpublished manuscript, University of Toronto, Department of Rehabilitation Medicine, Toronto, Ontario

Pact V, Sirotkin-Roses M, Beatus J 1984 The muscle testing handbook. Little, Brown and Company, Boston, MA

Palmer C E 1944 Studies of the center of gravity in the human body. Child Development 15(2-3): 99–180

Patterson R P, Baxter T 1988 A multiple muscle strength testing protocol. Archives of Physical Medicine and Rehabilitation 69: 366–368

Peacock B, Westers T, Walsh S, Nicholson K 1981 Feedback and maximum voluntary contraction. Ergonomics 24: 223–228

Pierson W R, Rasch P J 1964 Effect of knowledge of results on isometric strength scores. Research Quarterly 35: 313–315

Rheault W, Beal J L, Kubik K R, Nowak T A, Shepley J A 1989 Intertester reliability of the hand held dynamometer for wrist flexion and extension. Archives of Physical Medicine and Rehabilitation 70: 907–910

Riddle D L, Finucane S D, Rothstein J M, Walker M L 1989 Intrasession and intersession reliability of hand-held dynamometer measurements taken on brain-damage patients. Physical Therapy 69(3): 182–194

Saraniti A, Gleim G, Melvin M, Nicholas J 1980 The relationship between subjective and objective measurements of strength. Journal of Orthopedics & Sports Medicine 2: 15–19

Schafer M F, Dias L S 1983 Myelomeningocele: orthopaedic treatment. Williams and Wilkins, Baltimore, MD

Schenk J M, Forward E M 1965 Quantitative strength changes with test repetitions. Journal of the American Physical Therapy Association 45: 562–569

Schmidt R A 1988 Methodology for studying motor behavior. In: Schmidt R A (ed) Motor control and learning (2nd edn) Human Kinetics Publishers, Champaign, IL, p 45–73

Schneider J W 1985 Congenital spinal cord injury. In: Umphred D A (ed) Neurological rehabilitation, Vol. 3, C V Mosby, St Louis, MO, p 289–313

Scott O M, Hyde S A, Goddard C, Dubowitz V 1982 Quantitation of muscle function in children: a prospective study in Duchenne muscular dystrophy. Muscle and Nerve 5: 291–301

Sharrard W J W 1964 The segmental innervation of the lower limb muscles in man. Annals of the Royal College of Surgeons of England 35: 106–112

Shurtleff D B 1986 Myelodysplasias and extrophies: significance, prevention and treatment. Grune and Stratton, New York

Shurtleff D B 1991 Computer data bases for pediatric disability: clinical and research applications. Physical Medicine and Rehabilitation Clinics of North America 2: 665–687

Silver M, McElroy A, Morrow L, Heafner B K 1970 Further standardization of manual muscle test for clinical study: applied in chronic renal disease. Physical Therapy 50: 1456–1466

Smidt G L 1984 Muscle strength testing: a system based on mechanics. Smidt, Iowa

Smidt G L, Rogers M W 1982 Factors contributing to the regulation and clinical assessment of muscular strength. Physical Therapy 62: 1283–1290

Solgaard S, Kristiansen B, Jensen J S 1984 Evaluation of instruments for measuring grip strength. Acta Orthopaedica Scandinavica 55: 569–572

Steindler A 1955 Kinesiology of the human body under normal and pathological conditions. Charles C Thomas, Springfield, IL

Stuberg W A, Metcalf W K 1988 Reliability of quantitative muscle testing in healthy children and in children with Duchenne muscular dystrophy using a hand-held dynamometer. Physical Therapy 68: 977–982

Sullivan P E, Markos P D, Minor M A D 1982 An integrated approach to therapeutic exercise. Reston Publishing, Reston, VA

Surburg P R, Suomi R, Poppy W K 1992 Validity and reliability of a hand-held dynamometer applied to adults with mental retardation. Archives of Physical Medicine and Rehabilitation 73: 535–539

Sykanda A M, Armstrong R W, Rogers M J, Stewart S N 1988 Standards for evaluating muscle strength of children, using the myometer [Abstract]. Developmental Medicine & Child Neurology, 30(5) (Suppl. 57): 18–19

Taylor H L, Henschel A, Brozek J, Key A 1949 Effects of bedrest on cardiovascular function and work performance. Journal of Applied Physiology 2: 223–239

Thelen E 1985 The developmental origins of motor coordination: leg movements in human infants. Developmental Psychobiology 18(1): 1–22

Tornvall G 1963 Assessment of physical capabilities. Acta Physiologica Scandinavica 58 (Suppl. 201): 1–102

Tripp E J, Harris S R 1991 Test-retest reliability of isokinetic knee extension and flexion torque measurements in persons with spastic hemiparesis. Physical Therapy 71(5): 390–396

Unsworth A, Haslock I, Vasandakumar V, Stamp J 1990 A laboratory and clinical study of pneumatic grip strength devices. British Journal of Rheumatology 29: 440–444

van der Ploeg R J O, Fidler V, Oosterhuis H J G H 1991 Hand-held myometry: reference values. Journal of Neurology, Neurosurgery and Psychiatry 54: 244–247

van der Ploeg R J O, Oosterhuis H J G H 1991 The 'make /break test' as a diagnostic tool in functional weakness. Journal of Neurology, Neurosurgery and Psychiatry 54: 248–251

van der Ploeg R J O, Oosterhuis H J G H, Reuvekamp J 1984 Measuring muscle strength. Journal of Neurology 231: 200–203

Wadsworth C, Krishnan R, Sear M, Harrold J, Nielsen D 1987 Interrater reliability of manual muscle testing and hand-held dynametric muscle testing. Physical Therapy 67: 1342–1347

Weiss-Lambrou R, Dutil E 1986 The effect of differing feedback conditions on grip strength: a pilot study. The Occupational Therapy Journal of Research 6(2): 93–103

Westers B M 1982 Factors influencing strength testing and exercise prescription. Physiotherapy 68: 42–44

White M J, Davies C T M 1984 The effects of immobilization, after lower leg fracture, on the contractile properties of human triceps surae. Clinical Science 66: 277–282

Wikholm J B, Bohannon R W 1991 Hand-held dynamometer measurements: tester strength makes a difference. Journal of Orthopedics and Sports Physical Therapy 13(4): 191–198

Wiles C M, Karni Y 1983 The measurement of muscle strength in patients with peripheral neuromuscular disorders. Journal of Neurology, Neurosurgery & Psychiatry 46: 1006–1013

Wilk K 1990 Dynamic muscle strength testing. In: Amundsen L R (ed) Muscle strength testing: instrumented and non-instrumented systems. Churchill Livingstone, New York, p 123–150

Wright F V, Goldsmith C H 1988 Reliability of the modified sphygmomanometer for isometric testing of hip abductor strength in children [Abstract]. Physical Therapy 68: 817

Wright W 1912 Muscle testing in the treatment of infantile paralysis. Boston Medical Surgical Journal 167: 567

Zimny N, Kirk C 1987 A comparison of methods of manual muscle testing. Clinical Management 7(2): 6–11

8. Strength and aging: patterns of change and implications for training

Esko Mälkiä

INTRODUCTION

This chapter deals with changes in muscle strength associated with aging in adults. It begins with a review of research on the normal process of aging and on the many factors that may account for age related reduction in muscle strength. Because this reduction appears to follow a different pattern in men than in women, sex differences in strength also are examined. A subsequent section explores the problems that arise when normal losses of strength due to aging are combined with those from the pathology of diseases that become more common with advancing age. Two final sections review research of special concern to clinical physical therapists. The first of these discusses methods for assessing the muscle strength of aging subjects in relation to the physical demands of work and functional activities. The second presents a series of questions that provide the basis for many studies of muscle training, and suggests guidelines and precautions for strength training of older subjects suggested by the research literature.

1. SOME BASIC BIOLOGICAL FINDINGS APPLIED TO AGING

Most research on muscle performance in aging has been based on population studies. These have identified a wide variety of factors that are associated with maximal oxygen consumption. Many also have been found to be associated with other differences in muscle performance. These factors include various constitutional determinants; environmental influences, such as heat, cold and altitude; social and cultural characteristics, such as family size and occupation; and activity patterns as well as the presence of specific diseases (Shephard 1980).

Apart from population studies, many authors have tried to discover an etiology for age related changes in muscle strength based on laboratory studies in humans or animals. The ultimate result of aging, seen in muscular performance or strength measurements is a consequence of the varied biochemical and mechanical properties of different tissues. The aging performance is characterized by a slowing down of movements, a decrease in maximum strength and a loss of fine coordination (Skinner et al 1982). Behind these findings there are a number of physiological effects of aging having functional significance. There is a decrease in muscle mass, especially in fast twitch fibres (Larsson 1978). Larsson (1982) concluded that the etiology of age related muscle atrophy is very complex. According to Larsson, neuropathic and myopathic alterations are not primary factors in aging. Muscle atrophy is accompanied in many cases by nutritional deficiencies, the disuse of muscles or physical inactivity, a denervating process and endocrine alterations (Larsson 1982). Review studies present rather uniform conclusions about the reality of a type II atrophy in aging. Larsson's studies (1978) have shown type II fibres preferentially affected by aging. Secondary to the alterations in muscle mass atrophy is a decrease in muscle fibre number and size with aging (Larsson 1982, Grimby & Saltin 1983). Some studies have shown that among individual motor units the different fibre types form a continuum between slow and fast extremes (Thomason et al 1986, Staron & Pette 1987).

Recent studies in animals have shown the great importance of muscle connective tissue to the mechanical properties of muscle. At more advanced ages the concentration of total collagen and collagen in slow and fast muscles increases but this is more prominent in slow muscle (Kovanen 1989). This causes an increase in tensile strength, stiffness and elastic efficiency. Alterations in neurotransmission in aging have also been found (Knortz 1987). Studies by Larsson et al (1978) have shown changes in enzymatic activity with aging: anaerobic lactate dehydrogenase activity decreases while aerobic dehydrogenase activity remains unchanged.

In summary, the physiological effects of aging having functional significance in loss of strength and power are a decrease in muscle mass, in the number of type II fibres, in the size of motor units, in the action potential threshold, in total protein and nitrogen concentration (Brooks & Fahey 1985) and in the ratio between anaerobic and aerobic LDH activity. There is also an increase in collagen concentration (Kovanen 1989).

The natural effect of aging on muscle is difficult to differentiate from many factors relating to environmental differences and life style. In particular, the influence of physical activity on the physiological effects of aging has been investigated. Possible training-induced transformation of muscle fibres is one of the key questions of functional significance in the production of strength or power in aged muscle. Komi et al (1977) concluded that muscle fibre composition is genetically determined but Bouchard et al (1986) obtained a contradictory conclusion. Kovanen (1989) found that long-term endurance training accelerated the age related shift in muscle fibre composition towards more fatigue-resistant properties. The mechanism and nature of the stimulus responsible for the transformation is not clear, but changes in neural and muscle factors are both quantitative and qualitative (e.g. Kugelberg 1976, Pette & Vrbova 1985).

According to Kovanen (1989), both advancing age and life-long endurance training influence the slow-twitch and fast-twitch muscles with respect to their connective tissue and material properties. Grimby and Saltin (1983), in comparing differences in age related changes in rat and human muscles, postulated man's optimal life span to be 100–110 years.

The different effects of aging on strength and endurance may be due to loss of muscle mass, which has a direct impact on muscle strength, to changes in the proportions of type I and type II fibres, which enhance the endurance ability, and to complex changes in central and peripheral nerves, muscle tissue and circulation.

Apart from age related changes in muscle, there are many different reasons for a loss in strength and power which might occur concurrently with aging. From a neurophysiological viewpoint, Edwards (1981) summarized the reasons for muscle fatigue to be physiological mechanisms at the central or peripheral levels together with central or peripheral clinical mechanisms. Some diseases also directly influence the mechanisms of strength output. These include peripheral disturbances in blood circulation (Schersten 1977), acute infections (Friman 1977), the excessive use of alcohol (Carlsson 1967) and neuromuscular diseases (Brooke 1986).

2. STRENGTH AND HEALTH

Many diseases have a direct influence on the biology of muscular performance. Such pathological changes may be within muscle itself, e.g. abnormalities in fibre size, distribution, sarcolemmic nuclei, or regeneration; in the central or peripheral nervous system or in the circulation or connective tissue. The cure and care of many diseases demand rest, entailing disuse of muscles. A general trend towards a decrease in physical activity also occurs during aging (Mälkiä et al 1988, Mälkiä 1990). The selective atrophy of type II fibres may be present with muscle disuse as well as with myasthenia gravis, acromegaly, corticosteroid use, strokes and abnormalities of other pyramidal tracts, cachexia and denervation. The condition may also arise in normal adult women (Wheeler 1982, Larsson 1982). Muscular strength or performance has been quantified only for some disability groups.

Good self-rated health was positively associated with higher muscular strength in the study by Era et al (1992) in groups of 31–35 and 51–55-year-old men, but in the 71–75-year-old group the association was no longer significant.

Below normal muscular performance has been observed to accompany rheumatoid arthritis and osteoarthritis (Tiselius 1969, Beals et al 1985), multiple sclerosis (Gehlsen et al 1984), back pain (Nachemson 1989) and, of course, neuromuscular diseases (Brooke 1986). Mentally handicapped persons and those suffering from cerebral palsy also possess a lower muscular performance (Jansma et al 1988, Mälkiä et al 1987, Lahtinen 1986).

Table 8.1 Hand grip strength (Newtons) in sick (D) and healthy (H) men and women in different age groups (persons with cardiovascular risk or pain excluded). (Mälkiä 1983)

Age (years)	*Male* Mean (N) D	H	*Female* Mean (N) D	H
30–44	548	579	316	329
45–54	462	527	273	303
55–64	420	476	231	268
65–75	329	412	205	240
75 & over	274	322	172	206
	Mean difference of means: 87%		Mean difference of means: 88%	

D = Diagnosed disease according to own statement; H = healthy

Table 8.2 Number of sit-ups during 30 seconds for sick (D) and healthy (H) men and women (persons with cardiovascular risk or pain excluded). (Mälkiä 1983)

Age (years)	*Male* Mean (N) D (repeats in 30 s)	H	*Female* Mean (N) D (repeats in 30 s)	H
30–44	13	15	7	9
45–54	8	13	3	6
55–64	7	9	3	3
	Mean difference of means: 75%		Mean difference of means: 76%	

D = diagnosed disease according to own statement; H = healthy

Mälkiä (1983) showed significant differences in muscular performance in every age cohort for both sexes between persons who did and those who stated they did not have any lung, heart, vascular, joint, limb, back, mental or other disease diagnosed by a physician (Tables 8.1–8.3). When the differences between sick and healthy women were analysed disease by disease, muscular strength and performance did not differ significantly except in the group with vascular diseases. Sick and healthy men showed significant differences in muscular performance in many diseases. The most apparent and highly significant difference was between hand grip strength in men with and those without mental problems (Fig. 8.1).

Table 8.3 Number of back extensions during 30 seconds for sick (D) and healthy (H) men and women (persons with cardiovascular risk or pain excluded). (Mälkiä 1983)

Age (years)	*Male* Mean (N) D	H	*Female* Mean (N) D	H
30–44	15	16	12	14
45–54	11	15	9	11
55–64	10	13	8	10
	Mean difference of means: 80%		Mean difference of means: 85%	

D = diagnosed disase according to own statement; H = healthy

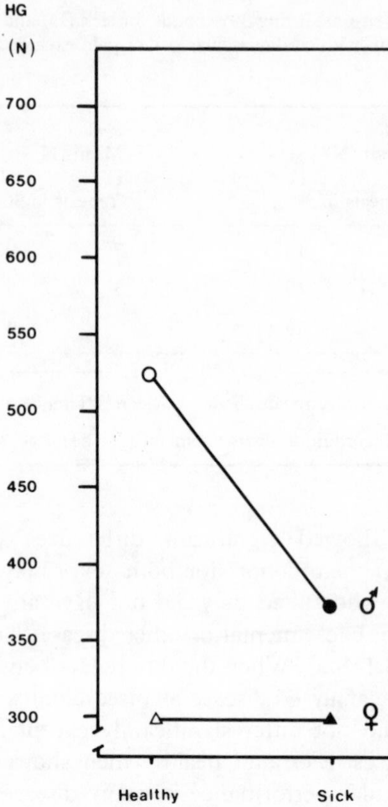

Fig. 8.1 Hand grip (HG) strength in men and women with and without mental problems. Age adjusted means. (n = 898).

3. ASSESSMENT OF STRENGTH IN THE ELDERLY SUBJECT

3.1 Strength and aging

Fundamental biological studies show that muscular strength decreases during aging. The question that remains is how and when muscular strength decreases, and whether there are any confounding factors apart from aging itself.

The results of muscular strength measurements are dependent on the method of evaluation adopted. Muscles tend to adapt specifically (Brooks & Fahey 1985). According to Edington and Edgerton (1976) the performance of muscle depends on speed, duration and load via energy pathways in movement. The relationship between muscle performance and aging, then, should only be studied in certain controlled movement conditions of speed, load and duration. In some studies, e.g. Aniansson et al 1984, Coyle et al 1981, Knapik and Ramos 1980, and Larsson 1978, it has been possible to evaluate muscle performance using apparatus to control speed, load and duration of movement. Modern isokinetic or variokinetic measurement systems are suitable for this purpose.

Most analyses of aging muscle performance are based on isometric measurements. In studies by Asmussen et al (1965) a high degree of correlation ($r = 0.8$) was observed between individual isometric and dynamic strength among a small group of active men. In Mälkiä's (1983) randomized sample of adult men and women ($N = 592$), however, correlations between hand grip strength and sit-ups (numbers repeated in 30 s) of 0.26 and between hand grip and back extensions (numbers repeated in 30 s) of 0.26 were found. The correlation between dynamic sit-ups and back extensions was 0.62. This demonstrates the existence of a positive correlation between isometric and dynamic measurements which, however, was lower than those between the dynamic measurements and too low to be of predictive value.

Many studies have shown that isometric and dynamic muscle strength are related to age and sex. The rate of the decline in strength between different age cohorts varies among different muscle groups, between isometric and dynamic tests, and between the strength and endurance (e.g. Asmussen & Heeboll-Nielsen 1962, Shock & Norris 1970, Larsson 1982, Mälkiä 1983, Heikkinen et al 1984). In their classical study, Asmussen and Heeboll-Nielsen (1962) (see also Larsson's review 1982) showed the age-related decline in muscle strength to be most conspicuous in the proximal muscles of the lower extremities, while back and hand grip muscles were less affected. Maximal muscle strength reaches its peak between 20–30 years of age depending on the muscles in question, whether the testing is isometric or dynamic and the sex of the subjects (Asmussen & Heeboll-Nielsen 1962). Studies of strength comparing females and males shows varying results with strength ratios from 36% to 97% (Pheasant 1983, Bishop et al 1987). In Laubach's (1976) review the sex differences in strength were similar for both dynamic and static strength measures. Considerable variation exists in the magnitude of the sex difference depending on age (Ikai & Fukunaga 1968), strength measurement technique and muscle group being tested (Bishop et al 1987).

Table 8.4 Dominant hand grip strength (Newtons) and decline during aging in different age cohorts of healthy men and women. (Data from Aromaa et al 1990; Mälkiä 1983)

Age (years)	Male Number	Male Mean (N)	Male decline % (30–34 y = 100%)	Female Number	Female Mean (N)	Female decline % (30–34 y = 100%)	Sex difference % from male
30–44	402	591	100	385	334	100	61
35–39	291	580	98	289	328	98	57
40–44	288	560	95	249	322	96	57
45–49	243	544	92	204	312	93	57
50–54	188	508	86	170	291	87	57
55–59	153	493	83	149	270	80	55
60–64	88	446	75	92	265	79	59
65–69	74	419	71	93	247	73	59
70–74	53	402	68	65	230	68	57
75–	41	335	56	62	205	61	61
Totals	1821			1758			

Table 8.5 Number of sit-ups during 30 seconds and decline in different age cohorts of healthy men and women. (Mälkiä 1983)

Age (years)	Male Number	Male Mean (repeats in 30 s)	Male decline % (30–34 y = 100%)	Female Number	Female Mean (repeats in 30 s)	Female decline % (30–34 y = 100%)	Sex difference % from male
30–44	139	14.8	100	120	9.4	100	64
45–54	41	12.8	86	49	6.3	67	49
55–64	16	8.8	59	24	2.9	31	33
Totals	196			193			

Hand grip has been one of the most used tests of isometric strength. Based on one of the largest health survey samples in the world (Aromaa et al 1990, Mälkiä 1983), Table 8.4 presents unpublished hand grip results of subjects who, in an inquiry, denied any illnesses. The decline in hand grip strength is fairly small and about 0.5% a year from the age 30 until age 45–49, when the decline starts accelerating to about 1% a year until an even bigger drop is registered at the age of 75 in both sexes. The sex difference in the strength results was very similar among all the age groups. These results bear a marked resemblance to the hand grip measurement results of men in studies by Heikkinen et al (1984), Viitasalo et al (1985) and Mathiowetz et al (1985). The female hand grip strength results of this study are quite comparable with Mathiowetz's results, except that Mathiowetz's study shows a difference of about 2% units less in the hand grip results of women and of men in USA compared to the Finnish studies.

Larsson (1982) concluded in his review that the isometric and dynamic strength of different muscles follows a similar pattern to that of hand grip, i.e. after attaining a peak value at about 30 years of age, a small or non-existent change occurs up until the fifth decade after which there is an accelerated decrease. The above mentioned results show a fairly clear linear change until 75 years of age. The main reason for the differences in results is, perhaps, the use of rather small samples in earlier studies, which have not demonstrated the 7–8% decline between the ages of 30 and 45 years. In any case, this decline is too small to be of importance in clinical practice. It is also not clear that all muscles behave with age in the same way. Tables 8.5 and 8.6 show that, in muscular performance tests, the results can differ considerably depending on muscle group, age and sex (Mälkiä 1983). The dynamic back extension test produces results similar to those of the hand grip test but the sit-up results of women decrease with age faster than hand grip. Women's strength in this sit-up test is also quite low.

In isokinetic measurements there have been problems comparing results obtained using different equipment. Results from tests where the same equipment was used, and performed in the same laboratory, can show up relative differences with regard to age and sex. The results in inclined bench press extension and flexion by 20° and 60° per second, and in leg extension and flexion by 60° and 180° per second (Ariel^{R}), show peak values at age 15–22 years in both sexes. The decline in torque is somewhat faster in men but about the same in women as in the decline in hand grip strength presented in Table 8.4. The rate of decline in bench press extensor strength in women compared to men is lower than the difference recorded for hand grip strength. On the other hand, the sex difference in leg extension and flexion is comparable with hand grip strength (Ariel 1990).

Many factors have been used to explain strength differences between the sexes, such as transverse muscles area, fat-free weight, fat-free cross-sectional areas in different muscles, stature, weight, body area, basal metabolic rate and body mass index (kg/m^2) (e.g. Asmussen & Heeboll-Nielsen 1962, Pheasant 1983, Mälkiä 1983, Bishop et al 1987). None of these factors either together or alone has been able to explain all the difference between the strength of men and that of women. Nonetheless, it appears to be the case that there is no qualitative difference between male and female muscles; such differences as exist relate to muscle mass and training effects.

In addition to age, physical activity during leisure time has also been related to muscular performance (Mälkiä 1983, Rikli & Busch 1986, Era et al 1990). High physical stress at work is associated with higher strength values in younger age groups and with corresponding lower strength values in older age groups in cross-sectional studies (Mälkiä 1974, 1983). In a 3.5 year longitudinal study, it was observed that men doing physical work showed the most significant decrease in musculoskeletal capacity (Nygård et al 1988). These observations were alike in both men and women. Mälkiä (1983) observed in a study of male subjects that men in sedentary occupations (< 3.5 MET*) who were fairly physically active in their

Table 8.6 Number of back extensions during 30 seconds and decline in different age cohorts of healthy men and women. (Mälkiä 1983)

Age (years)	Number	*Male* Mean (repeats in 30 s)	Male decline % (30–34 y = 100%)	Number	*Female* Mean (repeats in 30 s)	Female decline % (30–34 y = 100%)	Sex difference % from male
30–44	139	16.8	100	118	14.0	100	88
45–54	47	15.0	89	47	11.1	79	74
55–64	18	13.1	78	28	9.9	71	76
Totals	204			193			

*MET is a multiple of the resting rate of O_2 consumption:
1 MET = 3.5 ml x kg^{-1} x min^{-1} VO_2 at rest.

leisure time (> 5 MET) had higher dynamic back extensor strength compared to men in heavy (> 5 MET) or light manual occupations (< 5 MET) or no (< 2 MET) exercises in their spare time. Thus, physical stress at work is either not enough to stimulate the muscles in order to have an exercise effect or, in the case of heavy work, does not permit enough rest to allow muscles to regenerate or store neurogenic energy.

The profile of muscular endurance, which indicates the ability to hold maximum tension or submaximal tension or to make repetitions of dynamic exertions for more than a few seconds, is similar to that of muscle strength. In different studies it has been observed that isometric and isokinetic endurance values are not lower in older populations, at least up to 65 years of age (Larsson 1978, Johnson 1982).

3.2 Functional performance

The validity of muscle strength measurements in relation to physical ability in different age groups is an important issue for the clinician. Relatively few studies have been made on the association between muscle strength or performance and functional performance. Nonetheless, in most of the activities of daily living, and in most jobs, considerable muscular strength, at least in the hands, torso and legs is needed. How much muscular strength in needed at work, depends on the physical stress of the job.

In Mälkiä's cross-section study (1983) the physical ability of an adult Finnish population was tested using a battery of simple muscular performance tests together with self-estimated physical ability scales.

From the results it is apparent that muscular performance is related to subjective physical ability. The results showed quite good correlations between the strength measurements of dominant hand grip, isometric arm press, dynamic sit-ups, trunk extensions and those of self-estimated physical condition, the ability to manage job and the ability to run fairly short distances (Figs. 8.2–8.7). A similar association was found between muscular performance results and self-rated ability, scored by the same scale, for climbing one flight of stairs without pausing for a rest, for climbing several flights of stairs, for walking a distance of about half a kilometre and for running a fairly long distance. Men, in particular, showed a close relationship between muscular performance and the perceived

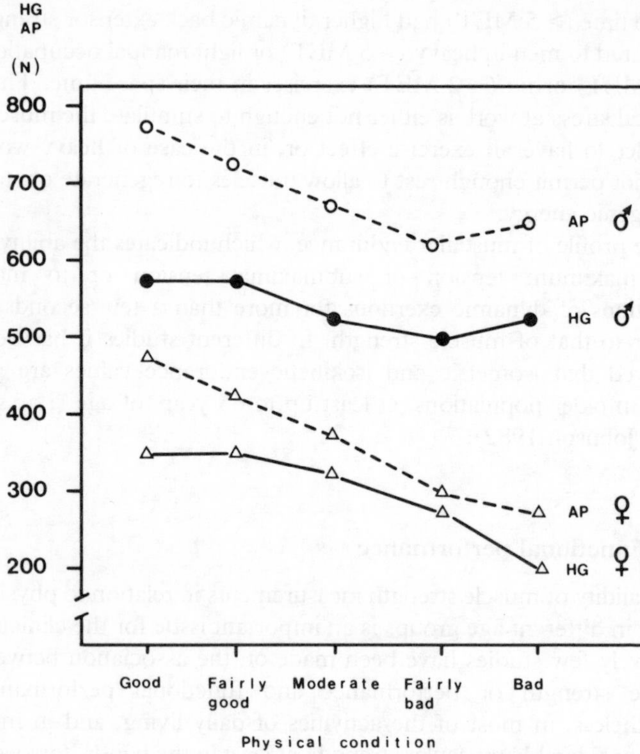

Fig. 8.2 Hand grip (HG) (n = 898) and isometric arm press (AP) (n = 601) strength in relation to self-estimated physical condition.

ability to accomplish daily tasks. Of the measurements used, the hand grip and abdominal muscle tests gave the best basis for the assessment of perceived physical ability. So muscular strength decreasing with age results in less perceived physical ability.

It seems realistic to suppose that in the future it will be possible to create reference-points for some of the most relevant muscular performance tests in evaluating physical ability in the activities of daily living or in certain job situations in the same way as it is possible to evaluate the aerobic working capacity from aerobic performance tests (e.g. Åstrand 1986, Grimby 1988).

4. RESEARCH ON TRAINING IN THE ELDERLY

The problems addressed by research on strength training can be summarized as follows:

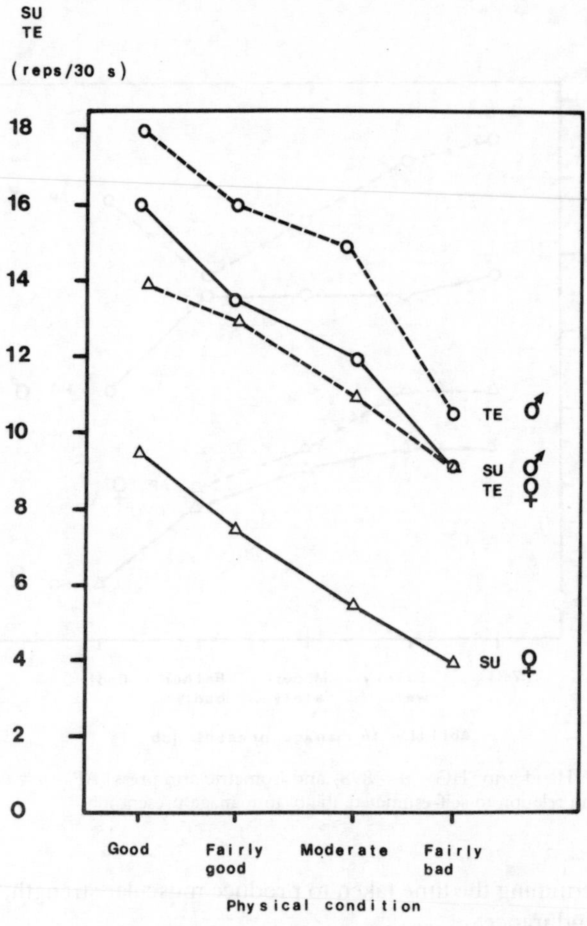

Fig. 8.3 Number of sit-ups (SU) ($n = 642$) and trunk extensions (TE) ($n = 638$) from 50° forward leaning position during 30 seconds, respectively, in relation to self-estimated physical condition.

— how to train 'strength' in different 'cells' — fast twitch and slow twitch fibres, connective tissue, the vascular bed, neurogenic components
— how to train energy sources and substrates
— how to choose speed, duration and resistance in movement in different strength training modalities
— the determination of the association between strength, power and endurance

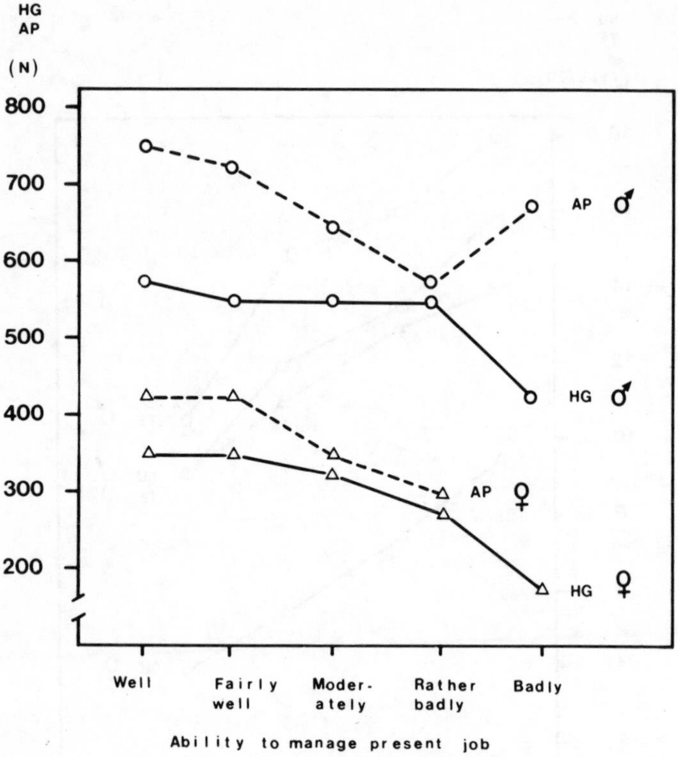

Fig. 8.4 Hand grip (HG) (n = 898) and isometric arm press (AP) (n = 601) strength in relation to self-estimated ability to manage present job.

— determining the time taken to produce muscular strength, power or endurance
— determining the effect of the duration of training
— the meaning (if any) of strength training for working capacity or for functional performance
— the possibilities of strength training in treating various disorders
— the possibilities of strength training at different ages
— the risks involved in strength training
— whether strength training is essentially biology, education or both.

There is now sufficient evidence from both animal and human studies to demonstrate the existence of a potential for the conversion of one fibre type to another (Kovanen 1989). Most studies have been based on training of a predominantly endurance character.

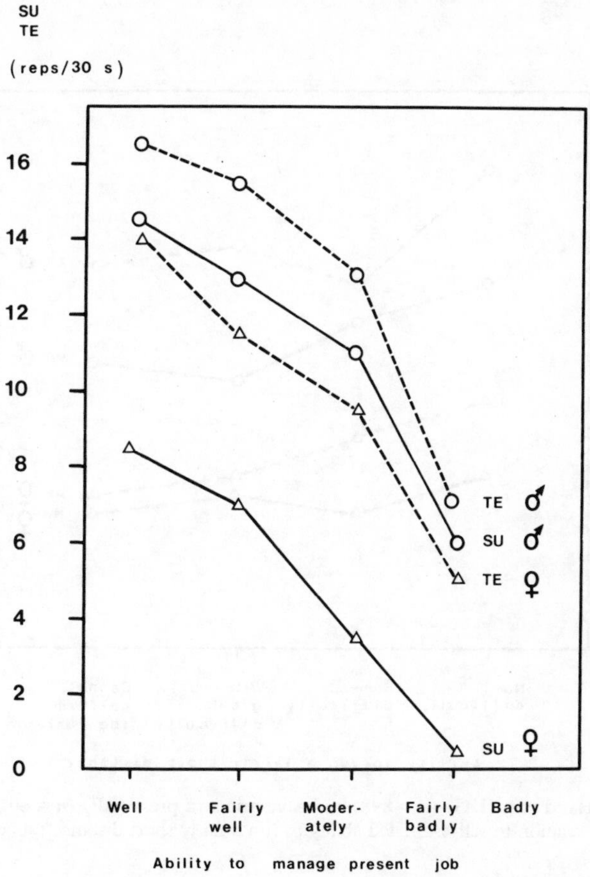

Fig. 8.5 Number of sit-ups (SU) (n = 642) and trunk extensions (TE) (n = 638) from 50° forward leaning position during 30 seconds, respectively, in relation to self-estimated ability to manage present job.

Nonetheless, all forms of training involve both endurance and explosive aspects, which are sometimes difficult to separate. Only in animal studies has it been possible to study the effects of life span physical training. These studies show that in endurance training, even at quite low intensities, transformations from fast to slow and from IIB to IIA fibre types take place (Green et al 1984, Kovanen 1989). In animal studies there is evidence for the increased utilization of substrates for oxidation by muscles after exercise or stimulation programmes which effects better fatigue resistant muscles (see Salmons & Henrikson 1981 in review). The capillary

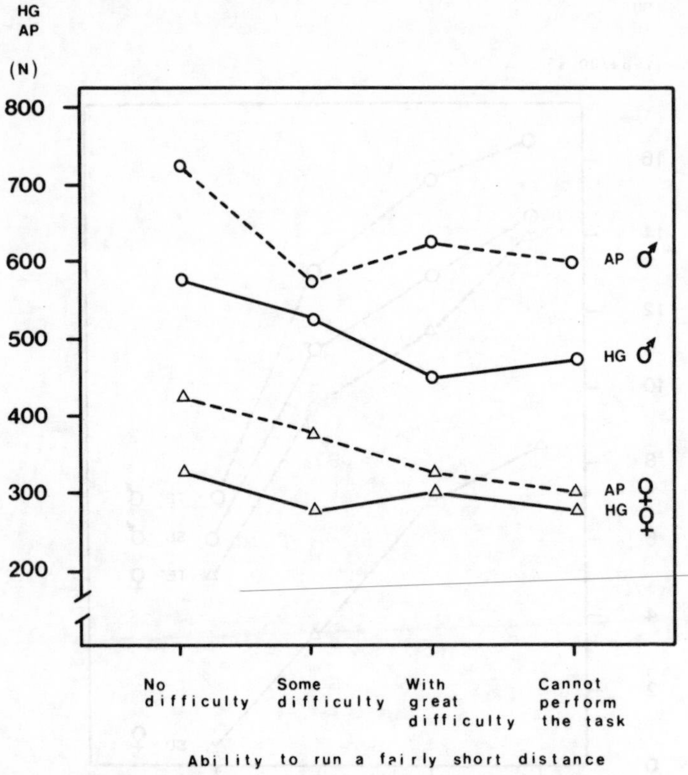

Fig. 8.6 Hand grip (HG) (n = 898) and isometric arm press (AP) (n = 601) strength in relation to self-estimated ability to run a fairly short distance (about 100 m).

density of skeletal muscle has also been shown to increase in response to endurance training (Salmons & Henrikson 1981). According to Kovanen (1989), collagen properties in muscles do not counteract the age-related changes after a life-long programme of endurance training. There is a paucity of studies of strength training in animals, nonetheless it seems to be the case that life-long training in rodents, even at relatively low intensity, helps these animals to increase fatigue tolerance. However, at the same time, training has effects which accelerate slowness and stiffness.

In humans, a number of studies have shown that, in training, the elderly muscle structure develops a maintained adaptability (Grimby 1988). There is also evidence of an increase in muscle strength, which can be similar to that observed in young individuals

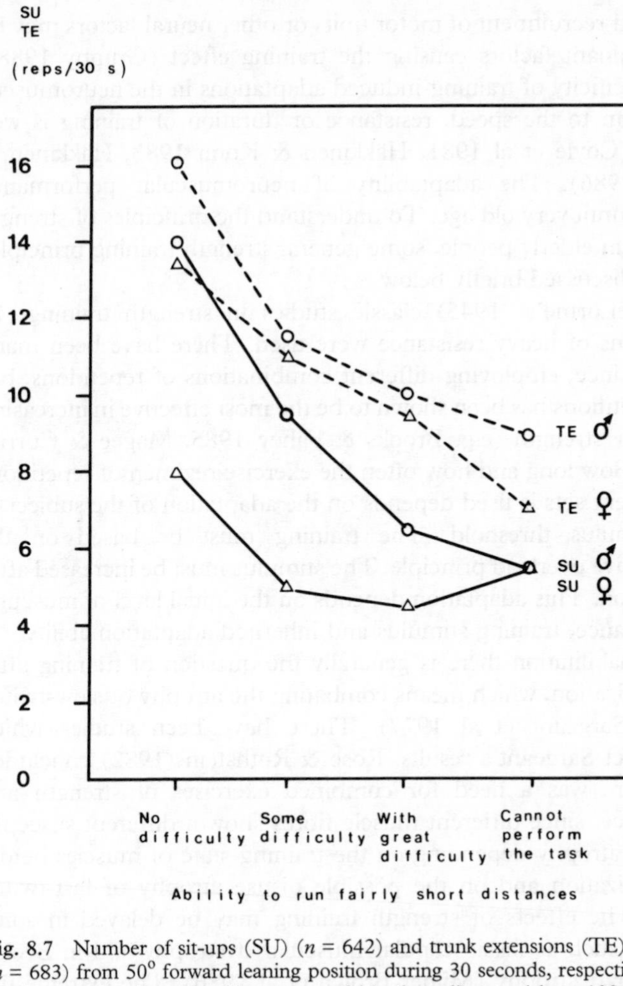

Fig. 8.7 Number of sit-ups (SU) ($n = 642$) and trunk extensions (TE) ($n = 683$) from 50° forward leaning position during 30 seconds, respectively, in relation to self-estimated ability to run a fairly short distance (about 100 m).

(Aniansson et al 1984, Vandervoot et al 1986). Life-long physical activity, of either endurance or power types, also influences the specificity of muscle function. Thus, power athletes at a mean age of about 50 years, who still trained, had higher hand grip and isometric trunk flexor strength values than either controls or endurance trained groups (Suominen et al 1989). Both endurance and power athletes seem to have better muscle quality after 30–70 years training than untrained athletes (Sipilä & Suominen 1991). Apart from muscle quality changes, most researchers agree that an increased recruitment of motor units or other neural factors may be the dominant factors causing the training effect (Grimby 1988). The specificity of training-induced adaptations in the neuromuscular system to the speed, resistance or duration of training is well known (Coyle et al 1981, Häkkinen & Komi 1983, Häkkinen & Komi 1986). The adaptability of neuromuscular performance persists until very old age. To understand the principles of strength training in elderly people, some general strength training principles will be discussed briefly below.

In DeLorme's (1945) classic studies in strength training, 10 repetitions of heavy resistance were used. There have been many studies since, employing different combinations of repetitions, but 4–8 repetitions has been shown to be the most effective in increasing muscular strength (e.g. Brooks & Fahey 1985, Magee & Currier 1986). How long and how often the exercise regimen of repetitions in different sets is used depends on the adaptation of the subject to the stimulus threshold. The training must be based on the progressive overload principle. The stimulus must be increased after adaptation. This adaptation depends on the initial level of muscular performance, training stimulus and inherited adaptation ability.

In rehabilitation there is generally the question of training after immobilization, which means combating the atrophy of slow-twitch fibres (Sargeant et al 1977). There have been studies which contradict Sargeant's results. Rose & Rothstein (1982) concluded that there was a need for combined exercises of strength and endurance, since different muscle fibres show a different susceptibility to atrophy depending on the training state of muscles before immobilization and on the possible disuse atrophy of fast-twitch fibres. The effects of strength training may be delayed in some diseases such as fascioscapular muscular dystrophy and in Becker muscular dystrophy (Milner-Brown et al 1986). The extreme use of the remaining muscle fibres in post-polio subjects can also have a training-like influence (Grimby et al 1989).

The specific use of muscular strength exercises in different diseases has not been evaluated in many studies. Except for cardiovascular risks and acute pain, there are few situations in which muscular exercise has been stated to be contraindicated. Heavy muscular exercises have been evaluated to be contraindicated in the case of muscular dystrophies (Schmalbruch 1989) and, in particular, Duchenne muscular dystrophy, but even here not all researchers agree (Bar-Or 1983). Exercise stress can also be adapted to the purpose of training and to the response of the client (Andersen et al 1989).

In training muscular performance the use of high-tension, low-repetition exercises or isometric contractions might be needed. Exercises of this kind result in increased systemic arterial blood pressure. This increases the work of the heart. Muscular exercises are often performed using the Valsalva manoeuvre, which causes a reduction in venous return and results in decreased blood flow to the heart and brain. High risk people should be encouraged to carry out dynamic low-weight exercises and training without breath-holding. Special attention should also be paid to sufficient warm-up and cool down, correct structural and functional body positions for lifting and the rhythmic performance of necessary movements (American College of Sport Medicine 1991; see also exact contraindications). In the case of rheumatics and arthritis, it is not possible to use weight bearing activities during active inflammation. To minimize risks the candidates for muscular performance training should be evaluated medically, certainly after the age of 40–45 years or even before, if they are at higher risk through, e.g. a history of high blood pressure, elevated cholesterol, cigarette smoking, abnormal ECG, risk factors in family history, diabetes mellitus, etc. (American College of Sport Medicine 1991). Medical evaluation should include a proper medical examination and laboratory tests, including exercise testing.

5. CLINICAL GUIDELINES FOR STRENGTH TRAINING OF ELDERLY PATIENTS

The effect of strength training can be adjusted by varying the speed, duration and resistance of different movements. This is possible by using strength training devices or by simple gymnastics. Training can be very simple. It is a question of teaching the right biomechanical movements to enable the client to carry out the correct motor activities according to load. Hence, the effect of loading exercises may be due to biological changes or to motor learning or to both. The question is how to choose exercises with 'optimal' benefit to the client or patient.

We know that exercise has a positive effect on people in old age and on those suffering from certain diseases or disorders. To induce an effect at the level of fast-twitch fibres we need to choose loads of high resistance for which a few repetitions only are enough. For slow-twitch fibres, a fairly low intensity with many repetitions is sufficient. We should combine high and low intensity training in order to achieve the most practical benefit in respect of the activities of daily living and work and to fight against the slowing effects of aging in modern societies. In exercise, the speed and acceleration of movements should also be trained on account of the importance of agility and the ability to maintain balance in avoiding accidents or incorrect loading of the kinetic chain. Obtaining the biological benefits and achieving correct motor learning from muscular exercise may involve negative effects on muscle connective tissue and in the joints, which lead to stiffness, in addition to the positive effects on the bones, cartilage, ligaments and tendons, which lead to increased tolerance of loading. Stretching and allied exercises are then necessary to avoid the disadvantages of exercise.

In aging and to counteract the effects of inactivity or bed rest, the training of the lower extremities and trunk muscles should be emphasized. Because there is a logarithmic relationship between increase in performance and risks of musculoskeletal or cardiovascular complications, the optimum exercise regimen should be chosen according to individual exercise abilities and motivation. At an exercise level of 75% VO_2max, optimal exercise frequency is 3–4 times a week lasting 20–30 minutes each. Exercise beyond 80% VO_2max rapidly increases the risks of cardiovascular complications (Vuori 1988).

Exercise has the greatest importance to everyday life in relation to aging, most diseases and positive health. The effects of exercise originate in biological processes, and can result in gains in functional abilities by maintaning sufficient strength to avoid the effects of impairment, and by learning effective patterns of activities of daily living and work, such as lifting or handling heavy objects, to avoid disability. Exercise also can provide an increase in social contacts and self esteem via better physical ability.

Choosing the right training regimen for older or sick people demands skill and experience. As well as questions of the training biomechanism involved or of the muscle groups to be trained, there is in addition the question of choosing the type and duration of training. Figure 8.8 summarizes the effects of strength training according to type of adaptation (modified from Frontera 1989, Komi 1990). Old untrained people can achieve faster gains in strength in the beginning of the training period than young untrained people. The optimal adaptation to strength training takes up to several months. The stimulus in strength must ensure the full

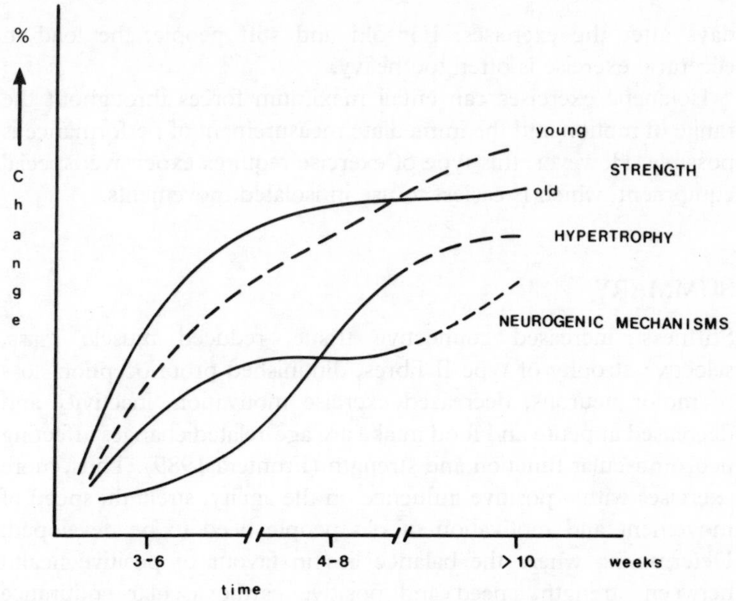

Fig. 8.8 Model of time course for changes in muscular performance from strength training in old and young people.

activation of all motor units. With this objective in mind, a descending pyramid strength training method has been used. This requires starting from one maximum RM and then descending to lighter loads using one or more RMs.

Different kinds of strength training have their own advantages and disadvantages. The specifity of the training should be kept in mind. People always do better on the type of task for which they have been trained (Delateur 1972).

Isometric exercises are easy to arrange, but they produce gains in strength mainly in the trained angles of the limbs. Besides, the training is not dynamic, unlike many situations in daily life. Isometric exercises may also create a high risk to the cardiovascular system.

Isotonic concentric exercises are flexible in programme designs and natural physiological movements can be used. The force production is not maximal throughout the range of motion. Risk factors depend on the load.

Eccentric exercises require high forces at low metabolic cost, but muscle soreness and weakness can be quite severe a few hours or days after the exercises. For old and stiff people, the load in eccentric exercise is often too heavy.

Isokinetic exercises can entail maximum forces throughout the range of motion and the immediate measurement of performance is possible. However, this type of exercise requires expensive, special equipment, which is easiest to use in isolated movements.

SUMMARY

Stiffness, increased connective tissue, reduced muscle mass, selective atrophy of type II fibres, diminished proprioception, loss of motor neurons, decreased exercise motivation, inactivity and decreased appetite and food intake are age-related changes affecting neuromuscular function and strength (Frontera 1989). Thus, more exercises with a positive influence on the agility, strength, speed of movement and motivation of old people need to be developed. Determining where the balance lies in favour of positive health between strength, speed and positive cardiovascular endurance training is a question of problem setting.

One of the most important challenges in the clinical use of exercise is to design appropriate programmes for preventing the effects of inactivity and for the promotion of health via physical activities. Studies in animals and humans of the effects of combined endurance, sprint and strength training throughout the whole life span provide considerable help in answering these questions.

REFERENCES

American College of Sports Medicine 1991 Guidelines for exercise testing and prescription. Lea & Febiger, Philadelphia

Andersen R, Mälkiä E, Fynbo Steffensen B 1989 Muskeldystrofi og traening — gavn eller skade. Ugeskr Laeger 151/123, Videnskab og praksis, 1483–1484

Aniansson A, Ljungberg P, Rundgren Å, Wetterqvist H 1984 Effects of a training programme for pensioners on condition and muscular strength. Archives of Gerontology & Geriatrics 3: 229–241

Ariel Tech Equipment (1990) Normative tables. LIFE Health and Fitness Center, State Highway 35S, Ocean Township, N J 07712

Aromaa A et al 1990 Health, functional limitations and need for care in Finland. Basic results from the mini-Finland health survey (in Finnish, English summary). Publications of the Social Insurance Institution, AL: 32, Finland

Asmussen E, Hansen O, Lammert D 1965 The relation between isometric and dynamic muscle strength in men. Communications from the Testing and Observation Institute of the Danish National Association for Infantile Paralysis, Nr 20. Hellerup, Denmark

Asmussen E, Heeboll-Nielsen K 1962 Isometric muscle strength in relation to age in men and women. Ergonomics 5: 167–169

Åstrand P O, Rodahl K 1986 Textbook of work physiology. McGraw-Hill, New York

Bar-Or O 1983 Pediatric sports medicine. Springer Verlag, New York

Beals C A, Lampman R A, Banwell B F, Brannstein E M, Albers J W et al 1985 Measurement of exercise tolerance in patients with rheumatoid arthritis and osteoarthritis. Journal of Rheumatology 12: 458–461

Bishop P, Cureton K, Collins M 1987 Sex difference in muscular strength in equally trained men and women. Ergonomics 30(4): 675–687

Brooke M H 1986 A clinician's view of neuromuscular diseases. Williams & Wilkins, Baltimore

Brooks G A, Fahey T D 1985 Exercise physiology. Macmillan Publishing Company, New York

Bouchard C 1978 Genetics, growth and physical activity. In: Landry F, Orban W A R (eds) Physical activity and human well-being. Symposia Specialists, Miami

Bouchard C, Simoneau J A, Lortie G, Boulay M R, Marcotte M, Tibault M C 1986 Genetic effects in human skeletal muscle fibre type distribution and enzyme activities. Canadian Journal of Physiology and Pharmacology 64: 1245–1251

Carlsson C 1967 Muskelkraft hos kroniska alkoholister. Nordisk Medicin 77(1): 17–19

Coyle E, Feiring C, Rotkis T, Cote R, Roby F, Lee W, Wilmore J 1981 Specificity of power improvements through slow and fast isokinetic training. Journal of Applied Physiology: Respirat. Environ. Exercise Physiology 51: 1437–1442

Delatour B, Lehmann J, Stonebridge J, Warren C 1972 Isotonic versus isometric exercise: double shift transfer of training study. Archives of Physical Medicine and Rehabilitation 53: 212–217

Delorme T L 1945 Restoration of muscle power by heavy-resistance exercise. Journal of Bone Surgery 26: 645–667

Edington D W, Edgerton V R 1976 The biology of physical activity. Houghton Mifflin Company, Boston

Edwards R H T 1981 Human muscle function and fatigue. In: Human muscle fatigue: physiological mechanisms. Ciba Foundation Symposium 82. Pitman Medical Publications, London, p 1–18

Era P, Lyyra A-L, Viitasalo J T, Heikkinen E 1992 Determinants of isometric muscle strength in men of different ages. European Journal of Applied Physiology 64: 84–91

Friman G 1977 Effect of acute infectious disease on isometric muscle strength. Scandinavian Journal of Clinical Laboratory Investigation 37: 303–308

Frontera W R 1989 Strength training in the elderly. In: Harris R, Harris S (eds) Physical activity, aging and sports. CSA-Albany, p 319–331

Gehlsen G M, Grigsby S A, Winant D M 1984 Effects of an aquatic fitness program on the muscular strength and endurance of patients with muscular multiple-sclerosis. Physical Therapy 64: 653–657

Green H J, Klug G A, Reichmann H, Seedorf U, Wiehrer W, Pette D 1984 Exercise-induced fibre type transitions with regard to myosin, parvalbumin, and sarcoplasmic reticulum in muscles of the rat. Pflügers Arch. 400: 432–438

Grimby G 1988 Physical activity and effects of muscle training in the elderly. Annals of Clinical Research 20: 62–66

Grimby G, Saltin B 1983 The aging muscle. Clinicial Physiology 3: 209–218

Grimby G, Einarsson G, Hedberg M, Aniansson A 1989 Muscle adaptive changes in post-polio subjects. Scandinavian Journal of Rehabilitation Medicine 21(1): 19–26

Heikkinen E, Arajärvi R-L, Era P, et al 1984 Functional capacity of men born in 1906–10, 1923–30 and 1946–50. Scandinavian Journal of Social Medicine, Suppl. 33

Häkkinen K, Komi P V 1983 Electromyographic changes during strength training and detraining. Medical Science of Sport and Exercise 15: 455–460
Häkkinen K, Komi P V 1986 Training-induced changes in neuromuscular performance under voluntary and reflex conditions. European Journal of Applied Physiology 55: 147–155
Ikai M, Fukunaga T 1968 Calculation of muscle strength per unit cross-sectional area of human muscle by means of ultrasonic measurement. Int. Z angew Physiol. einschl. Arbeitsphysiol 26: 26–32
Jansma P, Decker J, Ersing W, McCubbin J, Combs S 1988 A fitness assessment system for individuals with severe mental retardation. APAQ 5: 223–232
Johnson T 1982 Age related differences in isometric and dynamic strength and endurance. Physical Therapy 62: 985–989
Knapik J J, Ramos M V 1980 Isokinetic and isometric torque relationships in the human body. Archives of Physical Medicine and Rehabilitation. 61: 64–67
Knortz K A 1987 Muscle physiology applied to geriatric rehabilitation. Topics in Geriatric Rehabilitation 2(4): 1–11
Komi P 1990 Strength and power training: current issues and mechanism concepts. Paper in World Congress on Sport For All. Tampere
Kovanen V 1989 Effects of aging and physical training on rat skeletal muscle. Acta Physiologica Scandinavica 135, Suppl. 577
Kugelberg E 1976 Adaptive transformation of rat soleus motor units during growth. Journal of Neurological Science 27: 269–289
Komi P V, Viitasalo J T, Havu M, Thorstensson A, Sjödin B, Karlsson J 1977 Skeletal muscle fibres and muscle enzyme activities in monozygous and dizygous twins of both sexes. Acta Physiologica Scandinavica 100: 385–392
Lahtinen U 1986 Begåvningshandikappad ungdom i utveckling. En uppföljningsstudie av funktionsförmåga och fysisk aktivitet hos begåvningshandikappade ungdomar i olika livsmiljöer. Studies in Sport, Physical Education and Health 21. University of Jyväskylä, Jyväskylä
Larsson L 1982 Morphological and functional characteristics of the aging skeletal muscle in man. Acta Physiological Scandinavica, Suppl. 457
Larsson L 1982 Aging in mammalian skeletal muscle. In: Mortimer J A, Pirozzolo F J, Maletta G J (eds) Advances in neurogerontology, vol 3. The aging motor system. Praeger Publishers, New York, p 60–95
Larsson L, Sjodin B, Karlsson 1978 Histochemical and biochemical changes in human skeleton muscle with age in sedentary males age 22–65 years. Acta Physiologica Scandinavica 103: 31–39
Laubach L L 1976 Comparative muscular strength of men and women: a review of the literature. Aviation, Space and Environmental Medicine 47: 534–542
Mayee D J, Courier D P 1986 Effect of number of repetitions on isokinetic knee strength. Physiotherapy Canada 38:6: 377–392
Mathiowetz M S, Kashman N, Volland G, Weber K, Dowe M, Rogers S, 1985 Grip and pinch strength: normative data for adults. Archives of Physical Medicine and Rehabilitation. 66: 69–72
Milner-Brown H S, Mellenthin M, Miller M D 1986 Quantifying human muscle strength, endurance and fatigue. Archives of Physical Medicine and Rehabilitation 67: 530–535
Monod H 1972 How muscle are used in the body. In: Bourne G H (ed) The structure and function of muscle. Academic Press, New York, p 23–74
Mälkiä E 1974 The influence of age and physical performance on strain of the worker in making timber (in Finnish, English summary). Publications of Work Efficiency Association, no.173. Forssan kirjapaino, Helsinki
Mälkiä E 1983 Muscular performance as a determinant of physical ability in Finnish adult population (in Finnish, English summary). Publications of the Social Insurance Institution, AL: 23, Finland

Mälkiä E 1990 Physical activity of Finnish adults, studied according to age, sex, and place of residence. In: Doll-Tepper G, Dahms C, Doll B, von Seleam H (eds) Adapted Physical Activity, Springer-Verlag, Berlin, p 53–58

Mälkiä E, Impivaara O, Maatela J, Aromaa A, Heliövaara M, Knekt P 1988 Physical activity of Finnish adults (in Finnish, English summary). Publications of the Social Insurance Institution, ML:80, Finland

Mälkiä E, Rintala P, Nevala N, Rintala T 1987 Project for developing P E and sport for children with handicaps and chronic ailments. In: Jones D E, Cuddihy T (eds) Progress through refinement and innovation. IFAPA, Brisbane, p 11–16

Nachemson A L 1989 Exercise, fitness and back pain. In: Kvist M (ed) Paavo Nurmi Congress Book. The Finnish Society of Sports Medicine, Helsinki, p 136–145

Nygård C-H, Luopajärvi T, Ilmarinen J 1988 Musculoskeletal capacity of middle-aged women and men in physical, mental and mixed ocupations. European Journal of Applied Physiology 57: 181–188

Pette D, Vrbova G 1985 Invited review. Neural control of phenotypic expression in mammalian muscle fibres. Muscle & Nerve 8: 676–689

Pheasant S T 1983 Sex differences in strength — some observations on their variability. Applied Ergonomics 14(3): 205–211

Rikli R, Busch S 1986 Motor performance of women as a function of age and physical activity level. Journal of Gerontology 41: 645–649

Rose S J, Rothstein J M 1982 Muscle mutability. Physical Therapy 62(12): 1773–1787

Salmons S, Henriksson J 1981 The adaptive response of skeletal muscle to increased use. Muscle & Nerve 4: 94–105

Sargeant A J, Davies C T M, Edwards R H T et al 1977 Functional and structural changes after disuse of human muscle. Clinical Science and Molecular Medicine 52: 337–342

Schersten T 1977 Fysisk träning vid perifer arteriell insufficiens. Läkartidningen 74(44): 3897–3900

Schmalbruch H 1989 Muskeldystrofi og traening — gavn eller skade? Ugeskr Laeger 151/3: 179–180

Shephard R J 1977 Endurance fitness, 2nd edn. University of Toronto Press, Toronto

Shephard R J 1980 Population aspects of human working capacity. Annals of Human Biology 7(1): 1–28

Shock N W, Norris A H 1970 Neuromuscular coordination as a factor in age changes in muscular exercise. In: Brunner D, Jokl E (eds) Physical activity and aging. S. Karger, Basel, p 92–99

Sipilä S, Suominen H 1991 Ultrasound imaging of the quadriceps muscle in elderly athletes and untrained men. Muscle & Nerve 14: 527–533

Skinner J S, Tipton C M, Vailas A L 1982 Exercise, physical training and the aging process. In: Viidik A (ed) Lectures in gerontology, vol. I: on biology of aging. Part B, Academic Press, London, p 407–439

Staron R S, Pette D 1987 The multiplicity of combinations of myosin light chains and heavy chains in histochemically typed single fibres. Biochemistry Journal 243: 695–699

Suominen H, Rahkila P, Era P, Jaakkola L Heikkinen E 1989 Functional capacity in middle-aged male endurance and power athletes. In: Harris R, Harris S (eds) physical activity, aging and sports. Center for the Study of Aging, Albany, New York, p 213–218

Thomason D B, Baldwin K M, Herrick R E 1986 Myosin isozyme distribution in rodent hind limb skeletal muscle. Journal of Applied Physiology 60: 1923–1931

Tiselius P 1969 Studies on joint temperature, joint stiffness and muscle weakness in rheumatoid arthritis. Acta Rheumatologica Scndinavica, Suppl. 14

Vandervoot A A, Hayes K C, Belanger A Y 1986 Strength and endurance of skeletal muscle in the elderly. Physiotherapy Canada 38(3): 167–173
Viitasalo J T, Era P, Leskinen A-L, Heikkinen E 1985 Muscular strength profiles and anthropometry in random samples of men aged 31–35, 51–55 and 71–75 years. Ergonomics 28(11): 1563–1574
Vuori I 1988 Exercise prescription in medical practice. Annals of Clinical Research 20: 84–93
Wheeler S 1982 Pathology of muscle and motor units. Physical Therapy 62(12): 1809–1821
Young A 1986 Exercise physiology in geriatric practice. Acta Medica Scandinavica 711: 227–232

9. Evaluation and improvement of strength in competitive athletes

Birgitta Öberg

INTRODUCTION

Strength is a complex quality which can be measured and defined in many ways. Our knowledge about strength in relation to demands in sports and work is determined by the way we are able to measure and quantify strength and load. In this chapter I will try to highlight the research concerning muscle strength that has been reported in the field of sports medicine. Many aspects of muscle strength are not yet fully understood and the content of rehabilitation programmes and preventive programmes need to be developed. When discussing different goals for rehabilitation, the demands for different situations must be taken into consideration. It is obvious that different sports and different levels of performance put different demands on the athlete. The development of this field is a great challenge to physiotherapy (Fig. 9.1).

VARIATION IN STRENGTH AMONG ATHLETES IN DIFFERENT SPORTS

Strength in relation to sports activity has often been discussed and authors have stated that stronger athletes are better performers and have fewer injuries (Hage 1981). Different sports place different demands on the athletes and muscular capacity varies between categories of athletes. When male soccer players, cyclists, long distance runners and sprinters were compared with non active males in the same age groups with respect to thigh muscle strength, it was shown that the soccer players, sprinters and cyclists were stronger compared to the non active, and that the long distance runner was weaker (Ekstrand & Gillquist 1983, Öberg et al 1984a) (Fig. 9.2).

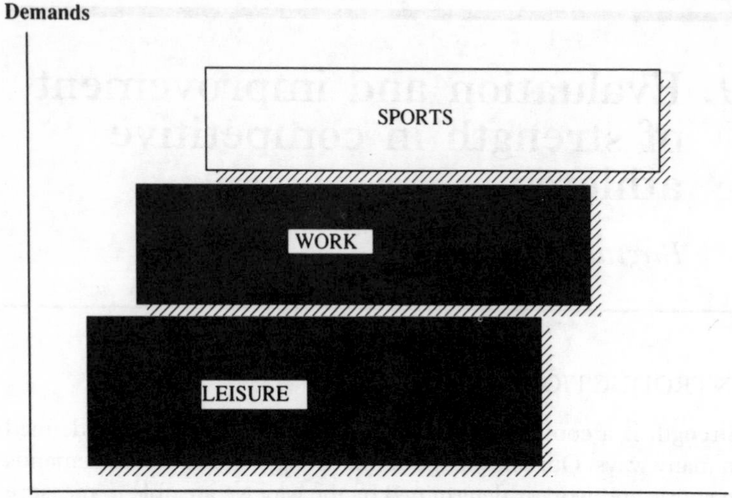

Fig. 9.1 Different levels of demands in leisure, work and sports.

Others have shown that alpine skiers are stronger compared to cross country and nordic combined skiers (Haymes & Dickinson 1980). Alpine skiers have been shown to be stronger in isometric strength while sprinters were stronger in dynamic strength (Thorstensson et al 1977).

For the soccer player, it has been shown that the higher the standard of soccer, the higher the muscle strength of the players. The player position has also been shown to influence differences between individuals. Goalkeepers and defenders were stronger compared to midfielders and forwards (Öberg et al 1984b). Coleman (1982) reported differences in knee flexor strength in baseball players at different positions and Gilliam et al (1979) found differences in knee flexor strength at slow speeds in linemen and backs in American high school football players. The results may reflect different training schedules; in soccer, the training for goal-keepers includes a lot of vertical jumping performance which might influence the thigh muscle strength more than ordinary soccer training.

Whether strength variations within different sports result from training effects, or whether they reflect a selection of athlete types

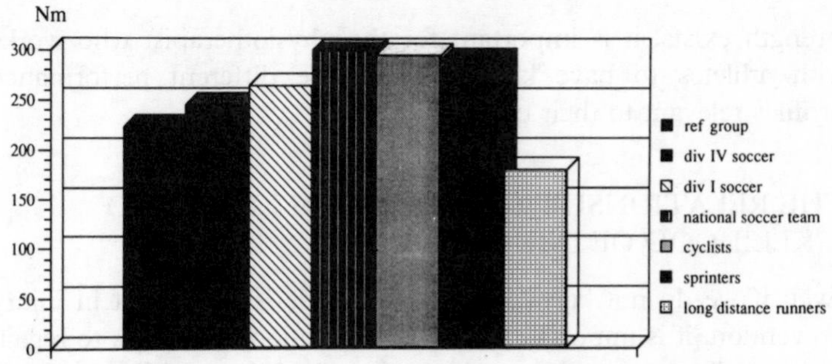

Fig. 9.2 Strength in the quadriceps tested at 30°/s in male athletes (soccer players, cyclists, sprinters, long distance runners) and non active men.

by certain sports, is not fully understood; however it is known to be easier to change from a fast to a slow capacity than vice versa.

In higher division soccer players it was found that the strength of the knee extensors and flexors at low speed was higher than normal, but the knee extensors of the non trained were stronger compared to lower division soccer players. The players from the national team showed, in addition, good muscle strength at high velocities. The differences were true even when body weight was taken into account (Öberg et al 1984a).

When testing strength at different angular velocities, the torque velocity ratio can be described. This ratio varies between muscle groups as well as between athletes. It was found that lower level soccer players had a lower fast/slow speed ratio for the knee extensors and plantar flexors. The players from the national team showed higher or the same ratios as the reference values, indicating that fast speed strength might be important in advanced levels of soccer. It is also known that the fast/slow speed ratio is higher in sprinters compared to long distance runners. It seems that high strength at high speeds is important for some sport activities, but not so important in those activities where the emphasis is on endurance.

One can conclude that both the type of sport, the level of performance and, in team sports, the player position can influence the results of isolated muscle strength testing. Since this variation of strength exists, it is important for the physiotherapist who works with athletes to have knowledge of the different performance profiles relevant to their clients.

THE RELATIONSHIP OF STRENGTH LEVELS TO LIKELIHOOD OF INJURY

Even if we do not know if strength per se is significant in injury prevention, it is important in the rehabilitation of athletes to regain near or full capacity of strength. As described above, different sports seem to put different demands on the individual and these demands are of a higher order than non-sporting requirements. Many reports show deficits remaining after injuries due to poor or no rehabilitation (Nicholas et al 1980, Noyes et al 1983, Tropp 1985) and if athletes are not fully rehabilitated there is a great risk of a reinjury that might be more severe than the original (Ekstrand & Gillquist 1982). The soccer players that had the greatest discrepancies in strength in the thigh muscle showed higher rates of reinjury than those with no muscle weakness.

For non contact soccer injuries, it was shown that muscle weakness was a risk factor and it was often caused by inadequate rehabiliation of previous injuries. In other injuries where contact and great force is involved, injury patterns that do not correlate with strength are present. There are some indications that in contact injuries the athlete who attacks is the one that will get injured more often. Some authors (Stafford & Grana 1984) have suggested that an abnormal strength relation in the hamstrings and quadriceps might lead to an increased risk of knee injuries, and therefore this would be important to consider when setting up rehabilitation goals.

Ankle injuries are one of the most usual injuries in teamsports and athletes often suffer from residual functional instability. For soccer players, it was shown that the players that suffered from many ankle injuries also had bad postural control as well as low strength in the ankle dorsiflexors and ankle pronators (Tropp et al 1985). Tropp showed that training of postural control, with daily exercises on a tilting board during 10 weeks for the players with functional instability, increased the strength in the ankle dorsiflexors as well as the pronators. Rehabilitation with the aid of a tilting board also influenced the postural control and the athletes suffered from fewer reinjuries after the training (Tropp & Askling 1988).

It has been suggested that previous injuries influence the mechanoreceptors in the ankle joint and therefore the individuals can not fully activate the muscles and, as a consequence of this, they are not able to stabilize the posture during standing. In strength testing of injured soccer players, the result was low muscle strength in the ankle dorsiflexors and pronators. The performance was improved by training of postural control. This shows that training on a tilting board, which is one way to improve the coordination of the muscles, will influence maximal isolated muscle strength. This highlights the importance of testing both functional movements and isolated muscle strength and the regime should be added to the isolated strength testing programme.

Coordination of muscle groups has also been shown to be important for shoulder injuries. It seems that without proper rehabilitation, an inhibition of activity in certain muscle groups remains. This appears to persist even after the acute, painful phase of injury. In sports, as well as in studies on the spine, it has been reported that when an individual is fatigued during performance the effect is a decrease in motor control (Asmussen 1979, Bates et al 1977). Many injuries occur when the athelete is fatigued, e.g. towards the end of a game in soccer or other team sports, therefore more knowledge about muscle endurance and injuries is needed.

STRENGTH IMPROVEMENT AS A COMPONENT OF REHABILITATION FOR INJURED ATHLETES

Implications of basic research for the design of exercise programmes

The specificity of training has been discussed and it has been shown that different training models give different training results with respect to the torque velocity ratio in separate muscle groups. The inclusion of trampoline exercises in soccer training increased strength at all velocities in the plantar flexors except for isometric and slow speed testing, whereas regular soccer training alone influenced the slow speed capability only (Öberg et al 1984b). Similar results have been shown by others. When isometric training is used, it has also been shown that the training effect can be angle-specific, which means that the strength improvement is not consistent throughout the whole range of motion (Lindh 1979) This indicates that the strength of different types of contraction can be influenced in different ways by training (Caiozzio et al 1981, Coyle et al 1981, Pipes & Wilmore 1975). To be able to create the proper training programme, exercises must be chosen which take into account the demands of the actual sport. If strength at high speed is important for the athlete, the physiotherapist must know how to create a programme with appropriate training exercises.

The agonist/antagonist ratio in a joint has been discussed mostly in relation to the knee joint. From isometric testing it has been suggested that the ratio should be 60% (Bender et al 1964, Burkett 1970) but when testing in isokinetic concentric contraction, this ratio varies with speed. The ratio between the hamstrings and quadriceps has been reported to be high in sprinters and a higher ratio has been found in soccer players compared to non-players; differences corresponding to player position were also recorded (Öberg 1984b). It would seem important to discuss agonist/antagonist ratios based on results from testing at different speeds. However, differences in testing procedures may produce results that are not due to muscle strength alterations alone.

It is important that the biomechanical adjustment of the testing equipment to the actual joint is performed properly because, if the axis of the measuring system does not coincide with that of the joint, the torque measurements in the agonist and antagonist can be influenced differently. This will affect the agonist/antagonist ratio (Öberg et al 1987). It is also important to take gravitational forces into account. Depending on the test position, the weight of the leg will influence the results. Further, the peak torque varies with angle and this variation is specific to individual muscle groups. Agonists and antagonists are activated at the same time during normal movements and therefore the ratio ought to be expressed as angle specific and not peak torque specific since the former resembles more the relation during normal movements.

The association between strength and injuries is not fully understood, perhaps suggesting that the strength testing models used do not test the parameters of performance that are important for the athletic demands actually being made. Recently, a testing device that can measure eccentric strength has been presented. The strength levels in eccentric contractions are known to be higher compared to concentric contractions. There seem to be differences in some reports between men and women (Colliander & Tesch 1989), but fewer reports have demonstrated differences in different sports. It has also been shown that the differences in vivo and in vitro torque velocity relationships is due to inhibition when testing eccentric contractions with dynamometers (Westing et al 1991). Perhaps the mechanical effect and loading in single joint testing are different during eccentric contractions compared to normal functional movements, when agonist and antagonist are activated together.

In functional movements there is almost always a combination of eccentric and concentric contractions. It has been shown that in jump performance the jump height is higher when a jump is performed with a counter movement jump, i.e. with an eccentric phase preceding the concentric phase (Komi & Bosco 1978). This eccentric phase produces a reservoir of energy that can be used during the execution of the concentric phase. In many other performances, such as throwing and running, the movements include stretch shortening cycles.

Strength testing equipment can be used in a similar way by carrying out combined testing to resemble the stretch shortening cycle. This will give higher torque values during the concentric contraction if it is preceded by an eccentric contraction, compared to a single concentric contraction alone (Svantesson et al 1991). When using only eccentric contraction, the torque output at higher velocities is low. We know that the speed in athletic movements often exceeds the limits for speed measurement in our testing equipment. The combined testing method might therefore be a better indication of 'explosive capability' than testing isolated contractions at high speed.

Setting goals for the level of strength to be achieved before athletes return to competition

The use of strength evaluation of athletes is often suggested. The best way to achieve this profiling is to carry out pre-season testing of different aspects of strength. This can be used as a base line if the athletes are injured during the season, and for detecting greater imbalances at an early stage. Isolated strength testing can be used to detect differences in specific muscle groups in bilateral comparison or sometimes to detect differences in comparison with reference values.

To detect discrepancies in strength bilateral comparison can be used in the thigh and upper shoulder since no (or only small) variations between sides have been reported (Öberg et al 1984a, Moffroid & Whipple 1970). For ankle muscle strength, there *is* a difference — the supporting leg is stronger (Öberg et al 1987, Fugl Meyer 1981) (Fig. 9.3). For hand muscle strength, hand dominance creates a difference.

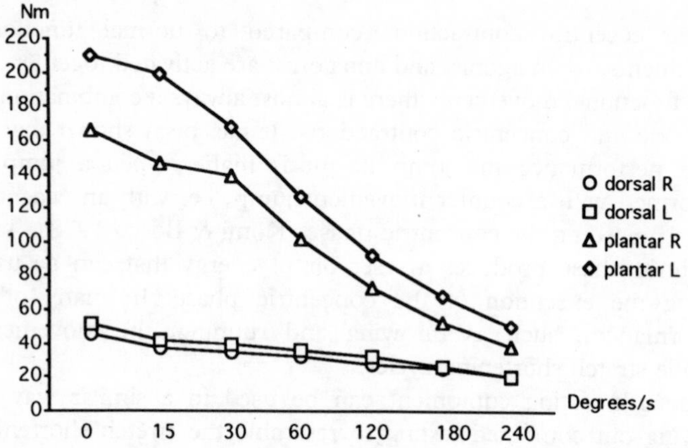

Fig. 9.3 Torque (Nm) tested at different velocities in the ankle dorsiflexors and plantarflexors on left (L) and right (R) sides.

The results from strength testing of athletes clearly demonstrates large variations of strength levels for different muscle groups. The physiotherapist must be aware of these levels when rehabilitation goals are being set up. The athlete loses strength very quickly if the activity level is lowered, as it will be if they are immobilized due to an injury. Therefore, a bilateral comparison might not give appropriate information about the strength level since there is an overall reduction of strength. In this situation, the physiotherapist can use that athlete's reference profile to decide whether the strength is lower than that needed for the sports activity.

In sports, the strength that is needed during a performance is dependent on the actions of many muscles activated in certain patterns, and the output is therefore dependent on the sum of these. To measure strength in a *single* joint and muscle group does not reflect this process and the torque output is probably affected. This is demonstrated by the fact that when carrying out two-leg testing, the torque output in the quadriceps is higher than in one leg testing (Schantz et al 1989). Tests of jump height, throwing and running produce more complex demands on strength, and in sports medicine this is important. Combining isolated muscle testing and functional perfomance will increase the knowledge of how these variables are connected.

Although muscle performance is complex, it is important to point out that standardized testing in functional movements can be of great value in gaining information about strength. Functional performance tested with jumping and running is correlated to the strength level in the thigh muscles. It has been shown that knee injured patients' subjective rating of their functional capability increases if the strength is improved (Tegner et al 1986, Andersson et al 1989). Therefore it is important that the strength is regained before the athletes are permitted to restart sports activities.

In the rehabilitation of knee injuries, the recommended levels in strength measurements to be achieved before resuming sports were suggested to be 80–90% of the value for the quadriceps of the uninjured leg (Tegner et al 1984). At the University Hospital of Linköping, Sweden, all knee patients are tested for strength but this is combined with testing of functional performance. One such test is the testing of a one legged jump, where the length of the jump with the injured leg is compared to that of the uninjured leg. The other test is performed by running in a figure of eight, where the total time, the time taken to turn and the time for straight ahead running are registered (Fig. 9.4). The patient's results are compared with reference values. If the patient is not fully rehabilitated, or if the instability is high, the time to turn is long but the straight ahead running can be normal (Tegner et al 1984).

It has been clearly demonstrated that long rehabilitation periods where the athlete is immobilized gives a fast decrease in strength; it has also been shown that long immobilization makes it harder to resume sports (Ekstrand & Gillquist 1982).

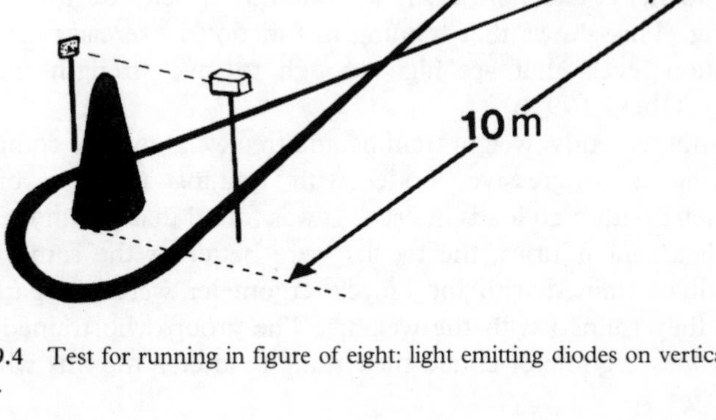

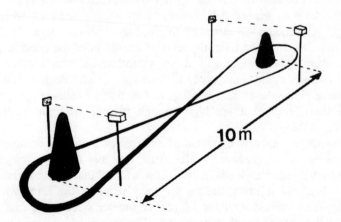

Fig. 9.4 Test for running in figure of eight: light emitting diodes on vertical sticks.

METHODS FOR ACHIEVING HIGH LEVELS OF MUSCLE ACTIVATION WITHOUT RISK OF OVERLOADING LIGAMENTOUS STRUCTURES

When designing rehabilitation programmes, the knowledge about activation of muscles in different situations can be used to create therapies where high activation levels are achieved without risk of overloading the injured structure. This has been important in the rehabilitation of knee ligament injuries. It is possible to use functional training movements that do not overload the ligaments in the early phases of rehabilitation (Arms et al 1984, Öberg 1991a, b, Renstrom et al 1986). This will shorten the rehabilitation period, and it has been shown that this model is important for soccer players. A rehabilitation programme that comprised mainly functional training exercises was tested on soccer players and showed that the players were able to resume soccer early and that the strength level of the injured leg was over 80% of that of the uninjured leg.

The major question for the training of anterior cruciate ligament injuries is how to find exercises with high activation levels in both the hamstrings and quadriceps, to achieve good training effects, but at the same time with low shear forces in the knee joint. Positions where the hamstrings are activated will lower the load on the anterior cruciate ligament. In a study on different training positions for the lower leg, it was found that training in semiflexed positions and with pulley exercises gave high activation levels for the thigh muscles. The activation levels registered with EMG were about 80% of the level in a maximal isometric contraction. Training with a bicycle ergometer was also seen to give high activation levels in the leg muscles. In these tests, the level of activation of the quadriceps was over 100% compared to the test contraction, which indicates that patients could more easily activate the muscles during bicycle training. This shows that training in functional exercises can give activation levels that are high enough to give strength training effects (Öberg 1991b).

In another study, weight training and free weights were compared following a progressive model with training using a bicycle ergometer with high loads interval. It was found that for unoperated knee ligament injuries, the results were better or the same when individuals trained with the bicycle ergometer were compared to when they trained with the weights. The group who trained with the bicycle ergometer ended their training after 2 months whereas the other groups had to continue for 3 months to achieve the same results (Öberg 1991a). These results have led to an increased use of functional training exercises in knee rehabilitation programmes and an example will be presented later in this chapter.

THE IMPORTANCE OF FLEXIBILITY

When discussing performance in sports it is important also to consider flexibility. Flexibility exercises like stretching are nowadays often included in warming up procedures and also after training. Flexibility can be defined as the active range of motion in a joint where the motion is restricted by the capsule, ligaments or the skeleton. In sport activities, the active range of motion is often restricted by the muscles and often by two joint muscles. Therefore when measurements of motion are made it is important to measure in a way that detects muscle stiffness. This must be performed, as in all types of measurements, in a standardized manner with careful positioning of the individual. A testing model for the lower leg, using goniometers, was devised by Ekstrand et al. The legs were placed in positions to detect the restriction of the range of motion that was caused by the muscles alone (Ekstrand et al 1982). To detect abnormalities in a range of motion, bilateral comparison and/or reference values can be used. The use of reference values has the same problem as the use of strength measurements: the variation is wide. In studies on soccer players, the mean value in the reference groups minus 2 standard deviations was used to define muscle stiffness. Soccer players were less supple than the reference group of non-athletes (Moller 1984) and in a study on injuries, there was a tendency towards a higher incidence of over-use injuries.

Many physiotherapists have experienced that athletes who train very intensively also develop muscle stiffness that might have negative influences on performance and also might increase the risk of injuries. In a study of the effect of strenuous muscle work on flexibility, it was shown that strength training and soccer training can give a decrease in range of motion lasting for 2 days after the training ended. The negative effect of strength training and soccer training was reduced if the training was combined with flexibility training. Prospective studies on soccer players showed that if the training schedule in soccer training was combined with stretching exercises, the flexibility of the players could be normalized (Moller 1984, Moller et al 1985).

Stretching exercises as a part of an injury prevention programme have been shown to decrease injuries in soccer (Ekstrand & Gillquist 1983). Therefore it is important that flexibility training is included in athletic training and also in rehabilitation programmes when strength training is performed to avoid development of muscle stiffness.

However it might be important in certain sports to have a certain degree of stiffness to be able to give maximal performance. A group of handball players were tested for strength in the thigh muscles, jump performance and flexibility before and after a set of stretching exercises. The strength, tested with isokinetic techniques, showed a decrease in torque in eccentric contractions and also in jump performance. This tells us that directly after a stretching procedure performance in, for instance, the high jump can be negatively influenced. The solution is to achieve a fine balance: to have a range of motions that do not create higher risk of injury and at the same time influence the performance favourably.

SAMPLE REHABILITATION PROGRAMME FOR PATIENTS WITH ANTERIOR CRUCIATE LIGAMENT INJURIES

In rehabilitation of knee injuries, the model for the programme must be decided in the light of the type of injury and type of operation. A model for the rehabilitation of anterior cruciate ligament injuries reconstructed with a fascia latae strip will be presented here.

The rehabilitation starts early and total immobilization of the knee is avoided. The programme is mostly based on training with loading of the leg in standing positions, and avoiding loading in extended positions, where there is a risk of high shear forces on the anterior cruciate ligament if the quadriceps is activated. The exercises in the different time periods listed below are examples to demonstrate an increasing loading of the knee joint and the leg muscles.

The programme is illustrated in Figure 9.5. Full details are not given here since the number of repetitions must be individualized. Pain, swelling and fatigue are factors that will influence the intensity of training.

Week 1

Directly after the operation, the patient is immobilized but during this period the patient should train with quadriceps contractions.

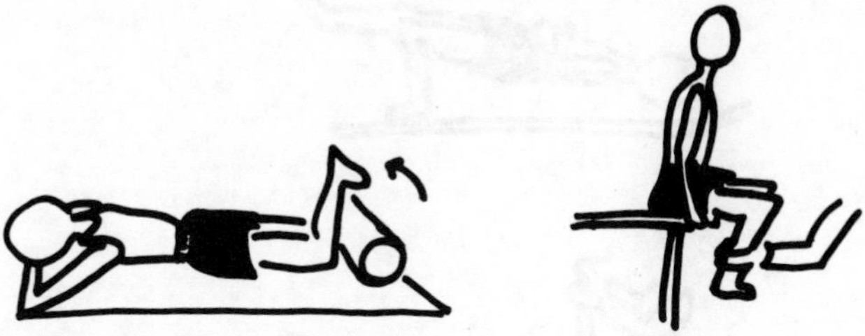

week 5 - 9

Fig. 9.5A–D Some of the exercises in the rehabilitation program for anterior cruciate ligament injuries. Left: active flexion exercises in limited range: Right: flexion exercises with manual resistance.

After approximately 5 days, the leg is stabilized with an orthosis that allows 30–60° of movement. The movements are made passively by the physiotherapist.

Weeks 2–5

The goal during this period is to minimize the inhibition of the muscles after the operation and to prevent any decrease in range of movement. The patient stays at home and attends the physiotherapy department 3 times weekly. Passive training of range of movement throughout 20–90° is undertaken. Weight bearing is not allowed and the patient walks with crutches.

Weeks 5–7

The goal during this period is to achieve a range of movement in flexion and to get coordination to prepare for 50% loading. The patient is allowed to actively flex the leg to 90° in sitting and forward leaning. The patient actively extends to 20° (Fig. 9.5A). The functional training starts in lying positions, with knees flexed, to begin training pelvis lift (Fig. 9.5B).

Weeks 7–8

Ergometer cycle training with low loading is added for the training of range of movement.

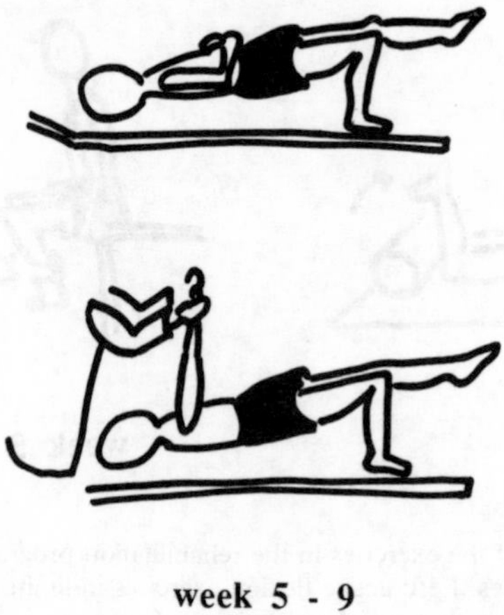

Fig. 9.5B Pelvis lift. Can be performed with loading on one or both legs. Resistance can be applied on the legs or arms by the physiotherapist.

Weeks 9–12

The goal during this period is to achieve a full range of movement and to achieve the strength and coordination to be able to tolerate full loading on the operated leg.

Full range of movement is allowed and the patient walks with one crutch. Functional training exercises are started in standing and stabilization is trained by sitting the patient on a big Bobath ball; the patient tries to maintain position with legs on the floor (Fig. 9.5C).

Weeks 12–14

The patient walks without crutches and is expected to have a normal range of movement. The functional training programme consists of training in standing with semiflexed knees, transferring the load from one leg to the other. Pulley exercises standing on two legs in semiflexed position and loading by the arms are introduced (Fig. 9.5D).

Use of the tilting board on two legs and easy jogging on the trampoline are performed.

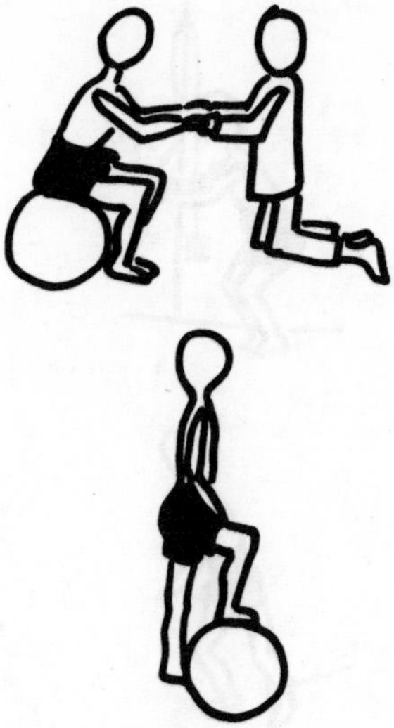

week 9 - 12

Fig. 9.5C Top: resistance is given in different directions by the physiotherapist; the patient tries to stabilize their posture. First both legs are used and later, loading on the operated leg only is used. Bottom: training starts with standing on the unoperated leg. At week 14, the operated leg can be stood upon.

Weeks 14–16

The goal during this period is to increase strength and coordination. Functional training exercises are started, standing on one leg in pulleys with resistance by arms or legs. Easy skipping rope exercise is introduced. Bilateral knee extension with loading (legpress) is performed and ergometer cycle exercises with higher loading are carried out.

Weeks 16–20

The goal during this period is to achieve full strength and coordination. Knee bending with loading and higher loading in functional exercises is used. After 20 weeks, strength training with isokinetic techniques sometimes can be combined with the functional training in jump performance and pulleys exercises.

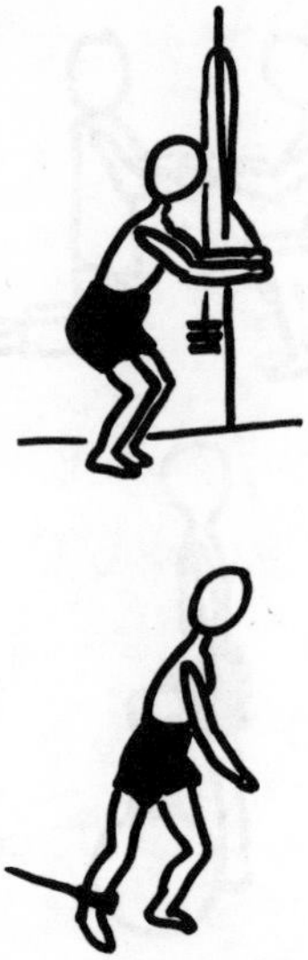

Fig. 9.5D Training in pulleys. The training starts standing on both legs in a semi-flexed position. The weights are used to give loading with the arms or with the leg from the medial and lateral side, as well as backwards and forwards. Standing on the operated leg begins at week 14.

The strength is tested and one legged jumps and running in a figure of eight are performed (Fig 9.4, p. 175). If the quadriceps and hamstring strength in the injured leg is 90% that of the uninjured leg, the athlete is allowed to start the schedule for regaining full performance.

UNANSWERED QUESTIONS AND NEEDS FOR FUTURE RESEARCH

Strength is a complex quality and more knowledge of testing procedures for isolated and combined movements is needed. Physiotherapists need to evaluate strength in standardized ways to be able to optimize rehabilitation and create profiles for different tasks. It is important to create new standardized tests which resemble natural movements in order to get better estimates of demands in real life, and especially to be able to include aspects of dynamic movements.

If better testing procedures are developed, we might be able to improve our understanding of how muscle strength is related to injuries.

It is important to continously evaluate the effects of different training programmes to gain better knowledge of how to train to produce best results in relation to the demands of different sports.

It is also important to understand the effect of strength training on structures like ligaments, and to find the limits for training.

REFERENCES

Agre C J 1985 Hamstring injuries. Sports Medicine 2: 21–33

Andersson C, Odensten M, Good L, et al 1989 Surgical or nonsurgical treatment of acute rupture of the anterior cruciate ligament. Journal of Bone and Joint Surgery 71A: 965–974

Arms S W, Pope M, Johnson R J, Fisher R A, Arvidsson I, Eriksson E 1984 The biomechanics of anterior cruciate ligament rehabilitation and reconstruction. American Journal of Sports Medicine 12: 8–18

Assmusen E 1979 Muscle fatigue. Medical Science of Sports 11: 313–321

Bates B T, Ostering L R, James S L 1977 Fatigue effects in running. Journal of Motor Behaviour 9: 203–207

Bender J A, Pierson J K, Kaplan H D, Johnson A J 1964 Factors affecting occurrence of knee injuries. JAMPR 18: 130–134

Burkett L S 1970 Causative factors in hamstring strains. Medical Science of Sports 2: 39–42

Caiozzo V J, Perrine J J, Edgerton R V 1981 Training-induced alterations of the in vivo force-velocity relationship of human muscle. Journal of Applied Physiology 51: 750–754

Coleman E 1982 Physiological characteristics of major league baseball players. Physical Sports Medicine 10: 51–57

Colliander E B, Tesch P A 1989 Bilateral eccentric and concentric torque of quadriceps and hamstrings muscles in females and males. European Journal of Applied Physiology 59: 227–232

Coyle E, Fering D, Rotkins T, Cote III R, Roby F, Lee W, Wilmore J 1981 Specificity of power improvements through slow and fast isokinetic training. Journal of Applied Physiology 51: 1437–1442

Ekstrand J, Gillquist 1982 The frequence of muscle tightness and injuries in soccer players. American Journal of Sports Medicine 10: 75–78

Ekstrand J, Gillquist J 1983 The avoidability of soccer injuries. International Journal of Sports Medicine 4: 124–128

Ekstrand J, Möller M, Öberg B, Gillquist J 1982 The reliability of some goniometric measurements. Archives of Physical Medicine and Rehabilitation 63: 171–175

Fugl-Meyer A R 1981 Maximum isokinetic ankle plantar and dorsal flexion torques in trained subjects. European Journal of Applied Physiology 47: 393–404

Gilliam T H 1979. Isokinetic torque levels for high school football players. Archives of Physical Medicine and Rehabilitation 60: 110–114

Hage P 1981 Strength: one component of a winning team. Physician Sports Medicine 9: 115–120

Haymes E M, Dickinson A I 1980 Characteristics of elite male and female ski racers. Medical Science of Sports 12: 153–158

Komi P V, Bosco C 1978 Utilization of stored elastic energy in leg extensor muscle by men and women. Medical Science of Sports 4: 261–265

Lindh M 1979 Increase of muscle strength from isometric quadriceps exercises at different knee angles. Scandinavian Journal of Rehabilitative Medicine 11: 33–36

Moffroid M, Whipple R H 1970 Specificity of speed of exercise. Physical Therapy 50: 1699–1700

Moller M 1984 Medical dissertation no. 182, Linkoping University, Sweden

Moller M, Öberg B, Gillquist J 1985 Stretching exercises and soccer. The effect of stretching on range of motion in the lower extremity in connection with soccer training. International Journal of Sports Medicine 6: 313–316

Nicholas J A, Strizak M A, Veras G 1980 A study of thigh muscle weakness in different pathological states of the lower extremity. American Journal of Sports Medicine 4: 241

Noyes F R, Matthews D S, Mooar P A et al 1983 The result of rehabilitation, activity modification and counselling on functional disability. Journal of Bone and Joint Surgery 65A: 163–173

Öberg B, Moller M, Gillquist J, Ekstrand J 1984a Isokinetic torque levels for knee extensors and knee flexors in soccer players. International Journal of Sports Medicine 5: 213–216

Öberg B, Ekstrand J, Moller M, Gillquist J 1984b Muscle strength and flexibility in different positions of soccer players. International Journal of Sports Medicine 5: 213–216

Öberg B, Bergman T, Tropp H 1987 Testing of isokinetic muscle strength in the ankle. Medical Science of Sports 19: 318–323

Öberg, B 1991a Strength training for anterior cruciate ligament injuries — a randomised study of different training programmes. Abstract Proceedings, WCPT, London

Öberg B 1991b EMG studies on training exercises for knee-injured patients. Abstract, Proceedings, WCPT, London

Pipes T V, Wilmore J H 1975 Isokinetic vs isotonic strength training in adult men. Medical Science of Sports 7: 262–274

Renstrom P, Arms S, Stanwyck T S, Johnson R J, Pope M 1986 Strain within the anterior cruciate ligament during hamstrings and quadriceps activity. American Journal of Sports Medicine 14: 83–87

Schantz P G, Moritani T, Karlsson E, Johansson E, Lundh A 1989 Maximal voluntary force of bilateral and unilateral leg extension. Acta Physiologica Scandinavica 136: 185–192

Stafford M G, Grana W A 1984 Hamstrings/quadriceps ratios in college football players: a high velocity evaluation. American Journal of Sports Medicine 12: 209–211

Svantesson U, Ernstoff B, Bergh P, Grimby G 1991 Use of Kin-Com dynamometer to study the stretch-shortening cycle during plantar flexion. European Journal of Applied Physiology 62: 415–419

Thorstensson A, Larsson L, Tesch P, Karlsson J 1977 Muscle strength and fibre composition in athletes and sedentary men. Medical Science of Sports 9: 26–30

Tegner Y, Lysholm J, Lysholm M, Gillquist J 1986 A performance test to monitor rehabilitation and evaluation of anterior cruciate ligament injuries. American Journal of Sport Medicine 4: 156–159

Tegner Y, Lysholm J, Gillquist J, Öberg B 1984 Two year follow-up of conservative treatment of knee ligament injuries. Acta Orthopaedica Scandinavica 55: 176–181

Tropp, H Askling C, Gillquist J 1985 Prevention of ankle sprains. American Journal of Sports Medicine 13: 259–262

Tropp H, 1988 Pronator muscle weakness in functional instability of the ankle joint. International Journal of Sports Medicine 7: 291–294

Tropp H, Askling C 1988 Effects of ankle disk training on muscular strength and postural control. Clinical Biomechanics 3: 88–91

Westing S H, Cresswell A G, Thorstensson A 1991 Muscle activation during maximal voluntary eccentric and concentric knee extension. European Journal of Applied Physiology 62: 104–108

10. Muscle strength in patients with brain lesions: measurement and implications

Richard W. Bohannon

INTRODUCTION

Most physical therapists probably take it for granted that muscle strength is worth measuring and that it has implications for clinical practice. When clinical practice involves patients with brain lesions, however, some therapists are of the opinion that muscle strength is not particularly important and that it is not an appropriate variable for measurement. Statements by Bobath[1] and by Daniels and Worthingham[2] characterize such opinions. Bobath provides four reasons why the testing of muscle strength is unreliable:

1. Weakness of muscles may not be real but relative to the opposition by spastic antagonists. If the latter's spasticity is reduced, the 'weak' muscles may show normal power.
2. A muscle which seems to be too weak to contract sufficiently when tested by itself as a prime mover may be capable of strong contraction when acting in a mass pattern or as part of abnormal tonic reflexes.
3. Weakness of muscles may be due to sensory deficit, either tactile or proprioceptive or both. With adequate and strong sensory stimulation, apparently weak muscles can be made to contract effectively.
4. The strength of contraction of specific muscle groups depends on synergistic fixation elsewhere, i.e. on adequate patterns of postural coordination. This fixation is lacking in patients with hemiplegia, whose muscles can only contract in abnormal mass patterns.

Daniels and Worthingham, although granting that muscle weakness exists in patients with brain lesions, cautioned that evaluation of voluntary movements in selected positions can be misleading because of altered reflex activity and changed states of tone in complete muscle synergies.[2] The concerns of clinicians, which have been summarized by Bobath and by Daniels and Worthingham, have some basis in fact. The concerns, however, do not obviate the measurement of muscle weakness, which is clearly the most common[3] and potentially disabling consequence of stroke. The perspective taken in this chapter, therefore, is that muscle strength is worthy of measurement.

In this chapter I will attempt to demonstrate that muscle strength has clear implications for patients with brain lesions and the therapists who work with them. The demonstration will be based primarily, albeit not exclusively, on studies of patients with stroke. The presentation will be organized under eight questions: What are we measuring when we measure muscle strength? Under what conditions can we measure muscle strength? With what and how can we measure muscle strength? What do measurements of muscle strength tell us about motor status? What do measurements of muscle strength tell us about motor recovery? What do measurements of muscle strength tell us about other measures of interest? Should we be treating muscle weakness? How should we treat muscle weakness?

WHAT ARE WE MEASURING WHEN WE MEASURE MUSCLE STRENGTH?

This question has been addressed to some degree in a previous section of this volume. What I will provide in this section is an emphasis on what we are measuring in patients with brain lesions. What we are measuring is the maximum short duration voluntary force or torque brought to bear on the environment.

When muscles connecting two limb segments contract, the force they impart on the segments can be measured externally, i.e. the force brought to bear on the environment can be measured. If the perpendicular distance from the axis of joint rotation to the point of force application is accounted for, torque can be measured. Whether the force or torque results in function (e.g. support during the single limb stance phase of gait) or subjective or objective measurements of strength, it represents the final output of the central nervous system.[4] What is actually measured, however, is resultant force or torque.

Resultant force or torque is the sum of agonist force or torque production minus antagonist restraint (force or torque).[5] Although antagonist restraint is probably not an issue during most activities in healthy individuals, it can influence (as Bobath has suggested) resultant force or torque in patients with brain lesions. Thus it will be addressed in the following review.

In keeping with Brooks and Stoneys' concept of resultant force being the product of agonist output minus antagonist restraint, Freund classified weakness in patients with brain lesions as resulting from reduced agonist output or from antagonist subtraction.[6] Reduced output paresis is the consequence of one or both of the following:

1. a decreased capacity of the motoneuron pool to drive the motor units of a target agonist muscle
2. a reduced capacity of the activated muscle fibres to generate force.

Whether the decreased capacity to drive motor units is secondary to cortical or subcortical lesions, it can be documented in the muscles of stroke patients through the use of electromyography (EMG). Reduced output appears to exist in limb and nonlimb muscles and to be manifest during both the isolated testing of specific actions and functional activities.[7–15] Consistent with Bobath's concern, reduced output can be manifested to a different extent depending on the circumstances of a muscle's activation. The quadriceps femoris muscles of some patients, for example, may have considerable output during the sit to stand manoeuvre but very little during resisted knee extension in sitting.[16]

Antagonist subtraction is also a documented reality in patients with stroke and other brain lesions. The subtraction can result even when the antagonist is electrically inactive. In such cases restraint to the agonist can result from passive resistance from the antagonist. Such resistance has been documented to be greater in the paretic ankle plantar muscles than in the nonparetic ankle plantar flexor muscles of stroke patients.[17–19] It has also been shown that resistance to dorsiflexion is greater when the knee is extended (and the gastrocnemius muscles are stretched) than when the knee is flexed.[17] Apparently, after brain lesions, the mechanical characteristics of paretic/spastic muscles can change. As a consequence, affected muscles sometimes demonstrate increased stiffness when stretched.[14, 17–21] Interventions aimed at reducing antagonist restraint, it should not be surprising to find, have been shown to increase resultant force production (strength).[22]

Although antagonist subtraction can be the consequence of passive antagonist restraint, it is probably more often the consequence of inappropriate coactivation of the antagonist, i.e. when the agonist alone should be electrically active, the antagonist is electrically active as well. Although inappropriate antagonist coactivation is by no means always present,[7,13,23,24] it can exist during both isolated joint testing[9, 23–27] and functional activities such as gait.[13, 28] Inappropriate antagonist coactivation, when present, is more likely during rapid and reciprocal contractions.[24, 25] During reciprocal contractions, antagonist restraint may be the consequence of continued (prolonged) activation of the antagonist after activation is no longer required.[9] For example, activation of the agonist knee extensor muscles during the knee extension phase of resisted reciprocal knee extension and flexion is necessary. Once knee extension is completed, however, the knee extensor muscles should become inactive antagonists while the agonist knee flexor muscles flex the knee against resistance. If activation of the knee extensor muscles persists, knee flexion will be restrained. Such persistence and/or restraint have been demonstrated in patients with brain lesions.[24] Consistent with such persistence in patients with multiple sclerosis, knee flexion torque immediately following knee extension has been shown to be significantly less than knee flexion torque not preceded by knee extension.[29]

Whether resultant force or torque is diminished secondary to reduced agonist output or antagonist restraint, muscle strength testing will reveal the loss in strength. Knutsson expressed a value for such revelations in stating that 'with correction for gravity and control of acceleration, isokinetic movements can be used for precise measurements of muscle force produced within a large range of movement speeds.'[30](p 205) What measurements of muscle strength do not reveal is 'an understanding of the neurophysiologic basis of functional impairment.'[27](p 106) To clarify the factors contributing to decreases in measured strength, Knutsson recommended the use of electromyography and other procedures to identify the role played by stretch reflexes, contractures and excessive coactivation.[30] Such a clarification may be important if clinicians intend to direct their interventions at the primary cause of reduced resultant force or torque.

UNDER WHAT CONDITIONS CAN WE MEASURE MUSCLE STRENGTH?

When muscle strength is measured in patients with brain lesions, it is typically measured out of context of function. This limitation, although potentially problematic, does not preclude the existence of significant correlations between muscle strength measurements and function (to be discussed later). Moreover, the contextual problem exists whenever muscle strength is measured in any type of patient. Presented in this section will be some of the different conditions under which muscle strength can be measured in brain lesioned patients. The conditions will be categorized as relating to the type of muscle contractions tested and issues of position during testing.

The muscle strength of patients with brain lesions can be tested statically (isometrically) or dynamically (during movement). Whether performed manually or with instruments, measurements of static muscle strength can be obtained during make tests or break tests. Although this distinction is not unique to patients with brain lesions, it may be of particular importance in such patients. During make tests patients use the tested muscle group to generate force against a fixed external object (e.g. the examiner's hand). During break tests patients use the tested muscle group to hold against an ever increasing externally applied force. Once the patients' capacity is exceeded and their contraction is 'broken' the muscle action becomes eccentric. In healthy persons the muscle force associated with a break test is greater than that associated with a make test. Bohannon demonstrated that the force of break tests of the elbow flexor muscles is 1.3 times the force of make tests in healthy young women.[31] Bohannon also demonstrated that the break test to make test force ratio was 1.3/1.0 on the nonparetic side of 22 patients with stroke.[32] On the patients' paretic side, however, the ratio of break test force to make test force was 1.7/1.0. Thus, relative to make test force, break test force is higher on the paretic side than on the nonparetic side of patients with stroke. The higher ratio can be explained in part by the resistance of the paretic muscles to stretch (spasticity).[32] Such resistance may be due, in part, to the relatively greater ability of hemiparetic patients to activate muscles that are being stretched while statically contracted rather than contracted isometrically only. Norton and Sahrmann showed, in patients demonstrating a stretch enhancement, that the EMG activity during voluntary isometric efforts with imposed stretches was greater than the EMG during voluntary isometric efforts alone.[33] More specifically, they demonstrated enhancements of 397% in the biceps brachia, 291% in the hamstring and 335% in the quadriceps femoris muscles. Given the potential influence of stretch and spasticity on break test force, make tests may be preferable for measuring purely voluntary isometric muscle strength in patients with brain lesions.

As described in an earlier section of this volume, the muscle strength (dynamic) demonstrated during joint movement can be measured concentrically (while the tested muscle shortens) or eccentrically (while the tested muscle lengthens). The strength varies depending not only on whether the contraction is concentric or eccentric, but on the speed of the movement and whether the movements are unidirectional (e.g. knee extension) or reciprocal (e.g. knee extension and flexion).

In stroke patients, as in healthy individuals, measured torque or force decreases as speed increases during concentric muscle contractions. Bohannon described percentage decreases in knee extension torque at 60°/s, 120°/s and 180°/s relative to torque at 30°/s.[34] On the paretic side the percentages were 17, 37 and 48. On the nonparetic side the percentages were 15, 35 and 46. The percentage decreases did not differ significantly between sides. Moreover, the torques at at speeds greater than 30°/s were significantly correlated with the torques at 30°/s. On the paretic side the Pearson correlations ranged from 0.74 to 0.95. On the nonparetic side the correlations ranged from 0.83 to 0.95. The results of other investigations of concentric strength-velocity relationships are similar, but not identical to those of Bohannon. The differences are probably a consequence of the severity of the patients' paresis and spasticity. Sjöström et al reported that three of the 19 subjects with stroke that they measured could not produce active static ankle plantar flexion torque.[35] Seven of the same subjects could not produce active plantar flexion torque at 30°/s. Nine could not produce plantar flexion torque at 90°/s. Nakamura et al demonstrated that isokinetic knee extension torque decreased with increased speed on both the paretic and nonparetic sides, but more on the paretic side.[36] More specifically, the ratio of paretic to nonparetic knee extension torque was 0.49 at 30°/s, 0.32 at 90°/s and 0.17 at 180°/s. Like Bohannon, Nakamura et al demonstrated a relationship between the torques at different speeds. The correlations ranged from 0.60 to 0.99 on the paretic side and 0.67 to 0.93 on the nonparetic side. In 24 patients with hemiparesis Knutsson and Martensson also showed decreases in concentric muscle torque with increased speed that were greater on the paretic than on the nonparetic side.[24] They reported that the knee extension torque on the paretic side of hemiparetic men was 38%, 36% and 25% of that of healthy men at 30°/s, 90°/s and 180°/s respectively. In a later study utilizing EMG, Knutsson et al demonstrated that EMG activity decreased in the agonist knee extensor muscles as speed increased during concentric contractions.[37] On the other hand, EMG activity increased in the agonist knee extensor muscles as speed increased during eccentric contractions.

The position of testing, like the type of muscle contraction, can influence the torque or force measured. Alterations in motor behaviour with position, which are not unique to patients with brain lesions, are often attributed to the influence of synergies on the patients.[38] Changes in muscle length with different positions, however, may offer a better explanation of differences in muscle strength in alternative positions. Sjöström et al stated that 'placement of the legs within patterns believed to facilitate (0° knee positions) or inhibit (90° knee position) extensor motoneurons did not give rise to systematic strength variations different from those of control subjects'.[35](p 58) Bourbonnais et al observed that EMG activity in the paretic elbow flexor muscles 'does not conform with established synergistic patterns'[39](p 85). Bohannon demonstrated that patients with hemiparesis had gravity-eliminated supine to sitting knee flexion torque ratios on the paretic and nonparetic sides that did *not* differ significantly.[40] On both sides knee flexion torque was greater when subjects were sitting (with the hips flexed and the hamstring muscles lengthened) than when subjects were supine (with the hips extended and the hamstring muscles shortened). The mean supine to sitting ratio was 0.70 on the paretic side and 0.56 on the nonparetic side. Bohannon concluded that the greater knee flexion torque with the hip flexed was largely the result of normal length-tension factors.

WITH WHAT AND HOW CAN WE MEASURE MUSCLE STRENGTH?

Numerous options exist for documenting muscle strength in patients, whether they have brain lesions or not. In this section the options to be addressed are ordinal scales, weights, hand dynamometers, fixed dynamometers, hand-held dynamometers and isokinetic dynamometers. The options will be described, and where possible, procedural issues addressed.

Ordinal scales

Two to 10 category scales of ordinal grades have been used to describe subjective measurements of muscle strength in patients with brain lesions.[41–80] Apparently, some of the scales that have been published were designed specifically for the studies in which they were used. Some such scales, although describing muscle strength, go beyond the mere description of strength alone. Two examples follow.

McDowell and Louis described motor deficits as absent, mild to moderate, or severe.[41] Patients with no motor deficit were described as having no weakness detectable on examination and little or no deficit of gait. Those with mild to moderate deficits demonstrated paresis on formal neurologic testing. Their gait was defective but they were able to walk alone without support or braces. Patients with severe deficits demonstrated complete paralysis of the leg with a need for braces, crutches or assistance for walking.

Bonita and Beaglehole described paresis as present or absent.[52] If present, paresis was categorized as mild, moderate, or severe. Mild paresis entailed 'functionally insignificant impairment of finer movement but with controlled movements through the full range.' Moderate paresis involved the 'presence of muscle contraction and movement against gravity or resistance but limited in range and not in a controlled fashion.' Severe paresis meant that there was 'little or no active movement on the affected side.'

Fullerton et al described a scale that is more typical and specific to muscle strength.[42] They characterized arm power and leg power using five level scales:

1 — no spontaneous movement,
2 — muscle flicker, no movement of limb,
3 — can move limb but not against gravity,
4 — weak but can move limb against gravity,
5 — full power.

Most ordinal scales used in monitoring muscle strength in patients with brain lesions are based on the six level Medical Research Council (MRC) scale.[81] The manual muscle testing grades in that scale and their descriptions are as follows:

0 = no contraction,
1 = palpable contraction, but no visible movement,
2 = movement without gravity,
3 = movement against gravity,
4 = movement against resistance lower than the resistance overcome by the healthy side,

5 = movement against resistance equal to the maximum resistance overcome by the healthy side.

A problem with rating 'movement against resistance equal to the maximum resistance overcome by the healthy side' is that the healthy side may not be normal either.[64]

Although ordinal scales might be used to measure a large number of muscle groups of the paretic and nonparetic sides of patients with brain lesions, they are normally applied to a limited number of muscle groups or actions. Demeurisse et al suggested that such limitations are necessary as 'it is impossible to make frequent detailed evaluations of muscle function because they are time consuming and fastidious for the medical staff and for the patient, whose cooperation during rehabilitation is essential.'[59] (p 388) Demeurisse et al, therefore, selected from 28 total movements one action from each joint (shoulder, elbow, hand, hip, knee, ankle) to include in a *motricity index*. Their selection of specific actions was justified by the high correlations (most > 0.90) between the manual muscle test scores of different actions measured at each joint. The actions they selected were shoulder flexion, elbow flexion, prehension (angual-tip pinch), hip flexion, knee extension and foot dorsiflexion. The manual muscle test score given to each action (0–5) was weighted. The total index score (maximum possible = 100) was equal to the sum of the weighted individual action scores. Demeurisse et al claimed the index 'given a rapid overall indication of a patient's progress in motor recovery, permits comparisons between different patients and the establishment of correlations with other clinical data.'[59] (p 382) Since the introduction of the index, its use has been reported in a number of publications.[43–46, 67, 71, 73, 74] When using the index, Wade and various colleagues have substituted shoulder abduction for shoulder flexion.[43–46, 73, 74] They have concluded that the motricity index is easy to use and that patients can be assessed with it anywhere, with a minimum of equipment, in a brief period of time.[67] They recommended it for 'routine use in assessing stroke patients.'[67] (p 53) Although the index will not describe specifically a patient's capacity to perform a nontested action (e.g. elbow extension), it will provide a reliable overall indication of motor loss and recovery. Collin and Wade reported interrater reliability coefficients of 0.88 and 0.77 for motricity scores of the paretic upper and lower extremities (respectively) of stroke patients.[45] They reported interrater reliability coefficients of 0.88 for total motricity scores of the paretic side.

Weights

Although not routinely used to quantify muscle strength in patients with brain lesions, weights can serve such a purpose. Inaba et al, for example, documented the amount of weight that stroke patients could move in a mass extension pattern on an Elgin^{R} table.[58]

Hand dynamometers

Hand dynamometers, which are grasped in the hand of the patient, provide a measurement of static grip strength. Although they have been used extensively in patients with brain lesions,[49, 76, 82–91] the specific devices and procedures vary. In some studies, the devices that were used to measure grip strength were not specified or were custom made for the study. Commercially available dynamometers that have been used to measure grip strength in patients with brain lesions are the Jamar dynamometer[90] and the MIE Medical Research Digital/Pinch Analyser.[91] Other devices are available, although all are not equally accurate or precise.[92, 93] Even different versions of the same dynamometer can provide different measurements of grip strength. Flood-Joy and Mathiowetz therefore recommended that 'the same dynamometer be used in pre and post testing of patients.'[94](p 242) For measuring grip strength in patients with brain lesions, the Jamar dynamometer is a reasonable choice given the availability of normative values obtained with it for subjects of 16 to 90 years of age.[95, 96]

The procedural variables most subject to differences between studies of hand grip strength are the position in which individuals are tested and the measurement used to indicate strength. The standardized position described by Mathiowetz et al[93] is worthy of recommendation. In that position the subject is seated, the shoulder is adducted and in neutral rotation, the elbow is flexed 90°, the forearm is in neutral and the wrist is extended 0–30° and ulnarly deviated 0–15°. The dynamometer handle is in the second position (Fig. 10.1). Smutok et al have used similar, albeit not identical, positions to test patients with traumatic brain injuries.[90] Patients who are unable to maintain sitting balance can be tested while supine, but can be placed in every other respect in the standardized position described by Mathiowetz et al. Typically patients are allowed one to three maximal grip efforts during a test session. Smutok et al requested their subjects to perform one maximal effort, but that was after one submaximal effort.[90] Haaland and Delaney,[87]

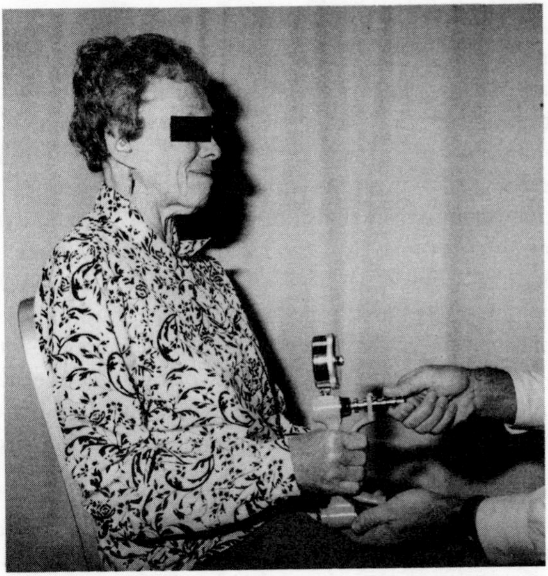

Fig. 10.1 Measurement of hand-grip in a stroke patient.

and Dodrill[88] had patients with brain lesions perform two maximal efforts. As a measurement the investigators used the mean of the two efforts. Sunderland et al had stroke patients squeeze the dynamometer as hard as possible three times.[91] They reported that the variability of the measurements was reduced only slightly by using the force of the first trial as a measurement rather than the mean force of the three trials as a measurement. They reported that the variability was reduced more when the mean force of three trials on the affected side was expressed as a percentage of the mean force of three trials on the unaffected side. They claimed that the 'percentage grip measure provides some control for the wide variations in strength which exist in the normal elderly population.' For the sake of time, my tendency during clinical testing is to allow patients two trials. Unless the second is substantially different from the first, I use the force of the first trial as a measurement.

Fixed dynamometers

Fixed dynamometers incorporate springs or strain gauges and are mechanically stabilized to prevent their movement during static strength testing. They have been used in numerous studies to document the strength of upper and lower extremity muscle groups in patients with stroke. Quinn used such a device to document shoulder abduction strength.[86] Colebatch and Gandevia used a fixed dynamometer to measure shoulder adduction strength.[97] In five different studies of stroke patients, fixed force gauges have been used to document wrist extension strength.[97–100] Fixed dynamometer measurements of elbow flexion and/or extension force have been reported more often.[7, 21, 23, 33, 97, 101, 102] Other investigators, however, have used fixed force gauges to measure muscle strength at the ankle[8, 103–109] and knee[33, 110–115] of patients with central nervous system lesions. It is noteworthy that because fixed dynamometers are fixed, they can be used to measure not only peak force but such time based measurements as time to peak force[113] and force consistency over time[7, 8] as well.

Hand-held dynamometers

Hand-held dynamometers are force measuring devices that are held in the hand of an examiner while the individual being tested exerts effort against the device. The devices can be used for both make tests and break tests. Given the possible contribution of spasticity to break test force measurements,[32] however, I recommend that only make tests be used with patients with brain lesions. A number of hand-held dynamometers are available commercially that incorporate either springs or strain gauges. One study of two spring and two strain gauge dynamometers that had been used extensively demonstrated that the two spring gauge dynamometers no longer provided accurate measurements of force.[116] Thus, strain gauge dynamometers may be preferable.

Whether employing spring or strain gauge hand-held dynamometers, numerous investigations of muscle strength in patients with brain lesions have been performed. With the exception of one study of the neck musculature[117] and three of the trunk musculature,[118–120] studies in which hand-held dynamometers have been used have focussed on limb muscle strength. Excepting a study by Riddle et al,[121] all hand-held dynamometer studies of limb muscle strength in stroke patients appear to have been performed by Bohannon and various colleagues.[32, 119, 120, 122–146]

Riddle et al and Bohannon and various colleagues used the same method to measure limb muscle strength in patients with brain lesions. Muscle groups were tested in gravity eliminated positions

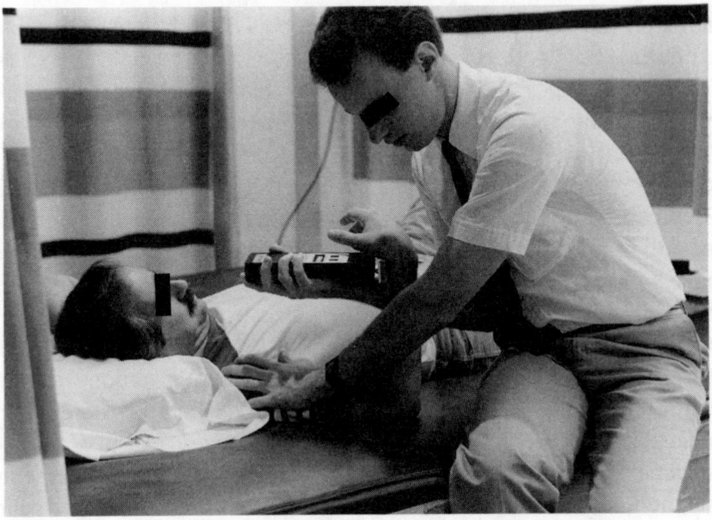

Fig. 10.2 Measurement of a stroke patient's elbow flexion strength with a hand-held dynamometer.

in the middle half of their range. Gravity eliminated testing is necessary to eliminate errors associated with the effects of gravity.[147] Testing in the middle half of range is performed so that the muscle is neither highly advantaged or disadvantaged by its length.

The knee flexor and extensor muscles are tested while patients sit upright. All other muscle groups are tested while patients are supine (Fig. 10.2). Make tests of four to six seconds are performed with the hand-held dynamometer. Patients are asked to take one to two seconds to come to maximal effort. Such a gradual increase in force makes it easier for the examiner to hold the dynamometer steady and perpendicular to the limb segment during testing. Specific joint positions and dynamometer placements are described in detail elsewhere.[123, 148] The reliability of muscle strength measurements obtained (from patients with brain lesions) as described heretofore has been investigated by Riddle et al,[121] Bohannon,[119, 139, 140] and Bohannon and Andrews.[136] All studies have demonstrated good to excellent intrasession reliability, with most reliability coefficients exceeding 0.90. Riddle et al also found excellent intersession reliability for measurements of muscle strength on the paretic side (ICC = 0.90 – 0.98).[121] The intersession reliability of measurements on the nonparetic side, however, was often below acceptable standards (ICC = 0.31 – 0.93).[121]

The advantages and disadvantages of hand-held dynamometers for measuring muscle strength in patients with brain lesions are closely tied to the fact that the devices are hand-held. Such portability expands the settings in which the devices can be applied. They can be applied, for example, to patients in their homes or at bedside in an institution. They can be used to rapidly test multiple muscle groups. I have been able to test routinely 10 muscle groups bilaterally (once) in about 10 minutes. Because the device is held in the examiner's hand and the patient is manually stabilized, the examiner can maintain a 'feel' for the patient's actions during testing. As a result, attempted substitutions can be noted and thwarted. Because hand-held dynamometers are grasped by the examiner, his or her strength and skill can influence measurements obtained. If the patient is stronger than the clinician, valid measurements of patient muscle strength will not be obtained. Measurements of such muscle groups (on the patients' nonparetic side) as the hip extensors and ankle plantar flexors can be problematic for all but the strongest of testers.

Isokinetic dynamometers

Isokinetic dynamometers are devices which are used primarily to measure dynamic muscular strength. Although the dynamometers are sometimes employed for isometric (static) testing, it is their ability to measure resultant force or torque at essentially constant angular velocities that sets them apart from other muscle strength testing options. When patients with brain lesions have limitations in muscle force or torque production at higher velocities, isokinetic dynamometers can help expose the limitations. When employed for reciprocal muscle testing (e.g. knee extension-knee flexion-knee extension), isokinetic dynamometers can help expose limitations in force or torque that are greater than present during unidirectional testing.[29] Numerous investigations of patients with brain lesions have been performed using the devices. Most of the investigations have involved the knee flexor and/or extensor muscles (Fig. 10.3),[24, 34, 36, 37, 64, 85, 140, 149–158] but the muscles of the ankle[35] and elbow[85] have also been tested. With one notable exception,[157] studies in which isokinetic dynamometers have been used for dynamic testing have not been accompanied by a verification of measurement reliability. In that study, reliability was demonstrated.

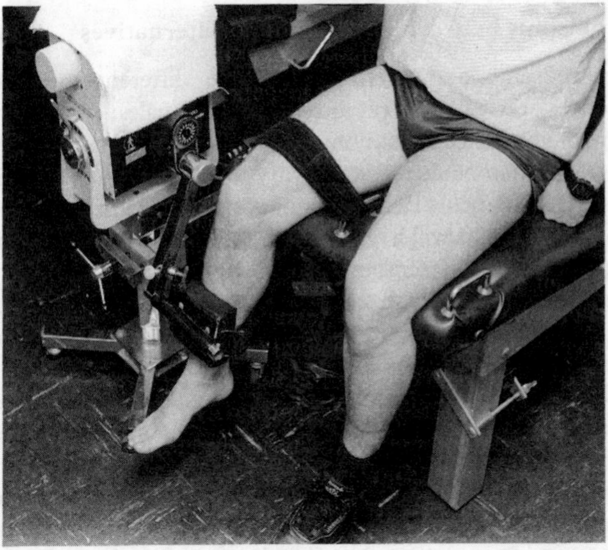

Fig. 10.3 Measurement of a stroke patient's knee extension strength with an isokinetic dynamometer.

Isometric measurements obtained from stroke patients using isokinetic dynamometers have been found to be reliable.[140, 149] Test-retest correlations exceeding 0.90 have been reported for isometric measurements repeated within and between sessions.

Although the ability to use isokinetic dynamometers for velocity spectrum testing may be advantageous, it may not be always necessary and may be outweighed by other disadvantages. Velocity spectrum testing may not be necessary because torque measurements at higher velocities, although less than at lower velocities, are correlated (as indicated previously) significantly with isometric torques and lower velocity torques.[34, 36] Regardless of the speed of testing, measurements obtained using the devices should be corrected for the effects of gravity.[30, 147, 159] A failure to make such corrections can lead to erroneous judgements about a patient's strength or recovery of strength. Disadvantages of isokinetic dynamometers include their cost (often in excess of $45,000 at the time of writing), the space they occupy and their lack of portability. The time required to set up the devices for testing many muscle groups is prohibitive.

Relationships between measurement alternatives

The practicality and usefulness of the different measurement alternatives reviewed heretofore (ordinal scales, weights, hand dynamometers, fixed dynamometers, hand-held dynamometers and isokinetic dynamometers) may vary depending on a clinician's practice environment. Regardless of which alternative is employed, however, the results will be indicative of the same variable — muscle strength. That different measurement alternatives may yield indications of muscle strength is suggested by the correlation between knee extension torque measured at different speeds.[34,36] That make and break tests of muscle strength obtained with a hand-held dynamometer are correlated significantly in patients with brain lesions also indicates that different measurements may be used to describe muscle strength.[32] Completely different measurements of muscle strength have also been shown to be correlated. Sunderland et al used hand-grip strength measurements and upper extremity motricity index scores to describe the arm function of 38 stroke patients.[91] The two measurements were significantly correlated on initial assessment ($r = 0.87$) and final assessment ($r = 0.83$). Inaba et al reported that the maximal resistance weight for 10 repetitions of a mass lower extremity extension movement was correlated highly with selective and patterned measurements of muscle strength.[58]

WHAT DO MEASUREMENTS OF MUSCLE STRENGTH TELL US ABOUT STATUS?

The purpose of measurements of muscle strength in patients with brain lesions is to establish the presence and extent of muscle weakness, one aspect of motor status. Because weakness is a deficit in muscle strength, it is typically expressed in relation to some norm or standard. That norm can be the strength of age matched healthy subjects or of the 'unaffected' side. Comparisons between patients with brain lesions and healthy subjects have demonstrated the expected, that the patients are weak in the limb muscles contralateral to their lesions.[8, 24, 35, 64, 89, 110, 111] Sjöström et al, for example, found that the ankle plantar flexion torques on the affected side of the hemiparetic subjects they tested were about 20% of those demonstrated by sedentary control subjects.[35] Jones et al found hand grip strengths in stroke patients (11 days postinfarction) that were 66% less on the paretic side than in control subjects.[89] The comparisons between patients with brain lesions and healthy subjects have sometimes also revealed the existence of a lesser weakness in the limb muscles on the side ipsilateral to the patients' lesions.[35, 64, 90] In the Jones et al study just cited, for example, the stroke patients were 13% weaker on their unaffected side than control subjects. In addition to outright reductions in maximum voluntary force of torque, brain damaged patients demonstrate other deficiencies in resultant force or torque relative to healthy subjects. Among such deficiencies are prolonged tension lag times (latency between the onset of EMG and the initial rise of tension),[110, 111] prolonged contraction times (latency between the initial rise of tension and maximal force production),[110] a decreased rate of tension development[110] and an inability to maintain constant levels of torque.[8]

The strength of the limb muscles of the 'affected' side (contralateral to the brain lesion) is sometimes compared to the strength of the same muscles of the 'unaffected' side (ipsilateral to the brain lesion). Such comparisons are imbedded in some measurements. For example, the MRC scale adapted by Demeurisse et al describes a strength score of '5' as 'movement against resistance equal to the maximum resistance overcome by the healthy side.'[59] Sunderland et al expressed the mean grip force of three trials on the affected side as a percentage of the mean force of three trials on the unaffected side of stroke patients to 'control for the wide variations in strength which exist in the normal elderly population.'[91] In several studies in which hand-held dynamometers were used, strength of the paretic side was described as percentage of or a deficit relative to the nonparetic side.[122, 124, 126, 127] Patients with brain lesions demonstrate deficiencies (other than reduced maximal voluntary force or torque) between sides, much like they do in comparison to healthy subjects. The deficiencies include increased tension lag times,[111] prolonged contraction times,[111, 155] a decreased rate of tension development[111] and lower electrically evoked twitch tensions.[113] Granting that expressing an 'affected' muscle group's strength relative to the contralateral side provides perspective and is convenient, clinicians should not ignore that the unaffected side of stroke patients may very well be affected, either by the patient's present stroke or by a previously undocumented or unrecognized stroke.

In addition to describing paresis relative to healthy individuals or the unaffected side, measurements of muscle strength have provided some indication of the relative involvement of different muscle groups. Bohannon and Smith reported that in 42 stroke patients the strength deficits of eight upper extremity muscle groups of the paretic side differed significantly.[126] In a later study, he and Andrews showed that among 69 stroke patients the elbow flexors were weakened relatively more than the elbow extensors, the shoulder abductors were weakened relatively more than the shoulder extensors, and the shoulder external rotators were weakened relatively more than the shoulder internal rotators.[130] Colebatch et al also have reported a greater reduction in elbow flexor than elbow extensor muscle strength in stroke patients.[23] In another study, Colebatch and Gandevia concluded that the patients with upper motor neuron lesions that they tested had shoulder muscles that were relatively spared but wrist and finger muscles that were relatively severely affected.[97] Knutsson and Martensson reported greater reductions in knee flexion torque than knee extension torque in 24 hemiparetic patients.[24]

The clinician wishing to document motor status in patients with brain lesions should realize that although alternatives exist, not all are equally sensitive. Watkins et al concluded from their manual muscle testing and Cybex isokinetic dynamometer testing of stroke patients that manual muscle testing was not sensitive enough to detect deficits on the 'unaffected' side.[64] Heller et al reported that 'recordable grip strength nearly always preceded other measurements of arm function during recovery' and suggested that it is the most sensitive test of initial status.[83] (p 717) Dodrill reported that hand grip dynamometry 'discriminated between normal and brain-damaged groups' as well as the tactual performance test and the tapping test.[88] Hand grip dynamometry was the procedure that correctly classified the largest number of brain damaged patients according to hemisphere involvement.

WHAT DO MEASUREMENTS OF MUSCLE STRENGTH TELL US ABOUT MOTOR RECOVERY?

Unlike motor status, which can be indicated by measurements of muscle strength at a given point in time, motor recovery is indicated by increases in muscle strength over time. Recovery is progress relative to a starting point or normal status.

Studies of patients with stroke clearly indicate that the patients tend to demonstrate increases in (a recovery of) muscle strength following the onset of their lesions, with the greatest recovery occurring early. The studies also demonstrate that measurements at a later time are significantly correlated with measurements obtained early after the stroke. Not all measures of muscle strength, however, are equally sensitive to changes in muscle strength.

Increases in muscle strength apparently occur spontaneously in patients with stroke. Increases, nevertheless, may be influenced by therapeutic interventions.[58, 104–106] Regardless of the factors underlying increases in muscle strength, they have been documented using ordinal scales,[41, 61, 67, 91] weights,[58] hand dynamometers,[89, 91] fixed dynamometers,[104–106, 109] hand-held dynamometers,[124–126, 135] and isokinetic dynamometers.[151] McDowell and Louis, who used an ordinal scale of motor performance, reported that between admission and discharge the percentage of stroke patients demonstrating various degrees of improvement were: marked (17%), moderate (20%), slight (14%) and none (12%). The remaining 34% died.[41] Andrews et al,[61] who also used an ordinal scale for strength, reported that maximal strength was reached by 58% of their patients in two weeks, 71% in three to eight weeks and 88% in 9–26 weeks. Of the 56 patients that Heller et al tested with a hand dynamometer, 23 (41%) had no measurable grip strength when first tested.[83] Thirteen of the 23 patients achieved measurable grip strength within three months. Of the 13, all actually achieved measurable grip within 24 days. Using a hand dynamometer Jones et al showed that the percentage deficit in grip strength demonstrated by stroke patients relative to healthy subjects decreased from 66% to 41% on the affected side and 13% to 4% on the unaffected side between 11 days and 12 months post stroke.[89] Hand-held dynamometer measurements of muscle strength in stroke patients also have demonstrated that the patients experience significant increases in strength during inpatient rehabilitation. Bohannon and Smith reported that one group of patients demonstrated a grand mean decrease in strength deficits (relative to the unaffected side) of 31%.[126] In another study the same authors reported the mean strength deficits of 10 upper extremity muscle groups decreased from initial values of 60–81% to discharge values of 39–58%.[124] Bohannon reported that the grand mean force produced by 16 affected paretic muscle groups of 38 stroke patients was 26% of the nonparetic side initially and 48% of the nonparetic side prior to discharge. Although Bohannon found that the muscle strength of all extremities (paretic and nonparetic, upper and lower) increased significantly after stroke, he did not find the increases in all muscle groups to be the same.[135] Percentage increases were greater in weaker muscle, albeit significantly in only two of seven of those tested. He questioned whether 'higher percentage increases in strength allow patients with weaker muscles to gain strength to a point that their muscles are as strong as those of patients who are stronger initially.' Nakamura et al, who measured the knee extension muscle strength of 18 hemiparetic stroke patients over an eight week period, reported that the strength of the paretic side was significantly greater at four weeks than initially, and greater at eight weeks than at four weeks.[151] They also reported that the strength of the nonparetic side did not increase significantly between the initial measurement and four weeks, but that it did increase significantly between four and eight weeks.

That measurements at a later time are related to measurements obtained earlier after a stroke has been demonstrated in several studies. Using the motricity index, Wade and Hewer showed that of surviving stroke patients who initially demonstrated severe upper limb paralysis, 73% were still severely paralyzed at three weeks and 55% were still severely paralyzed at six months; only 2% were normal at three weeks and only 10% were normal at six months.[67] Of the patients with severe upper limb paralysis at three weeks, 40% still had severe paralysis, 14% still had moderate paralysis, and 9% still had mild paresis at six months. Thirty-six percent had died by six months. None of the patients had recovered to normal strength in the upper limb. Logigian et al reported that final manual muscle test scores were significantly correlated ($r = 0.78$) with initial muscle test score in 42 stroke patients undergoing rehabilitation.[68] Bohannon demonstrated that the strengths of 16 muscle groups measured with a hand-held dynamometer on initial assessment were correlated significantly with the strength measured prior to discharge.[125] The correlations ranged from 0.56 to 0.83 depending on the muscle group. Bohannon and Smith demonstrated similarly that the strength deficits of paretic muscle groups of stroke patients measured on admission and discharge from rehabilitation were correlated.[124] The correlations ranged from 0.73 to 0.85 depending on the muscle group.

Not all measures of muscle strength are equally sensitive to changes in muscle strength. Basically, ordinal scales are less sensitive than all other alternatives which yield results in real numbers. This was demonstrated over 30 years ago in patients with poliomyelitis[160] and probably holds true for stroke patients as well. Sunderland et al reported that for the upper extremity, hand grip strength was sensitive to early as well as late changes.[91] They further stated that unlike the motricity index, hand grip dynamometry was effective for detecting small late improvements in strength.

WHAT DO MEASUREMENTS OF MUSCLE STRENGTH TELL US ABOUT OTHER MEASURES OF INTEREST?

Other measures of interest are primarily measurements of motor control and function (either specific or general). Numerous studies demonstrate that measurements of muscle strength are correlated with other measures of interest. Although the existence of significant correlations does not prove that weakness is the cause of diminished motor control or function, the correlations are consistent with such a possibility.

Measurements of muscle strength have been shown to correlate with the results of other assessments of motor status. Collin and Wade reported significant Spearman correlations between upper extremity motricity index scores and Rivermead motor assessment scores. The correlations were 0.76, 0.73 and 0.74 at 6, 12 and 16 weeks respectively.[45] They also reported correlations between lower extremity motricity index scores and Rivermead motor assessment scores of 0.81, 0.81 and 0.75 at 6, 12 and 18 weeks respectively. Sunderland et al found grip strength to be correlated with Motor Club assessment scores initially (r = 0.81) and at six months (r = 0.86).[91] Sjöström et al reported that isometric measurement of maximum strength of the affected lower extremity correlated significantly with Fugl-Meyer motor scores (r = 0.66).[35] Bohannon reported that the time required to perform alternating movements in the lower extremity was correlated significantly with the strength of several lower extremity muscle groups (adjusted R^2 = 0.495) measured with hand-held dynamometer.[131]

Performance of specific functions and functional index scores have both been shown to be correlated with muscle strength measured using various alternatives. Among the specific functional activities influenced by muscle strength are gait, transfer, standing and rolling.

Using a four level ordinal scale to describe the strength of straight leg raising and another ordinal scale to describe gait performance, Olesen et al demonstrated a significant relationship between muscle strength and gait (r = 0.89)[51] Secondary analysis of data reported by Wade and Hewer demonstrates a significant correlation between lower extremity motricity index scores and gait performance (γ = 0.860).[67] Wade and Hewer, however, noted that despite the apparent importance of muscle strength to gait performance, 11% of the patients with normal strength had difficulty walking and 15% of those with moderate weakness could walk alone. Bohannon has demonstrated in five different studies that various measures of gait performance are correlated with lower extremity muscle strength measurements obtained with a hand-held dynamometer. In the first study he demonstrated correlations between paretic muscle group forces and gait speed of 0.25 to 0.60.[123] The muscle groups demonstrating significant correlations were the hip extensors, knee flexors, and ankle dorsiflexors and plantar flexors. Gait cadence and muscle force correlations ranged from 0.26 to 0.65. Correlations with hip extensor and abductor, knee flexor and extensor, and ankle dorsiflexor and plantar flexor strengths were significant. Bohannon showed in another study that the sum of the strengths of seven paretic lower extremity muscle groups (normalized against body weight) was correlated significantly with gait speed ($r = 0.49$), cadence ($r = 0.51$), independence ($r = 0.37$) and appearance ($r = 0.42$).[128] The normalized strength of the nonparetic lower extremity was not correlated significantly with any gait measure ($r = 0.14 - 0.33$).[128] It should be noted that, motor control and balance, which were also measured in the study, were better predictors (than muscle strength) of gait performance. In a more recent study Bohannon demonstrated that the normalized strength of all seven measured lower extremity muscle groups of the paretic side correlated ($r = 0.56 - 0.85$) significantly ($p < 0.01$) with four gait (cadence, speed, distance, independence) measures.[137] The normalized strength of most of the seven measured lower extremity muscle groups of the nonparetic side correlated ($r = 0.31 - 0.70$) significantly ($p < 0.01$) with the four gait measures. These findings have been basically confirmed in two studies concerned only with knee extensor muscle strength and gait.[139, 161] Measurements of knee extension or flexion torque obtained with an isokinetic dynamometer have been shown in several studies to correlate significantly with gait performance. Hamrin et al demonstrated positive and significant correlations between locomotion and both knee extension and flexion torques measured at 60°/s on the paretic side ($r_s = 0.71 - 0.90$, $p < 0.001$).[85] The locomotion/torque correlations were lower on the nonparetic side ($r_s = 0.38 - 0.67$). Nakamura et al tested isometric as well as isokinetic knee extension strength in 11 patients with spastic hemiparesis.[36] They found that all strength measurements on the paretic side correlated significantly with gait cadence ($r = 0.61 - 0.85$) and that all but one strength measurement on the paretic side correlated significantly with gait speed ($r_s = 0.60 - 0.87$). None of the strength measurements of the nonparetic side correlated significantly with either gait measurement. In a follow up study, Nakamura et al found that the variance in gait speed explained by strength measurements on the paretic side increased from 0.25 to 0.50 during an eight week period of gait training.[151] Bohannon and Andrews, who tested isometric knee torque and gait speed on two consecutive days, found significant correlations between the two variables ($r = 0.57$ on day 1, $r = 0.57$ on day 2).[149] Bohannon obtained similar results in another study.[161] In that study he was unable to demonstrate any superiority of torque over force measurements or normalized over non-normalized strength measurements for predicting gait speed in stroke patients.

Besides gait performance; transfer, standing, rolling and stair climbing performance have been shown to correlate with measurements of muscle strength in hemiparetic stroke patients. Bohannon demonstrated that the strengths of seven paretic muscle groups of the lower extremity measured with a hand-held dynamometer were all correlated significantly with transfer independence at initial assessment ($r_s = 0.47 - 0.64$).[133] The correlations at final assessment and between assessment times, although positive, were rarely significant ($r_s = 0.30 - 0.48$). Bohannon demonstrated in 81 stroke patients that standing performance was correlated significantly with the strength of six of seven lower extremity muscle groups of the paretic and nonparetic sides ($r_s = 0.26 - 0.46$).[128] In a follow up study, Bohannon demonstrated that lower extremity muscle group strengths were correlated significantly with standing performance at initial and final assessment, as well as across assessment times.[138] The correlations ranged from 0.48 to 0.85 on the paretic side and from 0.42 to 0.70 on the nonparetic side. Rolling performance, i.e. independence in going from supine to nonparetic side lying, was shown by Bohannon to correlate with muscle strength of the nonparetic side measured with a hand-held dynamometer ($r = 0.51 - 0.75$).[134] Strength of the paretic side, on the other hand, did not correlate significantly with independence in rolling. Stair climbing scores, based on required assistance, rail use and pattern, have been shown to correlate significantly also with lower extremity muscle strength. Specifically, Bohannon and Walsh reported a Spearman correlation of 0.86 between the stair climbing scores and the sums of five lower extremity muscle strengths of 20 subjects.[144]

Various measures of muscle strength have also been found to correlate with different functional test and indexes. Measurements of muscle strength obtained using a number of ordinal scales have been described as related to function. Feigenson et al, who described weakness in stroke patients as mild, moderate or severe, found weakness to be one of the most powerful predictors of dressing, feeding and hygiene performance.[54] Fullerton et al found significant correlations ($p < 0.001$) between ordinal strength measurements ('arm power' and 'leg power') and outcome in 206 stroke patients.[42] Outcome at six months was categorized as: 1—complete recovery; 2—some disability, but regained independence in activities of daily living; 3—dependent in activities of daily living; and 4—dead. They concluded that the significance of 'measures of severity of weakness' in predicting outcome from stroke is not in question.[42] (p 158) Logigian et al reported significant correlations between manual muscle test scores and Barthel index scores obtained on admission and discharge as well as across time.[68]

Olsen, who used the Medical Research Council system to measure upper and lower extremity paresis, reported significant correlations between paresis and functional outcome (measured using various Barthel Index subscores).[75] The correlations ranged from $r = 0.53$ to $r = 0.58$. Olsen stated that as a predictor of function the initial Barthel Index score was only slightly better than the paresis score for predicting functional outcome. Friedman similarly reported that the degree of arm paresis described by the Medical Research Council System was a significant predictor of functional outcome measured with the Barthel Index.[78] He concluded that 'because evaluation of extremity paresis is easy, it appears to be useful as a preliminary predictor of outcome following stroke.' Demeurisse et al characterized comparisons of motricity and functional index scores as fruitful.[71] The findings of Wade and Hewer support the characterization. Wade and Hewer reported correlations between motricity index and Barthel index scores that were 0.75 on initial assessment, 0.77 at three weeks and 0.61 at six months.[67] Parker et al reported a significant correlation ($r = 0.90$) between upper extremity motricity index scores and Frenchay arm test scores.[46]

Objective measurements of muscle strength obtained with different devices have also been shown to correlate with general measures of function. Sunderland et al reported grip strength to be correlated significantly with Frenchay arm test scores at initial assessment ($r = 0.86$) and at six months ($r = 0.90$).[91] Hamrin et al found some but not all isokinetic measurements of elbow flexion and extension to be correlated significantly with primary activity of daily living functions such as personal hygiene, dressing and household work.[85] Wilson et al reported that wrist extension torque was among the significant predictor variables of upper extremity function in stroke patients.[100]

SHOULD WE BE TREATING MUSCLE WEAKNESS?

Considerable evidence has now been presented which substantiates a relationship between muscle strength and function in stroke patients. It is that relationship which I believe justifies the treatment of paresis. Further justification is provided by a limited number of studies of two types:

1. those which show improvements in function when compensations for weakness are applied,
2. those which show improvements in function when muscle performance is improved by various means.

Studies of the first type demonstrate that lower extremity weakness can be compensated for partly by the use of orthoses. Ankle foot orthoses, for example, have been shown to result in increased speed[162–164] and cadence during ambulation[164], increased stride length during ambulation[164] and increased stability of the paretic ankle joint during stance.[164]

Studies of the second type demonstrate that patients undergoing various treatments experience both increases in muscle performance and improvements in functional performance. Among the treatments shown to be accompanied by such results are resistance exercise,[58] functional electrical stimulation[108] and EMG biofeedback.[165]

HOW SHOULD WE TREAT MUSCLE WEAKNESS?

As an introduction to this section I must admit that it is far easier to identify muscle weakness as an appropriate target for treatment among stroke patients than it is to specify ways of bringing about increased muscle strength. Herein, two primary principles will be used to organize content. The first principle is that methods used to increase muscle strength should be feasible. The second principle is that methods used to increase muscle strength should incorporate existing information relative to muscle performance in stroke patients.

Feasible methods

By feasible methods, I mean methods that take both patient and nonpatient factors into account. Primary among patient factors are the goals and values that stroke patients and/or their families have for different activities. At least three studies have provided an indication of the value that patients have for functional activities. If it is activities such as walking and standing up and sitting down that patients most value,[166–168] then it follows that patients might participate more willingly and completely if such activities are the focus of treatment. The research of Yoder et al seems to support this contention. They found that added-purpose, occupationally embedded exercise elicited significantly more exercise repetitions than did rote exercise among female nursing home residents.[169] Although nonfunctional activities may be appropriate components of a strengthening regimen, they should not be used, in my opinion, in lieu of functional strengthening exercises. When the functional context of therapeutic interventions is not clear to a patient, I believe that an explanation of the functional relevance is in order.

Among the nonpatient factors of relevance to muscle strengthening are the amount of available time, the availability of equipment and the physical capacity of the clinician for working with the stroke patient. Evidently a substantial portion of the institutionalized stroke patient's time is spent simply sitting with no accompanying activity.[170, 171] Whether such a use of time is a matter of patient preference or not, it does represent time during which hands-on, supervised or independent activities could be engaged in to promote strengthening. The provision of opportunities to use 'down-time' for therapeutic ends would seem appropriate. Much, though of course not all, of what is done or might be done to strengthen stroke patients involves equipment. Characteristics that increase the feasibility that a piece of equipment will be used effectively in a variety of settings are simplicity, low cost, portability and adaptability. Some examples of how these characteristics are important will follow.

A simple biofeedback unit, that merely lets patients know when they have activated a target agonist muscle, may be better for independent use by patients than a computer bound device. Rather than using an expensive isokinetic dynamometer, chairs of varying heights can be used in conjunction with sit-stand-sit manoeuvres, to elicit varying amounts of concentric and eccentric activity in the quadriceps femoris muscles. A portable neuromuscular stimulator can be set up on patients, who then take the programmed unit with them for ongoing stimulation upon leaving the physical therapy department. A table top or cabinet unit could not be so used. Only if adaptable can some equipment be put to proper use. Unless a wheelchair's seat is low enough and its leg rests movable, it cannot be propelled by a stroke patient's lower extremities. A specific instance in which either equipment or assistance of another person is necessary to apply certain strengthening interventions, is when a clinician lacks the physical capacity to apply the intervention independently. Two such interventions could be the manual application of sufficient resistance during eccentric exercise or the provision of assistance during repeated sit to stand manoeuvres.

Methods incorporating research information

Like other therapeutic interventions applied to stroke patients, specific strengthening regimens have a very limited foundation in research. Nevertheless, some information exists which may be useful to clinicians who have available to them adequate time, equipment and or physical capacity. That information will be organized around the following working hypothesis: patients will only learn to generate more resultant force or torque when they are provided with experiences in which resultant force or torque is maximized.

Maximization of resultant force or torque with exercise

As the level of muscle's activation differs between exercise, I believe that functional exercises which maximize a muscle's activation should be sought. Electromyography can be used to determine the relative activation of a muscle group during various activities.[172] Bohannon has used EMG in this manner to demonstrate that the quadriceps femoris muscles are often activated more during sit to stand manoeuvres than during resisted knee extension in sitting. Asberg demonstrated that the sit to stand manoeuvre performed repetetively throughout the day had a significant effect on ADL independence measured during the first two weeks after stroke.[173] When a specific functional activity can not be used to activate a muscle group, a reasonable imitation of the movement may be adequate. Bohannon showed that resisted hip-knee extension patterns performed by supine stroke patients were relatively effective for activating the quadriceps femoris muscles.[16] Inaba et al found that a similar pattern performed against resistance by stroke patients on an Elgin^{R} table resulted in greater strength gains (13.5 lbs) than were demonstrated by a control group (7.0 lbs) or an active exercise group (4.3 lbs).[58] Other studies of the result of resistance exercise compared to alternatives, however, have not been so positive.[174] Because paretic agonist muscles are activated more and can generate greater resultant concentric force or torque at slow speeds,[24, 34, 37] training may need to be limited to such speeds until strength is adequately recovered. As stroke patients with spastic paresis activate their agonist muscles more and their antagonist muscles less, and generate greater resultant torque during eccentric than during concentric contractions,[37] eccentric exercise would appear to offer advantages over concentric exercise. When a stroke patient is unable to activate a paretic muscle in a shortened position, he may benefit from exercising the muscle in a lengthened position, where it can generate more resultant torque.[40] The efficacy of various techniques (e.g. brushing, vibrating, tapping) for augmenting muscle performance in stroke patients has been studied. Although such techniques may sometimes augment muscle performance during their application, they have no demonstrated residual effects.[175, 176] Thus, there may be little justification for their application beyond providing patients with a sense of using a muscle group.

Certain pharmacologic interventions can alter the stroke patient's ability to activate muscles during exercise. Their use, therefore, may of may not help to maximize resultant force or torque. Decisions about whether to use them should be made with knowledge of their influence on muscle performance. Tizandine appears to positively influence resultant torque through the enhancement of agonist activation and the inhibition of antagonist restraint.[150] Protirelin tartate[177] and thyrotropin-releasing hormone[178] also have been reported to affect strength positively. Baclofen and dantrolene sodium, on the other hand, appear to reduce resultant force.[110]

The influence of variables such as the frequency, intensity, duration and specificity of strength training on strength have not been investigated in stroke patients. They, nevertheless, may have as powerful an influence on the outcome of strengthening regimens in stroke patients as they do in healthy individuals. Thus, what is know about the variables[179] should be taken into account.

Maximization of resultant force or torque with electrical stimulation and/or biofeedback

Research studies indicate that electrical stimulation and/or biofeedback may be useful for maximizing resultant force or torque in stroke patients. Merletti et al investigated the effect of adding 20 minutes of peroneal nerve stimulation to one hour of traditional physical treatment for hemiparetic patients.[105] The recovery of ankle dorsiflexion torque was approximately three times greater in a group of subjects who received stimulation than in a group who did not. In another study Merletti et al provided patients with two months of traditional physical therapy.[104] During the second month they applied electrical stimulation to the ankle dorsiflexor muscles as well. The results of their study suggested that electrical stimulation had a positive effect on ankle dorsiflexion force during the second month, but that there was little residual effect from the stimulation two months later. Baker et al stated that patients with some active wrist extension at the beginning of a four week programme of passive cyclical electrical stimulation 'tended to develop stronger extension during the treatment program.'[98] The mean wrist extension torques demonstrated before (1.6 Newton metres) and after (2.5 Nm) the programme did not, however, differ significantly. Winchester et al showed that stroke patients who received feedback stimulation training and cyclical electrical stimulation to the knee extensor muscles for two hours per day made significant gains in voluntary knee extension torque over a four week period.[112] The mean increase in knee extension torque demonstrated by the stimulation group and a control group were 38 Nm and 19 Nm respectively. When electrical stimulation is used to increase strength in stroke patients the pattern of stimulation appears to matter. Because of the problem of muscle fatigue Packman-Braun recommended that 'a duty/cycle ratio of at least 1:5 should be used initially to enhance the effects of functional electrical stimulation to the wrist extensor muscles of patients with hemiparesis.'[99] Most electrical stimulation units should allow such a pattern. Lagasse and Roy showed an increase in the ratio of agonist to antagonist EMG following application of a specific pattern of stimulation.[26] That pattern, which is not possible with most commercially available units, consisted of a triphasic pattern with train frequencies adjusted to the natural firing frequency of the stimulated muscles.

Electromyographic feedback, like electrical stimulation, can be used to increase muscle strength. Basmajian et al found that strength and range of the ankle dorsiflexion motion increased about twice as much in an exercise and biofeedback group as in an exercise group.[106] Prevo et al also found EMG biofeedback to result in increased muscle strength.[101] When EMG biofeedback is used to increase muscle activation in stroke patients, greater residual effects may be realized if patients try to mimic the pattern of activation of the same muscles of their nonparetic side.[26] Such feedback, however, requires equipment that may not be available to most clinicians.

SUMMARY

Limitations in muscle strength are only one of many problems accompanying brain lesions. When defined as the maximum voluntary resultant force or torque that is brought to bear on the environment, muscle strength is a variable that can be measured manually or with instruments. Such measurements provide an indication of status, recovery and correlate with other important variables. Muscle strengthening, therefore, would appear to be an appropriate goal for interventions applied to many patients with brain lesions. Muscle strengthening programmes should incorporate feasible research based approaches.

REFERENCES

1. Bobath B 1970 Adult hemiplegia: evaluation and treatment (2nd edn.) William Heinemann Medical Books, London, p 18–19
2. Daniels L, Worthingham C 1986 Muscle testing techniques of manual examination (5th edn). W B Saunders, Philadelphia, PA, p 5
3. Wade D T, Hewer R L, Skilbeck C E, David R M 1985 Stroke. A critical approach to diagnosis, treatment, and management. Year Book Medical Publishers, Chicago, IL, p 23
4. Winter D A, White S C 1987 Cause-effect correlations of variables of gait. In: Jonsson B (ed) Biomechanics XA. Human Kinetics Publishers, Champaign, IL, p 363-368
5. Brooks V B, Stoney D 1971 Motor mechanisms: the role of the pyramidal system in motor control. Annual Review of Physiology 33: 337–392
6. Freund H J 1985 The pathophysiology of central paresis. In Struppler A, Weindl A (eds) Electromyography and evoked potentials. Springer-Verlag, Berlin, Federal Republic of Germany, p 19–20
7. Tang A, Rymer W Z 1981 Abnormal force — EMG relations in paretic limbs of hemiparetic human subjects. Journal of Neurology, Neurosurgery and Psychiatry 44: 690–698

8. Rosenfalck A, Andreassen S 1980 Impaired regulation of force and firing pattern of single motor units in patients with spasticity. Journal of Neurology, Neurosurgery and Psychiatry 43: 907–916
9. Sahrmann S A Norton B J 1977 The relationship of voluntary movement and spasticity in the upper motor neuron syndrome. Annals of Neurology 2: 460–465
10. Hammond M C, Fitts S S, Kraft G H, Nutter P B, Trotter M J, Robinson L M 1988 Cocontraction in the hemiparetic forearm: quantitative EMG evaluation. Archives of Physical Medicine and Rehabilitation 69: 348–351
11. Prezedborski S, Brunko E, Hubert M, Mavroudakis N, Zegers deBeyl D 1988 The effect of acute hemiplegia on intercostal muscle activity. Neurology 38: 1882–1884
12. Cruccu G, Fornarelli M, Manfredi M 1988 Impairment of masticatory function in hemiplegia. Neurology 38: 301–306
13. Knutsson E, Richards C 1979 Different types of disturbed motor control in gait in hemiparetic patients. Brain 102: 405–430
14. Dietz V, Berger W 1984 Interlimb coordination of posture in patients with spastic paresis. Brain 107: 965–978
15. Berger W, Horstmann G, Dietz V 1984 Tension development and muscle activation in the leg during gait in spastic hemiparesis: independence of muscle hypertonia and exaggerated stretch reflexes. Journal of Neurology, Neurosurgery and Psychiatry 47: 1029–1033
16. Bohannon R W 1990 Electromyographic activity of the quadriceps femoris muscles during four activities in stroke rehabilitation. International Journal of Rehabilitation Research 13: 80–82
17. Bohannon R W, Larkin P A 1987 Resistance to ankle dorsiflexions in hemiparetic stroke patients. Clinical Rehabilitation 1: 175–180
18. Halar E M, Stolov W C, Venkatesh B, Brozovich F V, Haley J D 1978 Gastrocnemius muscle and tendon belly length in stroke patients and able-bodied persons. Archives of Physical Medicine and Rehabilitation 59: 476–484
19. Thilman A F, Fellows S J, Ross H F 1991 Biomechanical changes at the ankle joint after stroke. Journal of Neurology, Neurosurgery and Psychiatry 54: 134–149
20. Hufschmidt A, Mauritz K H 1985 Chronic transformation of muscle in spasticity: a peripheral contribution to increased tone. Journal of Neurology, Neurosurgery and Psychiatry 48: 676–685
21. Lee W A, Boughton A, Rymer W Z 1987 Absence of stretch reflex gain enchancement in voluntarily activated spastic muscle. Experimental Neurology 98: 317–335
22. Reimers J 1990 Functional changes in the antagonist after lengthening the agonist in cerebral palsy I. Triceps surae lengthening. Clinical Orthopedics 253: 30–34
23. Colebatch J G, Gandevia S C, Spira R J 1986 Voluntary muscle strength in hemiparesis: distribution of weakness at the elbow. Journal of Neurology, Neurosurgery and Psychiatry 49: 1019–1024
24. Knutsson E, Martensson A 1980 Dynamic motor capacity in spastic paresis and its relation to prime mover dysfunction, spastic reflexes and antagonist co-activation. Scandinavian Journal of Rehabilitation Medicine 12: 93–106
25. Mizrahi E M, Angel R W 1979 Impairment of voluntary movement by spasticity. Annals of Neurology 5: 594–595
26. Lagasse P P, Roy M A 1989 Functional electrical stimulation and the reduction of co-contraction in spastic biceps brachii. Clinical Rehabilitation 3: 111–116

27. Hammond M C, Kraft G H, Fitts S S 1988 Recruitment and termination of electromyographic activity in the hemiparetic forearm. Archives of Physical Medicine and Rehabilitation 69: 106–110
28. Waters R L Garland D E, Perry J, Habig T, Slabaugh P 1979 Stiff-legged gait in hemiplegia: surgical correction. Journal of Bone and Joint Surgery 61[A]: 927–932
29. Duncan P W 1987 The effect of prior quadriceps contraction on knee flexor torque in normal subjects and multiple sclerosis patients with spastic paraparesis. Physiotherapy Practice 3: 11–17
30. Knutsson E 1985 Assessment for motor function in spastic paresis and its dependence on paresis and different types of restraint. In: Accles J, Dimitrijevic M R (eds) Upper motor neuron functions and dysfunctions. S Karger A G, Medical and Scientific Publishers, Basel, Switzerland, p 199–209
31. Bohannon R W 1988 Make tests and break tests of elbow flexor muscle strength. Physical Therapy 68: 193–194
32. Bohannon R W 1990 Make versus break tests for measuring elbow flexor muscle force with a hand-held dynamometer in patients with stroke. Physiotherapy Canada 42: 247–251
33. Norton B J, Sahrmann S A 1978 Reflex and voluntary electromyographic activity in patients with hemiparesis. Physical Therapy 58: 951–955
34. Bohannon R W 1987 Relative decreases in knee extension torque with increased knee extension velocities in stroke patients with hemiparesis. Physical Therapy 67: 1218–1220
35. Sjöström M, Fugl-Meyer A R, Nordin G, Wählby L 1980 Post-stroke hemiplegia, crural muscle strength and structure. Scandinavian Journal of Rehabilitation Medicine [Suppl. 7] 53–61
36. Nakamura R, Hosokawa T, Tsuji I 1985 Relationship of muscle strength for knee extension to walking capacity in patients with spastic hemiparesis. Tohoku Journal of Experimental Medicine 145: 335–340
37. Knutsson E, Gransberg L, Martensson A 1988 Facilitation and inhibition of maximal voluntary contractions by the activation of muscle stretch reflexes in patients with spastic paresis. EEG Clinical Neurophysiology 70: 37P–38P
38. Brunnstrom S 1970 Movement therapy in hemiplegia: a neurophysiological approach. Harper & Row, Hagerstown, MD, p 34–56
39. Bourbonnais D, Noven S V, Carey K M, Rymer W Z 1989 Abnormal spatial patterns of elbow muscle activation in hemiparetic human subjects. Brain 112: 85–102
40. Bohannon R W 1986 Decreased isometric knee flexion torque with hip extension in hemiparetic patients. Physical Therapy 66: 521–523
41. McDowell F, Louis S 1971 Improvement in motor performance in paretic and paralyzed extremities following nonembolic cerebral infarction. Stroke 2: 395–399
42. Fullerton K J, Mackenzie G, Stout R W 1988 Prognostic indices of stroke. Quarterly Journal of Medicine 66: 147–162
43. Wade D T, Hewer R L, David R M, Enderby P M 1986 Aphasia after stroke: natural history and associated deficits. Journal of Neurology, Neurosurgery and Psychiatry 49: 11–16
44. Wade D T, Hewer R L 1986 Stroke: associations with age, sex and side of weakness. Archives of Physical Medicine and Rehabilitation 67: 540–545
45. Collin C, Wade D T 1990 Assessing motor impairment after stroke: a pilot reliability study. Journal of Neurology, Neurosurgery and Psychiatry 53: 576–579
46. Parker V M, Wade D T, Hewer R L 1986 Loss of arm function after stroke: measurement, frequency, and recovery. International Journal of Rehabilitation Medicine 8: 69–73

47. Shiair R G, Champion S A, Freeman F R, Bugel H J 1979 Efficacy of myofeedback therapy in regaining control of lower extremity musculature following stroke. American Journal of Physical Medicine 58: 185–194
48. Jones H R, Millikan C H 1976 Temporal profile (clinical course) of acute carotid system cerebral infarction. Stroke 7: 64–71
49. Freund H J, Hummelsheim H 1988 Lesions of the premotor cortex in man. Brain 108: 697–733
50. Reding M J, Potes E 1988 Rehabilitation outcome following initial unilateral hemispheric stroke. Life table analysis approach. Stroke 19: 1354–1358
51. Olesen J, Simonsen K, Norgaard B, Gronback M, Johansen O S, Krogsgaard A, Andersen B 1988 Reproducibility and utility of a simple neurological scoring system for stroke patients (Cophenhagen Stroke Scale). Journal of Neurologic Rehabilitation 2: 59–63
52. Bonita R, Beaglehole R 1988 Recovery of motor function after stroke. Stroke 19: 1497–1500
53. Andrews K, Brocklehurst J C, Richards B, Laycock P J 1980 The prognostic value of picture drawings by stroke patients. Rheumatology and Rehabilitation 19: 180–188
54. Feigenson J S, McDowell F H, Meese P, McCarthy M L, Greenberg S D 1977 Factors influencing outcome and length of stay in a stroke rehabilitation unit: Part 1. Analysis of 248 unscreened patients—medical and functional prognostic indicators. Stroke 8: 651–656
55. Feigenson J S, McCarthy M L, Greenberg S D, Feigenson W D 1977 Factors influencing outcome and length of stay in a stroke rehabilitation unit: Part 2. Comparison of 318 screened and 248 unscreened patients. Stroke 8: 657–662
56. Adams R J, Meador K J, Sethi K, Grotta J C, Thomson D S 1987 Graded neurologic scale for use in acute hemispheric stroke treatment protocols. Stroke 18: 665–669
57. Dohrman G J, Nowack W J 1974 Relationship between various clinical signs in lesions of the descending motor system. Disease of the Nervous System 35: 375–377
58. Inaba M, Edberg E, Montgomery J, Gillis M K 1973 Effectiveness of functional training, active exercise, and resistive exercise for patients with hemiplegia. Physical Therapy 53: 28–35
59. Demeurisse G, Demol O, Robaye E 1980 Motor evaluation in vascular hemiplegia. Journal of European Neurology 19: 381–389
60. Smedley R R, Fiorino A J, Soucar E, Reynolds D 1986 Slot machines: their use in rehabilitation after stroke. Archives of Physical Medicine and Rehabilitation 67: 546–549
61. Andrews K, Brocklehurst J C, Richards B, Laycock P J 1981 The rate of recovery from stroke and its measurements. International Journal of Rehabilitation Medicine 3: 155–161
62. Andrews K, Brocklehurst J C, Richards B, Laycock P J 1982 The recovery of the severely disabled stroke patient. Rheumatology and Rehabilitation 21: 225–230
63. Verhas M, Schoutens A, Demol O, Patte M, Demeurisse G, Ganty C H, Rakofsky M 1975 Study in cerebrovascular disease: brain scanning with technetium 99m pertechnetate: clinical correlations. Neurology 25: 553–558
64. Watkins M P, Harris B A, Kozlowski B A 1984 Isokinetic testing in patients with hemiparesis: a pilot study. Physical Therapy 64: 184–189
65. Chalsen G G, Fitzpatrick K A, Navia R A, Bean S A, Reding M J 1987 Prevalence of the shoulder-hand pain syndrome in an inpatient stroke rehabilitation population: a quantitative cross-sectional study. Journal of Neurologic Rehabilitation 1: 137–141

66. Sheikh K, Smith D S, Meade T W, Brennan P J, Ide L 1980 Assessment of motor function in studies of chronic disability. Rheumatology and Rehabilitation 19: 83–90
67. Wade D T, Hewer R L 1987 Motor loss and swallowing difficulty after stroke: frequency, recovery, and prognosis. Acta Neurologica Scandinavica 76: 50–54
68. Logigian M K, Samuels M A, Falconer J, Zagar R 1983 Clinical exercise trial for stroke patients. Archives of Physical Medicine and Rehabilitation 64: 364–367
69. Merletti R, Acimovic R, Grobelnik S, et al 1975 Electrophysiological orthosis for the upper extremity in hemiplegia: Feasibility study. Archives of Physical Medicine and Rehabilitation 56: 507–513
70. Barer D H, Ebrahim S B, Mitchell J R A 1988 The pragmatic approach to stroke trial design: stroke register, pilot trial, assessment of neurological then function outcome. Neuroepidemiology 7: 1–12
71. Demeurisse G, Demol O, Robarge E 1979 Le bilan fontionnel dan l'hemiplegie vasculaire. Bruxelles Medical 59: 95–100
72. Dickstein R, Hockerman S, Pillar T, Shaham R 1986 Stroke rehabilitation: three exercise therapy approaches. Physical Therapy 66: 1233–1238
73. Wade D T, Skilbeck C, Hewer R L: 1989 Selective cognitive losses after stroke. Frequency, recovery, and prognostic importance. International Journal of Disability Studies 11: 34–39
74. Wade D T, Parker V, Hewer R L 1986 Memory disturbance after stroke: frequency and associated losses. International Journal of Rehabilitation Medicine 8: 60–64
75. Olsen T S 1990 Arm and leg paresis as outcome predictors in stroke rehabilitation. Stroke 21: 247–251
76. Knopman D S, Rubens A B 1986 The validity of computed tomographic scan findings for localization of cerebral functions. Archives of Neurology 43: 328–332
77. Visser S L, Aanen A 1981 Evaluation of EMG parameters for analysis and quantification of hemiparesis. Electromyographic Clinical Neurophysiology 21: 591–610
78. Friedman P J 1990 Spatial neglect in acute stroke: the line bisection test. Scandinavian Journal of Rehabilitation Medicine 22: 101–106
79. Allen C M C 1984 Predicting the outcome of acute stroke: a prognostic score. Journal of Neurology, Neurosurgery and Psychiatry 47: 475–480
80. Ee C H, Kwan P E, Tan E S 1991 Stroke rehabilitation of elderly patients in Singapore. Singapore Medical Journal 32: 55–60
81. Medical Research Council 1976 Aids to the investigation of peripheral nerve injuries. Her Majesty's Stationery Office, London
82. Nakamura R, Taniguchi R 1977 Reaction time in patients with cerebral hemiparesis. Neuropsychologia 15: 845–848
83. Heller A, Wade D T, Wood V A, Sunderland A, Hewer R L, Ward E 1987 Arm function after stroke: measurement and recovery over the first three months. Journal of Neurology, Neurosurgery and Psychiatry 50: 714–719
84. Wade D T, Hewer R L, Wood V A, et al 1983 The hemiplegic arm after stroke: measurement and recovery. Journal of Neurology, Neurosurgery and Psychiatry 46: 521–524
85. Hamrin E, Eklund G, Hillgren, A K, Borges O, Hall J, Hellström O 1982 Muscle strength and balance in post-stroke patients. Ups Journal Medical Science 87: 11–26
86. Quin C E 1971 Observations on the effects of proprioceptive neuromuscular facilitation techniques in the treatment of hemiplegia. Rheumatology and Physical Medicine 91: 186–192

87. Haaland K Y, Delaney H D 1981 Motor deficits after left or right hemisphere damage due to stroke or tumor. Neuropsychologia 19: 17–27
88. Dodrill C B 1978 The hand dynamometer as a neuropsychological measure. Journal of Consulting & Clinical Psychology 46: 1432–1435
89. Jones R D, Donaldson I M, Parkin P J 1989 Impairment and recovery of ipsilateral and sensory-motor function following unilateral cerebral infarction. Brain 112: 113–132
90. Smutok M A, Grafman J, Salazar A M, Sweeney J K, Jonas B S, DiRocco P J 1989 Effects of unilateral brain damage on contralateral and ipsilateral upper extremity function in hemiplegia. Physical Therapy 69: 195–203
91. Sunderland A, Tinson D, Bradley L, Hewer R L 1989 Arm function after stroke. An evaluation of grip strength as a measure of recovery and a prognostic indicator. Journal of Neurology, Neurosurgery and Psychiatry 52: 1267–1272
92. Sölgaard S, Kristiansen B, Jansen J S 1984 Evaluation of instruments for measuring grip strength. Acta Orthopedica Scandinavica 55: 569–572
93. Mathiowetz V, Weber V, Volland G, Kashman N 1984 Reliability and validity of grip and pinch strength evaluations. Journal of Hand Surgery 9 [A]: 222–226
94. Flood-Joy M, Mathiowetz V 1987 Grip-strength measurement: a comparison of three Jamar dynamometers. Occupational Therapy Journal of Research 7: 235–243
95. Mathiowetz V, Kashman N, Volland G, Weber K, Dowe M, Rogers S 1985 Grip and pinch strength: normative data for adults. Archives of Physical Medicine and Rehabilitation 66: 69–72
96. Agnew P J, Maas F 1982 Hand function related to age and sex. Archives of Physical Medicine and Rehabilitation 63: 269–271
97. Colebatch J G, Gandevia S C1989 The distribution of muscular weakness in upper motor neuron lesions affecting the arm. Brain 112: 749–763
98. Baker L L, Yeh C, Wilson D, Waters R L 1979 Electrical stimulation of wrist and fingers of hemiplegic patients. Physical Therapy 59: 1495–1499
99. Packman-Braun R 1988 Relationship between functional electrical stimulation duty cycle and fatigue in wrist extensor muscles of patients with hemiparesis. Physical Therapy 68: 51–56
100. Wilson D J, Baker L L, Craddock J A 1984 Functional test for the hemiparetic upper extremity. American Journal of Occupational Therapy 38: 159–164
101. Prevo A J H, Visser S L, Vogelaar T W 1982 Effect of EMG feedback on paretic muscles and abnormal co-contraction in the hemiplegic arm, compared with conventional physical therapy. Scandinavian Journal of Rehabilitation Medicine 14: 121–131
102. Ismail H M, Ranatunga K W 1981 Isometric contractions of normal and spastic human skeletal muscle. Muscle & Nerve 4: 214–218
103. Saltin B, Landin S 1975 Work capacity, muscle strength and SDH activity in both legs of hemiparetic patients and patients with Parkinson's disease. Scandinavian Journal of Clinical Laboratory Investigation 35: 531–538
104. Merletti R, Zelaschi F, Casale R, Sonetti L, Viola S 1978 Mid and long term variations of gross muscle force due to functional electrical stimulation in hemiparetic patients. Proceeding of 6th International Symposium on External Control of Human Extremities
105. Merletti R, Zelaschi F, Latella D, Galli M, Angeli S, Sessa M B 1978 A control study of muscle force recovery in hemiparetic patients during treatment with functional electrical stimulation. Scandinavian Journal of Rehabilitation Medicine 10: 147–154

106. Basmajian J V, Kukulka C G, Narayan M G, Takebe K 1975 Biofeedback treatment of foot drop after stroke compared with standard rehabilitation technique: effects on voluntary control and strength. Archives of Physical Medicine and Rehabilitation 56: 231–236
107. Teng E L, McNeal D R, Kralj A, Waters R L 1976 Electrical stimulation and feedback training: effects on the voluntary control of paretic muscle. Archives of Physical Medicine and Rehabilitation 57: 228–233
108. Carnstam B, Larsson L E, Prevec T S 1977 Improvement of gait following electrical stimulation. Scandinavian Journal of Rehabilitation Medicine 9: 7–13
109 Stefanovska A, Gros N, Vodovnik L, Rebersek S, Acimovic-Janezic R 1988 Chronic electrical stimulation for the modification of spasticity in hemiplegic patients. Scandinavian Journal of Rehabilitation Medicine [Suppl.17]: 115–121
110. Nakamura R, Tsuji I 1986 Effect of antispastic drugs on rapid force generation of spastic muscle. Tohoku Journal of Experimental Medicine 150: 447–453
111. Tsuji I, Nakamura R 1987 The altered time course of tension development during the initiation of fast movement in hemiplegic patients. Tohoku Journal of Experimental Medicine 151: 137–143
112. Winchester P, Montgomery J, Bowman B, Hislop H 1983 Effects of feedback stimulation training and cyclical electrical stimulation on knee extension in hemiparetic patients. Physical Therapy 63: 1096–1103
113. Tsuji I, Nakamura R 1988 Prolonged tension lag time of knee extensor muscle on twitch contraction in patients with spastic hemiparesis. Tohoku Journal of Experimental Medicine 156: 33–37
114. Moglia A, Arrigo A, Bejor M, Cattaneo S, Rascaroli M, Arrigo A, Scelsi R 1987 Surface EMG evaluation of quadriceps femoris muscle in hemiparetic patients. Functional Neurology 11: 181–187
115. Visser S L, Oosterhoff E, Hermens H J, Boon K L, Zilvold G 1985 Single twitch contraction curves in patients with spastic hemiparesis in relation to EMG findings. Electromyographic Clinical Neurophysiology 25: 63–71
116. Bohannon R W, Andrews A W 1989 Accuracy of spring and strain gauge hand-held dynamometers. Journal of Orthopaedic and Sports Physical Therapy 10: 323–325
117. Mastaglia F L, Knezevic W, Thompson P D 1986 Weakness of head turning in hemiplegia: a quantitative study. Journal of Neurology, Neurosurgery and Psychiatry 49: 195–197
118. Beevor C E 1909 Remarks on paralysis of movement of the trunk in hemiplegia. British Medical Journal 1: 881–885
119 Bohannon R W 1992 Lateral trunk flexion strength. Impairment, measurement reliability, and implications following brain injury. International Journal of Rehabilitation Research 15: 249–251
120. Bohannon R W 1991 Interrelationships of trunk and extremity muscle strengths and body awareness following unilateral brain lesions. Perception and Motor Skills 73: 1016–1018
121. Riddle D L, Finacune S D, Rothstein J M, Walker M L 1989 Intrasession and intersession reliability of hand-held dynamometer measurements taken on brain-damaged patients. Physical Therapy 69: 182–189
122. Bohannon R W, Larkin P A, Smith M B, Horton M G 1986 Shoulder pain in hemiplegia: statistical relationship with five variables. Archives of Physical Medicine and Rehabilitation 67: 514–516

123. Bohannon R W 1986 Strength of lower limb related to gait velocity and cadence in stroke patients. Physiotherapy Canada 38: 204–206
124. Bohannon R W, Smith M B 1987 Upper extremity strength deficits in hemiplegic stroke patients: relationship between admission and discharge and time since onset. Archives of Physical Medicine and Rehabilitation 68: 155–157
125. Bohannon R W 1987 Relationship between static strength and various other measures in hemiparetic stroke patients. International Journal of Rehabilitation Medicine 8: 125–128
126 Bohannon R W 1987 Assessement of strength deficits in eight paretic upper extremity muscle groups of stroke patients with hemiplegia. Physical Therapy 67: 522-525
127 Bohannon R W, Larkin P A, Smith M B, Horton M G 1987 Relationships between static muscle strength deficits and spasticity in stroke patients with hemiparesis. Physical Therapy 67: 1068-1071
128 Bohannon R W 1987 Gait performance of hemiparetic stroke patients: selected variables. Archives of Physical Medicine and Rehabilitation 68: 777-781
129. Bohannon R W 1987 Relationship between static standing capacity and lower limb static strength in hemiparetic stroke patients. Clinical Rehabilitation 1: 287–291
130. Bohannon R W, Andrews A W 1987 Relative strength of seven upper extremity muscle groups in hemiparetic stroke patients. Journal of Neurologic Rehabilitation 1: 161–165
131. Bohannon R W 1987 Relationship between strength and movement in the paretic lower limb following cerebrovascular accidents. International Journal of Rehabilitation Research 10: 420–422
132. Bohannon R W 1988 Relationship between shoulder pain and selected variables in patients with hemiplegia. Clinical Rehabilitation 2: 111–117
133. Bohannon R W 1988 Determinants of transfer capacity in patients with hemiplegia. Physiotherapy Canada 40: 236–239
134. Bohannon R W 1988 Rolling to the nonplegic side: influence of teaching and limb strength in hemiplegic stroke patients. Clinical Rehabilitation 2: 215–218
135. Bohannon R W 1988 Muscle strength changes in hemiparetic stroke patients during inpatient rehabilitation. Journal of Neurologic Rehabilitation 2: 163–166
136. Bohannon R W Andrews A W 1989 Influence of head-neck rotation on static elbow flexion force of paretic side in patients with hemiparesis. Physical Therapy 69: 135–137
137. Bohannon R W 1989 Selected determinants of ambulatory capacity in patients with hemiplegia. Clinical Rehabilitation 3: 47–53
138. Bohannon R W 1989 Correlation of lower limb strengths and other variables with standing performance in stroke patients. Physiotherapy Canada 41: 198–202
139. Bohannon R W 1989 Knee extension force measurements are reliable and indicative of walking speed in stroke patients. International Journal of Rehabilitation Research 12: 193–194
140. Bohannon R W 1990 Knee extension torque in stroke patients. Comparison of measurements obtained with hand-held and a Cybex dynamometer. Physiotherapy Canada 42: 284–287
141. Bohannon R W 1990 Significant relationships exist between muscle group strength following stroke. Clinical Rehabilitation 4: 29–32
142. Bohannon R W, Warren M E, Cogman K 1991 Influence of shoulder position on maximum voluntary elbow flexion force in stroke patients. Occupational Therapy Journal Research 11: 73–79

143. Bohannon R W, Warren M E, Cogman K 1991 Motor variables correlated with hand-to-mouth maneuver in stroke patients. Archives of Physical Medicine and Rehabilitation 72: 682–684
144. Bohannon R W, Walsh S 1991 Association of paretic lower extremity strength and balance with stair climbing ability in patients with stroke. Journal of Stroke and Cerebrovascular Disease 1: 129–133
145. Bohannon R W 1991 Relationship among paretic knee extension strength, maximum weightbearing, and gait speed in patients with stroke. Journal of Stroke Cerebrovascular Disease 1: 65–69
146. Bohannon R W 1991 Relationship between active range of motion deficits and muscle strength and tone at the elbow in patients with hemiparesis. Clinical Rehabilitation 5: 219–224
147. Winter D A, Wells R P, Orr G W 1981 Errors in the use of isokinetic dynamometers. European Journal of Applied Physiology 46: 397–408
148. Bohannon R W 1986 Upper extremity strength and strength relationships among young women. Journal of Orthopaedic and Sports Physical Threapy 8: 128–133
149. Bohannon R W, Andrews A W 1990 Correlation of knee extensor muscle torque and spasticity with gait speed in patients with stroke. Archives of Physical Medicine and Rehabilitation 71: 240–243
150. Knutsson E, Martensson A, Gransberg L 1982 Antiparetic and antispastic effects induced by tizanidine in patients with spastic paresis. Journal of Neurological Science 53: 187–204
151. Nakamura R, Watanabe S, Handa T, Morohashi I 1988 The relationship between walking speed and muscle strength for knee extension in hemiparetic stroke patients: a follow up study. Tohoku Journal of Experimental Medicine 154: 111–113
152. Stern P H, McDowell F, Miller J M, et al 1971 Factors influencing stroke rehabilitation. Stroke 2: 213–218
153. Stern P H, McCowell F, Miller J M, Robinson M 1970 Effects of facilitation — exercise techniques in stroke rehabilitation. Archives of Physical Medicine and Rehabilitation 51: 526–531
154. Bohannon R W 1991 Relationship between isometric torque and velocity of knee extension following stroke with hemiparesis. Journal of Human Muscle Performance 1(3): 40–46
155. Bohannon R W, Walsh S 1992 Nature, reliability, and predictive value of muscle performance measures in patients with hemiparesis following stroke. Archives of Physical Medicine and Rehabilitation 73: 721–725
156. Bohannon R W 1992 Knee extension power, velocity, and torque: relative deficits and relation to walking performance in stroke patients. Clinical Rehabilitation 6: 125–131
157. Tripp E J, Harris S R 1991 Test-retest reliability of isokinetic knee extension and flexion torque measurements in persons with spastic hemiparesis. Physical Therapy 71: 390–396
158. Katrak P H, Cole A M D, Poulos C J, McCauley J C K 1992 Objective assessment of spasticity, strength, and function with early exhibition of dantrolene sodium after cerebrovascular accident: a randomized double-blind study. Archives of Physical Medicine and Rehabilitation 73: 4–9
159. Bohannon R W, Larkin P A 1984 Knee flexion torque data. Opinions and comments. Physical Therapy 64: 959–960
160. Beasley W C 1956 Influence of method on estimates of normal knee extensor force among normal and postpolio children. Physical Therapy Reviews 36: 21–41
161. Bohannon R W 1991 Correlation of knee extension force and torque with gait speed in patients with stroke. Physiotherapy Practice 7: 185–190

162. Corcoran P J, Jebsen R H, Brengelmann G L, Simons B C 1970 Effects of plastic and metal leg braces on speed and energy cost of hemiparetic ambulation. Archives of Physical Medicine 51: 69–77
163. Lehmann J F, Condon S M, Price R, deLateur B J 1987 Gait abnormalities in the hemiplegic: their correction by ankle-foot orthoses. Archives of Physical Medicine and Rehabilitation 68: 763–771
164. Mojica J A P, Nakamura R, Kobayashi T, Handa T, Morohash I, Watanabe S 1988 Effect of ankle-foot orthosis (AFO) on body sway and walking capacity of hemiparetic stroke patients. Tohoko Journal of Experimental Medicine 156: 395–401
165. Binder S A, Moll C B, Wolf S L 1981 Evaluation of electromyographic biofeedback as an adjunct to therapeutic exercise in treating the lower extremities of hemiplegic patients. Physical Therapy 61: 886–893
166. Mumma C M 1986 Perceived losses following stroke. Rehabilitation Nursing 11: 19–24
167. Bohannon R W, Andrews A W, Smith M B 1988 Rehabilitation goals of patients with hemiplegia. International Journal of Rehabilitation Research 11: 181–183
168. Chiou I L, Burnett C N 1985 Values of activities of daily living. A survey of stroke patients and their home therapists. Physical Therapy 65: 901–906
169. Yoder R M, Nelson D L , Smith D A 1989 Added-purpose versus rate exercise in female nursing home residents. American Journal of Occupational Therapy 43: 581–586
170. Keith R A, Cowell K S 1987 Time use of stroke patients in three rehabilitation hospitals. Social Science and Medicine 24: 529–533
171. Tinson D J 1989 How stroke patients spend their days. International Journal of Disability Studies 11: 45–49
172. Wolf S L, Edwards D I, Shutter L A 1986 Concurrent assessment of muscle activity (CAMA): a procedural approach to assess treatment goals. Physical Therapy 66: 218–224
173. Asberg K H 1989 Orthostatic tolerance training of stroke patients in general medical wards. Scandinavian Journal of Rehabilitation Medicine 21: 179–185
174. Trombly C A, Thayer-Nason L, Bliss G, Girard C A, Lyrist A, Brexa-Hooson A 1986 The effectiveness of therapy in improving finger extension in stroke patients. American Journal of Occupational Therapy 40: 612–617
175. Matyas T A, Galea M P, Spicer S D 1986 Facilitation of maximum voluntary contraction in hemiplegia by concomitant cutaneous stimulation. American Journal of Physical Medicine 65: 125–134
176. Bohannon R W 1987 Hemiparetic elbow flexion force production before and after muscle belly tapping. Neurology Report 11: 75
177. Martinelli P 1990 Use of THR-T for symptomatic treatment of the pathology of the upper motoneurons and electrophysiologic evaluation of its efficacy. Annali Italiani di Medicina Interna 5: 262–269
178. Nakamura R, Fujita M 1990 Effect of thyrotropin-releasing hormone (TRH) on motor performance of hemiparetic stroke patients. Tohoku Journal of Experimental Medicine 160: 141–143
179. Bohannon R W 1990 Exercise training variables influencing the enhancement of voluntary muscle strength. Clinical Rehabilitation 4: 325–331

11. Low-back pain: strength tests and resistive exercises

Anne Elisabeth Ljunggren

I. INTRODUCTION

A. The impact of low-back trouble

Prevalence and incidence

Low-back trouble remains one of the most frequent and disabling conditions that affect people, especially during their productive years (Kelsey & White 1980). The prevalence (all cases at a certain time) and incidence (new cases during a defined time period) of low-back pain have been determined by retrospective, cross-sectional and prospective longitudinal studies in several countries, among which are the United States of America, Great Britain, the Netherlands and Scandinavia. The prevalence rates vary from a point prevalence of 14% (Biering-Sørensen 1982) to a month prevalence of 31% (Svensson & Andersson 1982). The life-time incidence values are higher and range from 49% (Hirsch et al 1969) to about 80% (Hult 1954), among which approximately 24% are of considerable severity (Frymoyer et al 1983). In a prospective study with questionnaires, Biering-Sørensen (1983) found that the one-year incidence in Copenhagen was 6% on average.

The rates of prevalence and incidence depend on the population studied, as well as the criteria used for definition of low-back pain. In particular, the frequency of reported pain is different from pain necessitating health care and hospitalization. It appears that the frequency of low-back *disability* as opposed to low-back pain has increased in the Western countries during the last three decades (Waddell 1987).

Natural course

Low-back problems have a differing prognosis in patients with acute, subchronic and chronic pain. The natural course of acute low-back pain favours recovery, and by two months about 90% of patients have resolution of the pain, irrespective of treatment given. However, 40–85% will experience recurring episodes; after six months 5% have persisting pain (Deyo & Tsui-Wu 1987) and 2% will be chronic (Åberg 1980). The reason might be that additional and cumulative trauma continues, even though initial musculoskeletal tissue injuries are healed. Postinjury deconditioning is frequently the major impediment to restoration of function. As the duration of disability approaches three months, the natural course of recovery from single episodes of low-back pain appears to change, the recovery curve becoming almost a flat line. Unfortunately, at this time a new pathophysiological diagnosis rarely can be made. Since many patients with chronic pain have combined biomedical, psychological and socioeconomic problems, determination of risk factors becomes of prime importance.

Consequences for working ability

Low-back disorders affect people in their most productive years. The trouble begins early in life, between 20–30 years of age, and the maximal frequency of symptoms appears in the age range of 30–60 years. As judged by health care utilization and time away from work, low-back pain causes the greatest problem in the middle working years of life, with a peak age of about 40 years (Kelsey et al 1979, Waddell 1987). Biering-Sørensen (1983) registered that among those gainfully employed at the time of the examination, 6.7% had taken days off within the past year because of low-back trouble, an absence rate which he calculates as corresponding to about two days per year per person. Low-back pain is considered second to the common cold as the major cause of work time lost (Kelsey & White 1980). In addition to loss of productivity, the inability to work creates suffering and diminished quality of life for the affected individuals.

Among those employees unable to work for more than six months because of low-back pain, only one half return to productive employment, and more than two years absenteeism due to back pain implies virtually no possibility of returning to work (Kelsey et al 1979). So, in the working population younger than 50 years, low-back pain is the second most frequent cause of disability pension (Kelsey et al 1979).

B. Muscle strength and etiology of low-back pain

Strength, pain and endurance

Measurements of trunk strength have been used to determine if there are differences between subjects with and without low-back pain. According to some investigations, patients with low-back pain have lower mean trunk strength than asymptomatic subjects (Nummi et al 1978, Addison & Schultz 1980, Hasue et al 1980, Karvonen et al 1980, MacNeill et al 1980, Nordgren et al 1980, Smidt et al 1983, Langrana et al 1984, Mayer et al 1985a, c). Lifting strength is also found to be decreased in persons disabled with chronic low-back pain (Chaffin & Park 1973, Biering-Sørensen 1984, Mayer et al 1988b). Pain itself is probably a strength reducing factor, as is the duration of back pain (Nachemson & Lindh 1969).

However, others have found no trunk strength difference between patients with low-back pain and controls (Pedersen et al 1975, Thorstensson & Arvidson 1982, Hemborg & Moritz 1985), and Suzuki & Endo (1983) noticed that duration of symptoms did not influence the strength of trunk muscles. Dehlin et al (1978) observed that nursing aides with back symptoms had lower quadriceps muscle strength than those with no current back symptoms or a history of them.

Most investigators have found trunk extensors to be weak compared to flexors in patients with low-back pain. However, Suzuki & Endo (1983) observed no such imbalance. Karvonen et al (1980) found that weak trunk extensors were associated with a history of sciatica and that weak trunk flexors were associated with back injuries and with current backache at work and exercise. In contrast, Nicolaisen & Jørgensen (1985) noticed that trunk strength was independent of the person's previous episodes of low-back pain. The findings are dependent upon the modes of tests used (see p. 231).

An association is indicated between low-back trouble and subnormal isometric endurance of the extensor trunk musculature (MacNeill et al 1980, Biering-Sørensen 1982, 1984; Nicolaisen & Jørgensen 1985), as well as isokinetic fatiguability (Suzuki & Endo 1983, Mayer et al 1985a). Differences in the distribution of slow and fast muscle fibres are suggested as an explanation of the endurance difference in patients and controls (Nicolaisen &

Jørgensen 1985). However, none of these studies clarifies whether a muscle weakness or imbalance is primary or secondary to low-back pain. In spite of this, the lack of muscle strength and endurance has frequently been cited as a suspected factor in the etiology of low-back pain.

Work demands

There appears to be a higher incidence of back pain in industries involving heavy work, the combination of a weak back and a low-back straining occupation greatly increasing the risk of low-back trouble (Chaffin 1974). This investigator together with Chaffin et al (1978) and Keyserling et al (1980) explored this relationship further using pre-employment isometric strength testing procedures with lifting. When the job requirements exceeded the strength capability of the person in an isometric test simulating the lifting job, the risk of a back injury was found to increase up to three fold. Davis & Dotson (1987) recommend that physical testing be required periodically, and not just used as a pre-employment assessment.

On the other hand, in a prospective study Troup et al (1987) found that none of the pre-employment screening tests, among these the maximal isometric lifting strength, were of value in predicting new cases of low-back pain.

Some studies of the isometric lifting strength even suggest that the strongest employees are at greater risk than the weaker ones (Battié et al 1989). High muscular forces give high compressive forces on the lumbar segments. In a Norwegian investigation in postal services (Nesse 1983), the strongest males had the highest frequency of back pain. This was explained by their generally reckless movement patterns, whereas the weaker male workers tended to omit loading activities.

To determine the importance of strength in preventing back pain one has to control for job demands, age, weight and sex (Biering-Sørensen 1984, Frymoyer et al 1983, Battié et al 1989), strength being important for specific tasks. Static strength is probably of less importance than dynamic strength and endurance in the development of low-back trouble. Only static strength has been tested in the pre-employment screening studies. However, Magora (1974) has already pointed out the problem of prolonged maintenance of a particular posture. Endurance capability of back extensor muscles seems to be of prime importance in withstanding postural stress, but even the most ideal and perfectly trained muscle can never adapt to static work. Muscle circulation, movement pattern and respiration also are important factors for working capacity and strength, especially in endurance (Sundsvold & Vaglum 1985).

It is still not clear whether back injury occurs as a result of poor match between job demands and the physical capabilities of the individual, poor use of body mechanics, or even fatigue and lack of coordination.

Other risk factors

People who are physically fit appear to have decreased incidence of low-back pain (Cady et al 1985). Prior history of back problems is established as a strong predictor of low-back trouble (Biering-Sørensen 1984, Troup et al 1987, Battié et al 1989). Weak trunk muscles are found with recurring or ongoing low-back trouble. Recurrent episodes of low-back pain probably represent a higher risk factor than first time episodes. Psychological aspects also have to be taken in to account: having a strong back is considered to be a sign of human strength; when afflicted with back pain, one is made to feel weak. Symptoms make themselves manifest to a greater or lesser degree depending on the psychological constitution. Braatøy (1965) included the trunk musculature among the mimic muscles, and even considered them to be the most important ones.

II. EVALUATION OF TRUNK STRENGTH AND ENDURANCE

The early methods for testing trunk strength are primitive when compared to the more recently developed varieties (Beimborm & Morrissey 1988). Today there is a great variation in equipment, methods and procedures, as well as type and speed of contraction recommended for testing.

A. Methods of measurement

There are several methods of muscular strength measurement: isometric, isokinetic (concentric or eccentric) and isoinertial, all except the first one referring to dynamic muscle work (Pitman & Peterson 1989). In addition to these one may include conventional functional tests, psychophysical testing and myoelectric registrations, and morphological measures. Lifting is a commonly used strength testing modality where isometric, isokinetic and isoinertial, as well as psychophysical, categories may be applied.

Isometric strength

Isometric strength is the ability to perform a static form of exercise against a constant resistance and with no observable joint movement. It has been tested using scales or strength gauges that are pulled on or pushed against. The first isometric strength tests of trunk flexion and extension were performed in the neutral, upright position. Later testing has been applied at different points in the range of motion. A summary of some studies of normal isometric strength is given in Table 11.1.

For testing isometric extensor trunk endurance, the method standardized by Biering-Sørensen (1984) is in widespread use. The so-called 'Sørensen test' measures the period of time the unsupported upper part of the body of the prone lying person can be kept horizontal (up to 240 seconds). Hasue et al (1980) and Smidt et al (1983) noticed that trunk flexors fatigue faster than trunk extensors. However, to date no standardized method for the testing of isometric flexor trunk endurance has been published.

Isokinetic strength

During the last decade the concept of isokinetic movement has been diligently used. These movements are performed at a constant speed, selected by the clinician, and with totally accommodating resistance throughout the entire range of motion. The subject can never exceed the set speed, no matter how much effort is exerted, increased effort resulting in increased resistance, not faster speed. The force output is displayed as a curve (Fig. 11.1). For trunk flexion, extension and rotation the curve illustrates the torque at each point in the range of motion. By examining the shape of the curve throughout the range of motion it is possible to locate problem areas that may be due to pain, fatigue, muscular weakness or mechanical dysfunction (Fig. 11.1 c and d).

With the advent of isokinetic testing, accurate analysis of the concentric and eccentric torque producing performance of the muscles has been achieved. This method can demonstrate endurance factors as well as coordination factors (Mayer & Gatchel 1988). Rapid motion seems to be much more discriminating than slow motion in terms of loss of muscular function in patients with low-back pain, whereas isokinetic tests at slow speeds are considered to reveal articular problems. A summary of some studies of normal isokinetic strength is given in Table 11.2.

Measurement of isokinetic strength requires special equipment providing selective training and measurement. As always in testing, control of subject position is vital so that comparison from one occasion to another may be accomplished. Further, physiologic movement is not simulated, as might be the case with measurement of isoinertial strength.

Isoinertial strength

The most recent advance in the area of functional assessment of the spine is the testing of isoinertial muscle contraction (Parnianpour et al 1988, 1989). In an isoinertial contraction, muscles work against a constant load. If the muscle generated torque is equal to or less than the resistance, the muscle length remains unchanged; however, if the muscle torque is greater than the resistance, the muscle shortens and the surplus torque will determine the acceleration of the body part (Kroemer 1983).

The spine represents complex spatial joints, giving simultaneous motion in three planes. This requires a three-axial measurement system. Most dynamometers in use are uni-axial, and thus treat the joints as planar hinge joints. Equipment testing trunk strength in three-dimensional motion may give added insight into spinal injury and rehabilitation. Such information is obtained through the Isostation B200 device, which measures the torque, angular position and velocity for all three axes simultaneously (Parnianpour et al 1988, 1989). In these studies fatigue is reflected by changes of position noted isodynamically, the mode of muscle contraction being isoinertial. A summary of normal isoinertial strength is given in Table 11.3.

Conventional functional tests

Since the demands for muscle torque change throughout a movement, muscle tension must *adapt*, and the term 'isotonic muscle contraction' in its truest sense does not exist (Pitman & Peterson 1989). However, in trunk testing and exercising, isotonic contractions are still considered to occur when using constant resistance, such as dumb-bells, or simply the weight of the trunk alone. In these situations, the number of sit-ups and spinal extension arches completed have been used as indicators of trunk flexor and extensor strength, respectively. Among others, Nummi et al (1978) used methods for evaluating back and abdominal dynamic muscle performance capacity. They considered as normal at least seven repetitions without jerks.

With traditional isotonics, there is no way to accommodate for biomechanical leverage changes that increase and decrease muscular efficiency throughout the range of motion, therefore the dynamically contracting muscle is only loaded maximally at its weakest point in the range of motion. Smidt et al (1983) and Smidt & Blanpied (1987) conclude that conventional clinical tests of trunk strength are inadequate as they are poor discriminators and lack the range or resistance necessary to cover the spectrum of human strength capability.

A subcategory of isotonics, called 'variable resistance exercise,' was designed in response to this problem. These exercises are performed on specially designed weight machines. With the use of a cam, resistance varies throughout the range of motion, even though the specific amount of weight being lifted remains constant. This varying resistance does help accommodate for biomechanical leverage changes. However, because of differences in individual size and strength, the muscle may still not be loaded to its full capacity throughout the entire range of motion.

Lifting

Lifting has been diligently used as a mode of strength testing in isometric (Chaffin & Park 1973, Chaffin 1974, Chaffin et al 1978), isokinetic (Mayer et al 1985c, 1988b) and isoinertial (Mayer et al 1988a, 1990) regimes.

With respect to isometrics, a single exertion in a given lifting position usually allows fairly precise prediction of the subjects' mean strength in that position (Zeh et al 1986, Chaffin et al 1978, Keyserling et al 1980). If several positions are to be tested, it is recommended to do only one lift in a given position to minimize the risk of injury during strength testing. However, using two lifts in a given position improves precision of the strength assessment and may therefore be warranted if only one or two positions are to be tested. The testing of isometric lifting does not reflect natural lifting. Marras et al (1984) showed prominent differences in trunk muscle recruitment patterns during static and isokinetic lifting exertions.

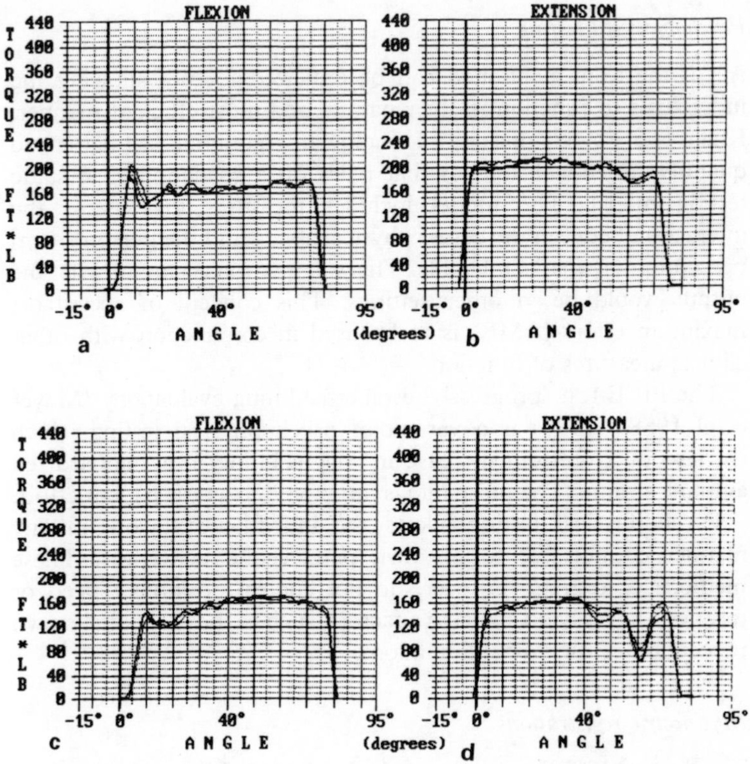

Fig. 11.1 Flexion (a and c) and extension (b and d) curves with three repetitions of isokinetic (Cybex TEF) contractions maximum at 60°/second in two well-trained males, both in their forties: a and b are normal curves; in c and d the curve shapes indicate spine pathology, in this case probably a pattern of insufficient segmental control ('instability').

They conclude that work recommendations based upon isometric tests can be misleading. Concerning manual lifting tasks, Mital et al (1986) warn that even high frequency lifting (three times or more per minute) is not strength oriented.

In isokinetics, faster speeds are considered to accompany decreased joint compressive forces. However, Hall (1985) demonstrated that the faster lifting significantly increases compressive and shear forces at the L5/S1 level and generates a higher external moment to be balanced by the muscles and other structures of the back.

Psychophysical testing

All of the tests mentioned can be criticized for not allowing the individuals to function in their natural and most efficient manner. Khalil et al (1987) decided to employ an ergonomic test battery to quantify functional abilities that relies on a psychophysical static testing model. The model includes measures that assess the interaction between the actual physical ability and the person's own perception of what is tolerable. This will give a measure of what the output would be in other settings. This concept of acceptable maximum effort (AME) is to be used in conjunction with other clinical measures of function.

The PILE test (progressive isoinertial lifting evaluation) (Mayer et al 1988a, 1990) is a variant of psychophysical testing which carries out a uniform increase in weight lifting in a standardized amount of time. The pulse rate is monitored to assess patient effort.

Psychophysical testing allows the individual to work in any manner comfortable to his own perceived effectiveness. These methods of testing, however, do not control positions, speed or torque. They rely on subjective factors, such as the individual's own perception of functional limitations.

Myoelectric registrations

Trunk muscle fatigue also can be evaluated through myoelectric testing (Kondraske et al 1987). It has been shown that a fatiguing muscle will reduce the frequency of discharge, and therefore there will be a shift of the median or mean signal frequency level to a slower rate.

A difference in EMG curves has been demonstrated between those who develop back pain during prolonged postural stress and those who do not (DeVries 1968). Using sustained isometric contraction at different force levels, Roy et al (1989) pointed out that specific median frequency variables of the surface EMG correctly classified patients with low-back pain versus controls. However, Mayer et al (1989b) found no significant correlation between myoeletric spectral analysis for endurance assessment and isokinetic trunk strength measures.

Morphological measures

Mayer et al (1989a) report significant correlations between increased isokinetic extensor muscle strength and greater extensor muscle density on CT scan. Laasonen (1984) revealed atrophy in the paraspinal and psoas muscles in patients with multiple operations on the lower back. Thus, it is possible that morphological measures can be used as indicators of strength loss and gain.

B. Variables that influence selection of a method of measurement

Strength is a complicated quality which has to be measured through a number of characteristics. There is no one test which alone allows optimal evaluation of strength testing in the lumbar spine, either for prediction of failure, assigning normal function or assessing rehabilitation progress (Mayer et al 1985c, Mayer & Gatchel 1988). Such a test would, however, be very useful in terms of cost-effectiveness analyses.

It also remains difficult to understand fully what should be measured. With computer technology it is possible to measure many variables, such as peak torque, average torque, torque at specific angles and velocities, power, rate of fatigue, work and strength ratios, e.g. for flexors versus extensors. Current evidence suggests that average power and total work produced probably are very useful measures, as is the average points variance, which serves as a measure of consistency between sets of curves taken at the same speed (Mayer & Gatchel 1988). Parnianpour et al (1990) have shown that velocity and power are better discriminators of the patient's capability than torque, even the isoinertial torque variety. The shapes of curves showing torque/position angle relationships are informative in functional assessment, the consistency of curves being of particular value (see Fig. 11.1, p. 235). Hazard et al (1988) conclude that clinical judgement is required in evaluating effort during tests as maximal and submaximal isokinetic trunk and lifting strength. The working technique of the patient might be a significant, but rather problematic variable to measure.

Evaluation of functional abilities still needs to be standardized. Currently it is nearly impossible to compare results from different studies on treatment outcomes in view of the widely divergent methods used to measure progress (Tables 11.1–11.3). The subject's motivation is of major importance for the results of strength tests. As an example, in a test-retest situation of the rectus abdominal muscle, a learning effect was found to represent an isometric flexion increase of 17% (Stokes et al 1989).

Table 11.1 Summary of some studies concerning normal isometric muscle strength of trunk flexors (F) and extensors (E).

Authors	Subjects (n)	Testing position	Testing equipment	Mean peak torque (Nm) F (SD)	E (SD)	Mean ratio F/E
Smidt et al 1983	Males (12)	Sitting	Iowa	290	350	0.83
	Females (12)	Sitting	Iowa	150	200	0.75
Langrana et al 1984	Males (50)	Sitting	Cybex II	130(45)	239(85)	0.54
	Females (26)	Sitting	Cybex II	64(22)	123(57)	0.52
Reid & Costigan 1987	Males (20)	Sitting (F) Kneeling(E)	KIN/COM KIN/COM	120(31)	143(31)	0.85
Addison & Schultz 1980	Males (27)	Standing	Harness	149	210	0.71
	Females (30)	Standing	Strain-gauge	87	117	0.74
Parnian-pour et al 1988	Males (20)	Standing	Isostation B200	198(55)	200(46)	0.99
Smidt et al 1980	Males (11)	Side-lying	Iowa	194(33)	293(62)	0.66
Nordin et al 1987	Females (101)	Lying: Supine (F) Prone (E)	Cybex II	61(19)	98(23)	0.62

Muscle synergies

In testing trunk strength it is difficult to separate the hip and the lower back. Thorstensson & Nilsson (1982) observed maximum torque output to be larger with the axis at the trochanter major than when the pivot point was at L2–3 (Table 11.2). They also found that with the centre of rotation at the hip joint, the relative contribution of the hip muscles to the total torque produced was larger for the flexors than for the extensors, and that it varied with velocity and position. Accordingly, a strength difference between patients and controls was only found in the initial part of isokinetic trunk flexion (Thorstensson & Arvidson 1982).

The interaction of the hip and spine in trunk extension refers especially to lifting. The order of recruitment in standing trunk extension is as follows: hamstrings muscles and the glutei, and then the paravertebral muscles (Örtengren & Andersson 1977). Forward

Table 11.2 Summary of some studies concerning normal isokinetic muscle strength of trunk flexors (F) and extensors (E)

Authors	Subjects (n)	Testing position	Testing equipment	Speed (°/sec)	Mean peak torque (Nm) F (SD)	E (SD)	Mean ratio F/E
Langrana et al 1984	Males (50)	Sitting	Cybex II	30	137(43)	212(66)	0.65
	Females (26)	Sitting	Cybex II	30	60(15)	98(46)	0.61
Nordin et al 1987	Females (101)	Sitting	Cybex II	30	111(28)	122(40)	0.90
				60	107(38)	108(41)	0.99
Thorstensson & Nilsson 1982	Males (14)	Side-lying (axis at L2–3	Cybex II	15	91(23)	250(51)	0.36
					86(20)	242(50)	0.36
				30			

bend in standing position is primarily controlled by an eccentric contraction of the trunk extensors (Morris et al 1962). In trunk flexion the firing sequence is less clear.

Consequences of contraction modalities, speed and inertia

It is possible to generate more torque isometrically than concentrically (Tables 11.1 and 11.2), and still more eccentrically. Moreover, increased velocity gives increased eccentric torque and decreased concentric torque. However, there appears to be a physiological inhibition to maximal eccentric contractions. This safety switch implies that we can never obtain a true maximal effort with testing of voluntary eccentric force output (Westing et al 1988).

Table 11.3 Summary of normal isoinertial trunk muscle strength in different planes using Isostation B200

Authors	Subjects (n)	Resistance level % of MVC	Maximum torque (Nm) Sagittal (SD)	Coronal (SD)	Transverse (SD)
Parnianpour et al 1989	Males (9)	100	160(46)	126(40)	107(41)
		70	148(29)	102(14)	135(45)
		50	121(27)	87(20)	106(46)
		30	83(20)	61(19)	45(32)

Smidt et al (1980) found eccentric contractions of both trunk flexors and extensors to be stronger than concentric contractions. Smidt et al (1980) and Thorstensson & Nilsson (1982) observed isometric contractions to be strongest with the muscle in a stretched position near the end of the range of motion. In such positions isometric torques even exceeded those in eccentric contractions (Smidt et al 1980).

Parnianpour et al (1987) found poor correlations between normal isometric and isokinetic trunk strength and endurance, thus making dynamic strength assessment indispensable in the clinical setting.

In trunk testing the significance of gravitational force on the upper body increases with speed. Several studies (Troup & Chapman 1969, Smidt et al 1980, Thorstensson & Arvidson 1982, Torstensson & Nilsson 1982) have used apparatus that allows gravity to be eliminated or considered in data analysis. As inertia tends to assist flexion and hinder extension in most testing conditions, these studies show flexion/extension ratios to be lower than in studies performed without the elimination of gravity.

Effect of position

Strength testing has been performed with the person in the seated position (Smidt et al 1983, Langrana et al 1984, Reid & Costigan 1987), or standing (Addison & Schultz 1980, MacNeill et al 1980, Mayer et al 1985a, c, Smith et al 1985, Parnianpour et al 1988), or in the prone or supine position (Smidt et al 1980, Thorstensson & Nilsson 1982, Suzuki & Endo 1983, Nordin et al 1987).

Pedersen & Staffeldt (1972) compared four different back muscle strength tests and found the standing maximal isometric test to be the most reliable and best suited for untrained persons. Recent testing systems adopt the standing position, which is supposed to reflect functional vertebral body positioning and maintain normal orientation of the spinal curves. However, Kumar (1989) found that the trunk strength in the sitting position was higher than in the standing, and that lying position gave the lowest strength values. He recommends a seated posture to be adopted as the standard for functional evaluation, whereas strength testing for occupational purposes should be performed in job simulated postures.

Pain

Studies comparing strength in normals versus patients with low-back pain require special consideration because of the influence of the pain itself on the force-producing capacity of the individual patient. Pain can greatly hinder maximal effort and, as a result, testing of patients with low-back pain may actually be tests of their pain level and tolerance. In addition to the effects of pain on effort, the pathologic problems that occur in low-back pain patients may result in reflex inhibition of the surrounding musculature. In light of these confounding factors, precise analysis of pain level is important and must be controlled when comparing trunk force production in patients with low-back pain.

C. Normal muscle torque values

Training goals and effects have to be related to normal values. In peripheral joint injury, muscle torque in the injured extremity is often determined relative to the uninjured extremity. As a criterion for return to sports in knee injuries, some authors recommend the strength of the injured knee extensors should be at least 80% of the uninjured leg. These values may differ in various muscle groups (Beimborn & Morrissey 1988).

In the trunk we may relate the muscle strength of the injured individual to preinjury values. However, such information is usually not available. In these circumstances we are restricted to comparing strength values in the individual patient to normative values for the muscle group and motion in question in uninjured subjects of the same sex, similar age and activity level. A criterion of 80–90% may then prove useful for return to activities such as sports and heavy work.

The generated muscle torques result from at least the following factors: sex, age, height, weight and activity level of the individual, muscle mass and length, length of the muscle's lever arm, the testing apparatus used, subject position, rotation axis, speed, duration of measurement, repetitions and rest allowed between successive trials. The instructions given represent another influence, human strength being the result of many motivational and psychological processes. These factors may affect trunk flexion, extension, lateral flexion and rotation differently. Summaries of some studies giving normal isometric, isokinetic and isoinertial muscle strength in trunk flexors and extensors are given in Tables 11.1–11.3.

The muscle strength given in torque has to be related to body weight. Mayer et al (1985a, b, c) and Smith et al (1985) give torque/body weight ratios. For trunk extensors these ratios (Nm/kg) should amount to a value of about 2, to comply with ordinary work demands (Harstad et al 1990).

Muscle strength ratios

The relative ranking of the normal strength of the muscle groups for trunk motions is as follows: trunk extensors, flexors, lateral flexors and rotators (Beimborn & Morrissey 1988). Greater normal trunk extension force compared to flexion has been noted in all modes of testing: isometric (Asmussen & Heebøll-Nielsen 1959, Troup & Chapman 1969, Addison & Schultz 1980, MacNeill et al 1980, Heebøll-Nielsen 1982, Portillo et al 1982, Nicolaisen & Jørgensen 1985), as well as isokinetic (Hasue et al 1980, Smidt et al 1980, 1983, Davies & Gould 1982, Thorstensson & Arvidson 1982, Thorstensson & Nilsson 1982, Suzuki & Endo 1983, Langrana et al 1984, Mayer et al 1985a, c, Smith et al 1985, Nordin et al 1987), isoinertial (Parnianpour et al 1988), and non-specific dynamic (Flint 1958, Nachemson & Lindh 1969).

As is shown in Tables 11.1 and 11.2, the trunk peak torque flexor/extensor ratio changes with the different investigations. This is primarily due to various methods of testing and background variables used in the analyses. The ratio shows larger variations in isokinetics than in isometrics. It is suggested that trunk extensors should be 30% stronger than the flexors, i.e. a ratio of about 0.70.

It seems that the normal ratio of left/right lateral flexion (MacNeill et al 1980, Portillo et al 1982, Thorstensson & Arvidson 1982) as well as left/right transversal rotation (Mayer et al 1985b, Smith et al 1985) is approximately 1. However, the torque of right side bending is found to be slightly higher than left side bending (Addison & Schultz 1980, Parnianpour et al 1988).

Sex differences

As shown in Table 11.1, the female/male ratio for isometric trunk strength varies between 0.49 and 0.58. Chaffin (1974) found isometric lifting strength in females to be 58% of that in males, whereas Troup & Chapman (1969) report 64%. According to Smith et al (1985), total isokinetic trunk strength for females is about ⅔ that of males. The ratio found by Langrana et al (1984) with isokinetic testing is lower (Table 11.2).

Smith et al (1985) calculated torque to body weight ratios (ft lb/lb) for males and females, and found the ratios in males to be 67–95 in flexion and 110–124 in extension. In females the corresponding values were 40–70 and 79–94.

Static back muscle endurance is observed to be less in males than in females (Biering-Sørensen 1984, Nicolaisen & Jørgensen 1985), which might explain the preponderance of reported low-back trouble in males. The latter authors suggested that this difference is explained by larger intramuscular pressures in men.

Age differences

In proportion to age it is found that both trunk flexors and extensors become markedly weaker after the age of 40 years (Hasue et al 1980). In males the weakening was at the same pace for flexors and extensors; in females muscle balance was influenced by the aging process, abdominal muscles becoming weaker than extensors. However, Smith et al (1985) found that trunk extensor and flexor strength remain equivalent between persons in their third and fourth decades.

III. CONTRAINDICATIONS TO TESTING AND TRAINING

Prior to any test, indications and contraindications relative to musculoskeletal, neuromuscular, cardiovascular and other physical conditions should be carefully assessed. Patients with acutely injured discs and other recent trauma should not be tested or exercised for strength purposes. This is also essential in case of neurological signs and peripheralizing pain. In cases of recent back surgery and chemonucleolysis, trunk strength testing and training are to be avoided. Patients should not be tested routinely until two to six months post-surgery and six weeks to three months after chemonucleolysis. In the United States, glaucoma, pregnancy and hypertension are included in the list of relative contraindications to strength testing and training. Other considerations for contraindication include osteoporosis, spinal tumours, inflammatory disease and impaired circulation.

IV. TRAINING GOALS AND EFFECTS

A. Goals

The cause of low-back pain in the individual patient is often elusive, and an understanding of the anatomy and pathophysiology is frequently insufficient to direct effective prevention and treatment (Flor & Turk 1984). The primary training goal is to avoid first time episodes of low-back trouble. Goals of physical rehabilitation programmes for a patient with low-back trouble are to prevent recurrences of low-back pain and return the patient to work and normal activities. The prevention of back pain, rather than treating the resultant disability, represents a cost saving effort.

Even patients undergoing simple discectomy have substantial functional deficits in lumbar spine capacity. These may subject the postoperative patient to recurrences of injuries that produce a vicious circle, leading to permanent disability (Mayer & Gatchel 1988). In patients with failed back syndrome an estimation of rehabilitative potential is probably equally important as an assessment of specific therapeutic interventional needs. Inherent in this type of assessment should be an effort to identify symptom amplifiers as well as motivational factors.

Exercise for trunk muscles is one of the most commonly prescribed treatment modalities for patients with low-back pain. The purpose of physical training is to stress the body systematically so that it improves its capacity to withstand physical stress.

Training goals should be concrete and, preferably, possible to evaluate in an objective way. Training programmes should be systematically progressive. Quantification of human performance is not only helpful in tracing response to treatment, it also provides a basis for prevention by identifying the physical functional deficits compared to the demands of occupation and environment. It is probably more important for such quantification of physical performance to be matched against the demands of the individual occupation and environment rather than to some set of normative values. Adequate muscular strength in the trunk appears mandatory for a return to function and employment following a back injury and pain. Usually the job itself does not provide sufficient stimulus to maintain fitness. Therefore a physical fitness programme should be an integral part of the daily schedule (Davis & Dotson 1987). Also the relative importance of trunk versus whole body performance in relation to future low-back injury risk should be defined.

B. Effects

Strength

Data indicate that commonly prescribed strengthening and flexibility exercise programmes may not be helpful (Jackson & Brown 1983a). Smidt et al (1983) and Smidt & Blanpied (1987) demonstrate that conventional clinical resistive exercises do not provide appropriate resistance for improving trunk muscle strength in most people. In examining six different abdominal muscle exercises, Ekholm et al (1979) found that the curl-up variant activated the rectus and oblique muscles most, but only to 50% of the values for maximum isometric contraction as measured by integrated EMG.

According to this, several clinical trials found that abdominal strengthening and back flexibility exercises for low-back pain did not assist patients in getting over symptoms or returning sooner to normal activities (Bergquist-Ullman & Larsson 1977, Davies et al 1979, Kendall & Jenkins 1968a, Lidström & Zachrisson 1970, Martin et al 1986). Abdominal strengthening and flexibility exercises also are often poorly tolerated, and the patient drop-out rate is high. Partial sit-up exercises impose considerable mechanical stress on the back (Kendall & Jenkins 1968b, Nachemson & Elfström 1970). There are even indications that these exercises actually can delay the patient's recovery (Kendall & Jenkins 1968a). Additionally, there is little justification for recommending trunk strengthening exercises to increase intra-abdominal pressure (Hemborg et al 1985).

On the other hand, Gracovetsky et al (1985) advocate the strengthening of muscles acting on the thoracolumbar fascia, finding this fascia to be important in stabilizing the lumbar spine. Anatomical and biomechanical analyses (Macintosh et al 1987) point out the importance of the back muscles, but question the relevance of the abdominal muscles in trunk stabilization. In agreement with this, Manniche et al (1988) have shown excellent results in patients with chronic low-back pain with intensive dynamic back extensor exercises, ad modum Plum & Rehfeld (1985), over a period of three months. Manniche et al (1988) stress the importance of lifelong exercising. Among others Mayer et al (1985c) found increased trunk extensor strength to be correlated with working capability.

Fitness

The concept of *fitness* has been emphasized strongly for patients with low-back pain, fitness being a broad term, including in its definition strengthening exercises and cardiovascular status. Aerobic conditioning exercises appear to offer the greatest benefit for all types of patients with low-back pain (Jackson & Brown 1983b, Liemohn et al 1988). In jogging, the way you run and where you run are important considerations.

Conditioning exercises seem to prevent back injuries and decrease pain intensity and duration. Cady et al (1985) found that a regular fitness programme significantly reduced the number of back injuries in a healthy population of American firemen. Moderate physical exercise improves intervertebral disc metabolism and nutrition (Holm & Urban 1987). It is also found to decrease muscular tension, relieve depression, reduce stress and facilitate sleep. An effect on cognitive function has even been observed (Young 1979). Pain experience is reduced by prolonged exercise (Colt et al 1981, Scott & Gijsbers 1981). Hoffman et al (1990) even showed that, in rats, the effect of running on cerebrospinal fluid levels of immunoreactive β-endorphin remained for up to 48 hours.

Combined programmes

Among the intensive training regimens and activation progammes, is the so-called 'work hardening' which is a prescriptive, individually structured, productivity developed scheme, including carefully progressive biomechanical, cardiovascular and even psychophysical intervention strategies (Matheson 1988). A comprehensive programme, including work exercises in simulated postures with extensive psychological support, has been shown to be effective in the treatment of the deconditioning syndrome of the lumbo-pelvic functional unit (Mayer et al 1985c, Mayer & Gatchel 1988). The results of the Dallas group show that among chronically disabled low-back pain patients, 80% of programme graduates returned to work. These outcomes have been reproduced in the northern part of the United States (Hazard et al 1989). However, neither of these studies have a true control group. It is also problematic to compare studies using different outcome variables and populations. Work status as an outcome criterion is influenced by many factors beyond the control of any rehabilitation programme, such as cultural factors, the social insurance system, the local job market and work satisfaction. The results of the Dallas group have not been replicated in Scandinavian countries (Alharanta et al 1992).

Varieties of intensive training and activation programmes exist in many places. Several studies have been published where variants of this model were applied, including studies in Sweden, designed after the Norwegian variant at Hernes Institute of Rehabilitation (Åberg 1980), and in Hawaii (Lichter et al 1984), the United States of America (Fredrickson et al 1988), Denmark (Manniche et al 1988), Norway (Harstad et al 1989), Ontario (Mitchell & Carmen 1990) and Finland (Estlander et al 1991).

Graded activity seems to be of utmost importance in the rehabilitation of low-back pain. Medical exercise therapy, which has been developed in Norway (Faugli 1987), aims at treating physical impairment. It is a carefully progressive regimen, starting even with negative loads and aiming at training stabilization, control and coordination as well as mobility and endurance.

According to the principles of Fordyce (1991), a behavioural approach seems to be most promising. In Gothenburg a randomized prospective intervention study in blue collar workers with idiopathic low-back pain sick-listed for more than eight weeks has been carried out (Lindström et al 1992). An individually designed, submaximal, gradually progressive activity programme was set up, according to the results of physical and behavioural tests and the demands of work. The programme strongly supported a return to work; it encouraged patient performance and improvement of capacity. Compared to the control group, the patients in the activity programme returned significantly earlier to their ordinary work, and were significantly less sick-listed even during the second follow-up year.

V. TRAINING PRINCIPLES

Wolff's law refers to bone as well as to soft tissue and the annuli fibrosi (Brickley-Parsons & Glimcher 1984). Systematically increasing the resistive capacities of muscles, ligaments, discs and bony tissues is essential in returning the system to productive levels following injury (Porterfield 1985). Treatment of soft tissue injuries remains a balance between the immobilization required for primary healing of the tissues and the motion and stress-dependent homeostatic response (Tammi et al 1987).

A. Information

Proper information is always essential. It will motivate, prevent injuries and enable patients to help themselves. Ideally, preprinted handouts should not be used; however, it is practical to have some basic material to be modified for each individual patient. Use of specific exercise should be governed by sound scientific principles (Jackson & Brown 1983b).

During the period of acute symptoms it is justifiable to advise patients to avoid sitting, also that they should take several walks per day to combat the debilitating effects of bed rest. Bed rest should not exceed one week (Deyo et al 1986).

Before starting strength exercises, the patient is advised to engage in a short cardiovascular warm-up to raise muscle temperature. Strength training is always to be followed by stretching of the actual muscles.

B. Motivation

Feedback is essential in all human relationships. Asfour et al (1990) showed that EMG biofeedback techniques can be an effective add-on therapeutic modality for increasing muscle strength.

Perhaps the most efficient training principle is the evaluation and testing itself (Harstad et at 1990). Testing should be systematic and preferably objective, showing the patients that they are being taken seriously, thereby increasing their motivation to cope. People should be inspired to exercise with heart and soul.

C. Progression in types of contractions

In postoperative discectomy patients, Kahanovitz et al (1989) observed at least 30% loss of expected normal strength, except in male isokinetic flexion. Electrical stimulation may be a valuable treatment in the early care of low-back pain patients in helping to maintain and increase strength and endurance of back muscles when a more active exercise programme is too painful to perform (Kahanovitz et al 1987).

To reduce the load on the back during muscle strengthening exercises, it has been recommended that isometrical contractions are emphasized initially (Nachemson & Elfström 1970), progressing to movements only when isometric contractions can be performed without pain. Isometric exercises seem to be valuable in teaching the patient to avoid vulnerable positions and movements and improve balance.

Isometric exercises and other slow speed resistance exertions are effective in achieving an increase in maximal strength. Exercises at high rates of repetition will probably increase the training capacity of muscles for aerobic adaptation as well as facilitating the function of the neuromuscular reflex system (Lee 1986).

The idea of eccentric exercises for the trunk extensors makes sense, since that is how they normally function most of the time. Smidt et al (1989) found that for gain in trunk extensor strength and endurance, the eccentric form of exercise was superior to other types. Maximal eccentric contractions represent advanced exercising. In training with machines, there are ways to set torque limits, and patients can use a break-out button to escape painful loading.

Cardiovascular training also has to be increased progressively. Fortunately, activities for cardiovascular endurance training, such as speed walking, cycling, swimming, or even jogging at therapeutic intensities, can usually be incorporated early in the recovery period.

D. Progression in muscle groups

Training in one plane only is probably not very functional. In the early phase of a rehabilitation regimen, however, this may be necessary to keep and improve control mechanisms. Controlling transversal rotation seems to be of the utmost importance for active stabilization of the trunk with training of deep muscle layers. On the other hand, the lumbar spine is vulnerable to torsion (Farfan 1984). In sitting, it is suggested that the knees are kept high to stabilize the lumbosacral column.

Programmes to develop the trunk extensor musculature are essential to restore normal function. The most substantial strength deficit is in the trunk extensors: they show a more significant and faster decrement from normal and a more rapid decline over the speed spectrum than noted in the flexors (Mayer et al 1985a). In abdominal muscle training, a certain flexion in the hip joint is recommended. Particular attention should be given to the quadriceps muscles (Dehlin et al 1978). If these muscles are weak or fatigued, the movement pattern will change, and load in the lumbar spine may increase (Trafimow et al 1989). Also, during jogging, leg strength is shown to be effectively trained and maintained (Gettman et al 1979). To keep spinal loading as symmetrical as possible, it is of the utmost importance that impairments such as extremity pareses are dealt with before recommending running and vigorous walking.

There is a specific role for medical exercise therapy in the early phase of back injury. Training can be progressed to simulate work postures, movements and loads and other activity varieties, and the resistance adapted to the inner and outer parts of the motion range. In all cases sequence training may be applied (Gunnari et al 1983). The alternation between different muscle groups, optimally five in a sequence, gives a general fatigue, governing the duration of the training period. Sequence training can be performed with conventional equipment as well as without, and is preferably performed in groups. An all-round training is considered to be of prime importance in low-back trouble.

Muscle training for back problems should also include a mode of self-exercising; this should be simple to carry out and be functional, especially when the exercise programme is going to be performed for a longer period of time. Group exercising is time and cost saving and can give mutual inspiration and motivation. Outdoor training in the fresh air might be preferred.

VI. SUMMARY AND CONCLUSION

Disorders of the lumbar spine are among the most common medical problems in western countries. The strength of trunk extensors is frequently found to be reduced in patients with chronic low-back pain. The association between reduced endurance and back trouble does not suggest a causative explanation. Mismatch between strength and job demands increases the risk of back injury.

The relative ranking of normal trunk strength is as follows: extension, flexion, lateral flexion, transversal rotation. The generated torques are dependent on several factors: sex, age, height, weight and activity level, muscle mass, joint position, length of the muscle lever arm, testing apparatus used, subject position, rotation axis, speed, duration of measurement, repetitions, rest allowed during successive trials, as well as instructions given, motivational factors and pain.

General physical fitness is of prime importance. The combined training of trunk strength with skeletal stabilization, increasing trunk muscle endurance and aerobic capacity seems to be appropriate in the functional restoration of spinal disorders. Dynamic training should be a lifelong activity. Work satisfaction and training is the best medicine for low-back trouble.

There is still a great need for further research in the area of trunk muscle performance, especially as it relates to spinal pathology. Many unanswered questions remain concerning the relationship between back pain and muscle strength and endurance. As these studies progress, standardized protocols for testing and exercise have to be worked out and guidelines developed for the selection of measuring devices and for methods of quantifying muscle strength.

REFERENCES

Åberg J 1980 Hur framgångsrik är ryggrehabilitering? Utvärdering av verksamheten vid Rygginstitutet i Sundsvall. Socialmedicinsk tidsskrifts skriftserie 44

Addison R, Schultz A 1980 Trunk strengths in patients seeking hospitalization for chronic low-back disorders. Spine 5: 539–544

Alharanta H, et al 1992 Intensive physical and psychosocial training program had no success in preventing retirement compared to more passive rehabilitation program: a controlled clinical trial of 293 chronic low back pain patients with two year follow up. The International Society for the Study of the Lumbar Spine, Chicago, Abstract 78

Asfour S S, Khalil T M, Waly S M, Goldberg M L, Rosomoff R S, Rosomoff H L 1990 Biofeedback in back muscle strengthening. Spine 15: 510–513

Asmussen E Heebøll-Nielsen K 1959 Posture, mobility and strength of the back in boys, 7 to 16 years old. Acta Orthopaedica Scandinavica 28: 174–189

Battié M C, Bigos S J, Fisher L D, Hansson T H, Jones M E, Wortley M D 1989 Isometric lifting strength as a predictor of industrial back pain reports. Spine 14: 851–856

Beimborn D S, Morrissey M C 1988 A review of the literature related to trunk muscle performance. Spine 13: 655–660

Bergquist-Ullman M, Larsson U 1977 Acute low back pain in industry. Acta Orthopaedica Scandinavica (Suppl. 170): 1–117

Biering-Sørensen F 1982 Low back trouble in a general population of 30, 40, 50 and 60-year-old men and women. Danish Medical Bulletin 29: 289-99

Biering-Sørensen F 1983 A prospective study of low back pain in a general population. III. Medical service — work consequence. Scandinavian Journal of Rehabilitation Medicine 15: 89–96

Biering-Sørensen F 1984 Physical measurements as risk indicators for low-back trouble over a one-year period. 1983 Volvo Award. Spine 9: 106–119

Braatøy T 1965 De nervøse sinn. Medisinsk psykologi og psykoterapi. Cappelen, Oslo

Brickley-Parsons D, Glimcher M J 1984 Is the chemistry of collagen in intervertebral discs an expression of Wolff's law? 1984 Volvo Award. Spine 9: 148–163

Cady L D, Thomas P C, Karwasky R J 1985 Program for increasing health and physical fitness of firefighters. Journal of Occupational Medicine 27: 110–114

Chaffin D B, Park K S 1973 A longitudinal study of low-back pain as associated with occupational weight lifting factors. American Industrial Hygiene Association Journal 134: 513–525

Chaffin D B 1974 Human strength capability and low-back pain. Journal of Occupational Medicine 16: 248–254
Chaffin D B, Herrin G D, Keyserling W M 1978 Preemployment strength testing: an updated position. Journal of Occupational Medicine 20: 403–408
Colt E W D, Wardlaw S L, Frantz A G 1981 The effect of running on plasma β-endorphin. Life Sciences 28: 1637–1640
Davies J E, Gibson T, Tester L 1979 The value of exercises in the treatment of low back pain. Rheumatology and Rehabilitation 18: 243–247
Davies G J, Gould J A 1982 Trunk testing using a prototype Cybex II isokinetic dynamometer stabilization system. The Journal of Orthopaedic and Sports Physical Therapy 3: 164–170
Davies P O, Dotson C O 1987 Job performance testing: an alternative to age discrimination. Medicine and Science in Sports and Exercise 19: 179–185
Dehlin O, Berg S, Hedenrud B, Andersson G, Grimby G 1978 Muscle training, psychological perception of work and low-back symptoms in nursing aides. Scandinavian Journal of Rehabilitation Medicine 10: 201–209
DeVries H A 1968 EMG fatigue curves in postural muscles. American Journal of Physical Medicine 47: 175–181
Deyo R A, Diehl A K, Rosenthal M 1986 How many days of bed rest for acute low back pain? The New England Journal of Medicine 315: 1064–1070
Deyo R A, Tsui-Wu Y-J 1987 Descriptive epidemiology of low-back pain and its related medical care in the Unites States. Spine 12: 264–268
Ekholm J, Arborelius U, Fahlcrantz A, Larsson A-M, Mattson G 1979 Activation of abdominal muscles during some physiotherapeutic exercises. Scandinavian Journal of Rehabilitation Medicine 11: 75–81
Estlander A-M, Mellin G, Vanharanta H, Hupli M 1991 Effects of follow-up of a multimodal treatment program including intensive physical training for low back pain patients. Scandinavian Journal of Rehabilitation Medicine 23: 97–102
Farfan H F 1984 The torsional injury of the lumbar spine. Spine 9: 53
Faugli H-P 1987 Medizinische Trainingstherapie. In: vanOw D, Hüni G (eds) Beurteilung motorischer Funktionen Patientengerechte Übungs- und Trainungs-Konzepte. Perimed mbH, Erlangen, 125–133
Flint M 1958 Effect of increasing back and abdominal strength on low-back pain. Research Quarterly 29: 160–171
Flor H, Turk D C 1984 Etiological theories and treatments for chronic back pain, I. Somatic models and interventions. Pain 19: 105–121
Fordyce W E 1991 Behavioral factors in pain. Neurosurgery Clinics of North America 2: 749–759
Fredrickson B E, Trief P M, vanBeveren P, Yuan H A, Baum G 1988 Rehabilitation of the patient with chronic back pain. A search for outcome predictors. Spine 13: 351–353
Frymoyer J W, Pope M H, Clements J H, Wilder D G, MacPherson B, Ashikaga T 1983 Risk factors in low-back pain. An epidemiological survey. The Journal of Bone and Joint Surgery 65A: 213–218
Gettman L R, Ayres J J, Pollock M L, Durstine L, Grantham W 1979 Physiologic effects on adult men of circuit strength training and jogging. Archives of Physical Medicine and Rehabilitation 60: 115–120
Gracovetsky S, Farfan H, Helleur C 1985 The abdominal mechanism. Spine 10: 317–324
Gunnari H, Evjenth O, Brady M 1983 Sekvenstrening med og uten utstyr. Norges Bedriftsidrettsforbund, Dreyer, Oslo
Hall S 1985 Effect of attempted lifting speed on forces and torque exerted on the lumbar spine. Medical Science in Sports and Exercise 17: 440–444
Harstad H, Alvsaker K, Nessiøy I 1989 Attføringssenteret i Rauland. Trenings- og behandlingseffekter. Tidsskrift for den Norske Lægeforening 109: 212–215

Harstad H, Tveiten G, Peltonen K 1990 Ryggtrening ved Attføringssenteret i Rauland. Report

Hasue M, Fujiwara M, Kikuchi S 1980 A new method of quantitative measurement of abdominal and back muscle strength. Spine 5: 143–148

Hazard R G, Reid S, Fenwick J W, Reeves V 1988 Isokinetic trunk and lifting strength measurements. Variability as an indicator of effort. Spine 13: 54–57

Hazard R G, Fenwick J W, Kalisch S M et al 1989 Functional restoration with behavioral support. A one-year prospective study of patients with chronic low-back pain. Spine 14: 157–161

Heebøll-Nielsen K 1982 Muscle strength of boys and girls, 1981 compared to 1956. Scandinavian Journal of Sports Science 4: 37–43

Hemborg B, Moritz U 1985 Intra-abdominal pressure and trunk muscle activity during lifting. II. Chronic low-back pain patients. Scandinavian Journal of Rehabilitation Medicine 17: 5–13

Hemborg B, Moritz U, Hamberg J, Holmström E, Löwing H, Åkesson I 1985 Intra-abdominal pressure and trunk muscle activity during lifting. III. Effect of abdominal muscle training in chronic low-back patients. Scandinavian Journal of Rehabilitation Medicine 17: 15–24

Hirsch C, Jonsson B, Lewin T 1969 Low-back symptoms in a Swedish female population. Clinical Orthopaedics and Related Research 63: 171–176

Hoffman P, Terenius L, Thoren P 1990 Cerebrospinal fluid immunoreactive beta-endorphin concentration is increased by voluntary exercise in the spontaneously hypertensive rat. Regulatory Peptides 28: 233–239

Holm S H, Urban J P G 1987 The intervertebral disc: factors contributing to its nutrition and matrix turnover. In: Helminen H J, Kiviranta I, Sääminen A-M, Tammi M, Paukkonen K, Jurvelin J (eds) Joint loading. Wright, Bristol, p 187–226

Hult L 1954 The Munkfors investigation. Acta Orthopaedica Scandinavica (Suppl. 16)

Jackson C P, Brown M D 1983a Is there a role for exercise in the treatment of patients with low back pain? Clinical Orthopaedics and Related Research 179: 39–45

Jackson C P, Brown M D 1983b Analysis of current approaches and a practical guide to prescription of exercise. Clinical Orthopaedics and Related Research 179: 46–54

Kahanovitz N, Nordin M, Verderame R et al 1987 Normal trunk muscle strength and endurance in women and the effect of exercises and electrical stimulation. Part 2: Comparative analysis of electrical stimulation and exercises to increase trunk muscle strength and endurance. Spine 12: 112–118

Kahanovitz N, Viola K, Gallagher M 1989 Long-term strength assessment of postoperative discectomy patients. Spine 14: 402–403

Karvonen M J, Viitasalo J T, Komi P V, Nummi J, Järvinen T 1980 Back and leg complaints in relation to muscle strength in young men. Scandinavian Journal of Rehabilitation Medicine 12: 53–59

Kelsey J L, White A A III, Bisbee G E 1979 The impact of musculoskeletal disorders on the population of the United States. The Journal of Bone and Joint Surgery 61-A: 959–964

Kelsey J L White A A III 1980 Epidemiology and impact of low-back pain. Spine 5: 133–142

Kendall P H, Jenkins J M 1968a Exercises for backache: a double-blind controlled trial. Physiotherapy 54: 154–157

Kendall P H, Jenkins J M 1968b Lumbar isometric flexion exercises. Physiotherapy 54: 158–163

Keyserling W M, Herrin G D, Chaffin D B 1980 Isometric strength testing as a means of controlling medical incidents on strenuous jobs. Journal of Occupational Medicine 22: 332–336

Khalil T M, Goldberg M L, Asfour S S, Moty E A, Rosomoff R S, Rosomoff H L 1987 Acceptable maximum effort (AME). A psychophysical measure of strength in back pain patients. Spine 12: 372–376

Kondraske G V, Deivanayagam S, Carmichael T, Mayer T G, Mooney V 1987 Myoelectric spectral analysis and strategies for quantifying trunk muscular fatigue. Archives of Physical Medicine and Rehabilitation 68: 103–110

Kroemer K H 1983 An isoinertial technique to assess individual lifting capability. Human Factors 25: 493–506

Kumar S 1989 Rationale for standardization of back strength measurement. The International Society for the Study of the Lumbar Spine, Kyoto. Abstract 21

Laasonen E M 1984 Atrophy of sacrospinal muscle groups in patients with chronic, diffusely radiating lumbar back pain. Neuroradiology 26: 9–13

Langrana N A, Lee C K, Alexander H, Mayott C W 1984 Quantitative assessment of back strength using isokinetic testing. Spine 9: 287–290

Lee C K 1986 The use of exercise and muscle testing in the rehabilitation of spinal disorders. Clinics in Sports Medicine 5: 271–276

Lichter R L, Hewson J K, Radke S J, Blum M 1984 Treatment of chronic low-back pain. Clinical Orthopaedics and Related Research 190: 115–123

Lidström A, Zachrisson M 1970 Physical therapy on low-back pain and sciatica: an attempt at evaluation. Scandinavian Journal of Rehabilitation Medicine 2: 37–42

Liemohn W, Snodgrass L B, Sharpe G L 1988 Unresolved controversies in back management — a review. Journal of Orthopedic Sports Physical Therapy 9: 239–244

Lindström I et al 1992 The effect of graded activity on patients with subacute low back pain: a randomized prospective clinical study with an operant-conditioning behavioral approach. Physical Therapy 72: 279–293

Macintosh J E, Bogduk N, Gracovetsky S 1987 The biomechanics of the thoracolumbar fascia. Clinical Biomechanics 2: 78–83

MacNeill T, Warwick D, Andersson G, Schultz A 1980 Trunk strength in attempted flexion, extension, and lateral bending in healthy subjects and patients with low-back disorders. Spine 5: 529–538

Magora A 1974 Investigation of the relation between low back pain and occupation. 6. Medical history and symptoms. Scandinavian Journal of Rehabilitation Medicine 6: 81–88

Manniche C, Hesselsøe G, Bentzen L, Christensen I, Lundberg E 1988 Clinical trial of intensive muscle training for chronic low-back pain. Lancet 2: 1473–1476

Marras W S, King A I, Joynt R L 1984 Measurements of loads on the lumbar spine under isometric and isokinetic conditions. Spine 9: 176–187

Martin P R, Rose M J, Nichols P J R, Russell P L, Hughes I G 1986 Physiotherapy exercises for low-back pain: process and clinical outcome. International Rehabilitation Medicine 8: 34–38

Matheson L N 1988 Integrated work hardening in vocational rehabilitation: an emerging model. Vocational Evaluation and Work Adjustment Bulletin 22: 1–9

Mayer T G, Smith S S, Keeley J, Mooney V 1985a Quantification of lumbar function. Part 2: Sagittal plane trunk strength in chronic low-back pain patients. Spine 10: 765–772

Mayer T G, Smith S S, Kondraske G, Gatchel R J, Carmichael T W, Mooney V 1985b Quantification of lumbar function. Part 3: Preliminary data on isokinetic torso rotation testing with myoelectric spectral analysis in normal and low-back pain subjects. Spine 10: 912–920

Mayer T G, Gatchel R J, Kischino N et al 1985c Objective assessment of spine function following industrial injury. A prospective study with comparison group and one-year follow-up. 1985 Volvo Award. Spine 10: 482–493

Mayer T G, Gatchel R J 1988 Functional restoration for spinal disorders. The sports medicine approach. Lea & Febiger, Philadelphia

Mayer T G, Barnes D, Kishino N D et al 1988a Progressive isoinertial lifting evaluation. I. A standardized protocol and normative database. Spine 13: 993–997

Mayer T G, Barnes D, Nichols G et al 1988b Progressive isoinertial lifting evaluation. II. A comparison with isokinetic lifting in a disabled chronic low back pain industrial population. Spine 13: 998–1002

Mayer T G, Vanharanta H, Gatchel R J et al 1989a Comparison of CT scan muscle measurements and isokinetic trunk strength in postoperative patients. Spine 14: 33–36

Mayer T G, Kondraske G, Mooney V, Carmichael T W, Butsch R 1989b Lumbar myoelectric spectral analysis for endurance assessment. A comparison of normals with deconditioned patients. Spine 14: 986–991

Mayer T, Gatchel R, Barnes D, Mayer H, Mooney V 1990 Progressive isoinertial lifting evaluation. Erratum notice. Spine 15: 5

Mital A, Channaveeraiah C, Fard H F, Khaledi H 1986 Reliability of repetitive dynamic strengths as a screening tool for manual lifting tasks. Clinical Biomechanics 1: 125–129

Mitchell R I, Carmen G M 1990 Results of a multicenter trial using an intensive active exercise program for the treatment of acute soft tissue and back injuries. Spine 15: 514–521

Morris J M, Benner G, Lucas D B 1962 An electromyographic study of the intrinsic muscles of the back in man. Journal of Anatomy 96: 509–520

Nachemson A, Lindh M 1969 Measurement of abdominal and back muscle strength with and without low back pain. Scandinavian Journal of Rehabilitation Medicine 1: 60–65

Nachemson A, Elftström G 1970 Intravital pressure measurements in lumbar discs. A study of common movements, maneuvres and exercises. Scandinavian Journal of Rehabilitation Medicine (Suppl. 1): 1–40

Nesse T 1983 Helse og arbeidsmiljø i transportavdelingen. Del V Belastningslidelser, Postverkets bedriftshelsetjeneste, nr.12

Nicolaisen T, Jørgensen K 1985 Trunk strength, back muscle endurance and low-back trouble. Scandinavian Journal of Rehabilitation Medicine 17: 121–127

Nordgren B, Schele R, Linroth K 1980 Evaluation and prediction of back pain during military field service. Scandinavian Journal of Rehabilitation Medicine 12: 1–8

Nordin M, Kahanovitz N, Verderame R et al 1987 Normal trunk muscle strength and endurance in women and the effect of exercises and electrical stimulation. Part 1: Normal endurance and trunk muscle strength in 101 women. Spine 12: 105–118

Nummi J, Järvinen T, Stambej U, Wickström G 1978 Diminished dynamic performance capacity of back and abdominal muscles in concrete reinforcement workers. Scandinavian Journal of Work Environment & Health 4 (Suppl. 1): 39–46

Örttengren R, Andersson G B J 1977 Electromyographic studies of trunk muscles, with special reference to the functional anatomy of the lumbar spine. Spine 2: 33–52

Parnianpour M, Nordin M, Moritz U, Kahanovitz N 1987 Correlation between different tests of trunk strength. Proceedings of Musculoskeletal Disorders at Work, University of Surrey. Taylor & Francis, London, p 234–238

Parnianpour M, Nordin M, Kahanovitz N, Frankel V H 1988 The triaxial coupling of torque generation of trunk muscles during isometric exertions and the effect of fatiguing isoinertial movements on the motor output and movement patterns. 1988 Volvo Award. Spine 13: 982–992

Parnianpour M, Li F, Nordin M, Kananovitz N 1989 A database of isoinertial trunk strength tests against three resistance levels in sagittal, frontal, and transverse planes in normal male subjects. Spine 14: 409–411
Parnianpour M, Nordin M, Sheikhzadeh A 1990 The relationship between torque, velocity, and power with constant resistive load during sagittal trunk movement. Spine 15: 639–643
Pedersen O F, Staffeldt E S 1972 The relationship between four tests of back muscle strength in untrained subjects. Scandinavian Journal of Rehabilitation Medicine 4: 175–181
Pedersen O F, Petersen R, Staffeldt E S 1975 Back pain and isometric back muscle strength of workers in a Danish factory. Scandinavian Journal of Rehabilitation Medicine 7: 125–128
Pitman M I, Peterson L 1989 Biomechanics of skeletal muscle. In: Nordin M, Frankel V H (eds) Basic biomechanics of the musculoskeletal system (2nd edn). Lea & Febiger, Philadelphia, p 89–111
Plum P, Rehfeld J 1985 The treatment of acute and chronic back pain by muscular exercise. Lancet 1: 453–454
Porterfield J A 1985 Dynamic stablization of the trunk. The Journal of Orthopaedic and Sports Physical Therapy 6: 271–277
Portillo D, Sinkora G, MacNeill T, Spencer D, Schultz A 1982 Trunk strengths in structurally normal girls with idiopathic scoliosis. Spine 7: 551–554
Reid J G, Costigan P A 1987 Trunk muscle balance and muscular force. Spine 12: 783–786
Roy S H, deLuca C J, Casavant D A 1989 Lumbar muscle fatigue and chronic lower back pain. Spine 14: 992–1001
Scott V. Gijsbers K 1981 Pain perception in competitive swimmers. British Medical Journal 283: 91–93
Smidt G L, Amundsen L R, Dostal W F 1980 Muscle strength at the trunk. The Journal of Orthopaedic and Sports Physical Therapy 1: 165–170
Smidt G, Herring T, Amundsen L, Rogers M, Russell A, Lehmann T 1983 Assessment of abdominal and back extensor function. A quantitative approach and results for chronic low-back patients. Spine 8: 211–219
Smidt G L, Blanpied P R 1987 Analysis of strength tests and resistive exercises commonly used for low-back disorders. Spine 12: 1025–1034
Smidt G L, Blanpied P R, White R W 1989 Exploration of mechanical and electromyographic responses of trunk muscles to high-intensity resistive exercises. Spine 14: 815–830
Smith S S, Mayer T G, Gatchel R J, Becker T J 1985 Quantification of lumbar function. Part 1: Isometric and multispeed isokinetic trunk strength measures in sagittal and axial planes in normal subjects. Spine 10: 757–764
Stokes I A F, Maffroid M, Rush S, Haugh L D 1989 EMG to torque relationships in rectus abdominis muscle. Results with repeated testing. Spine 14: 857–861
Sundsvold M Ø, Vaglum P 1985 Muscular pains and psychopathology: evaluation by the GPM method. In: Michels T H (ed) Pain. International Perspectives in Physical Therapy. Churchill Livingstone, Edinburgh, p 18–47
Suzuki N, Endo S 1983 A quantitative study of trunk muscle strength and fatigability in the low back – pain syndrome. Spine 8: 69–74
Svensson H-O, Andersson G B J 1982 Low back pain in forty to forty-seven year old men. I. Frequency of occurrence and impact on medical services. Scandinavian Journal of Rehabilitation Medicine 14: 47–53
Tammi M, Paukkonen K, Kiviranta I, Jurvelin J, Sääminen A-M, Helminen H J 1987 Joint loading-induced alterations in articular cartilage. In: Helminen H J, Kiviranta I, Sääminen A-M, Tammi M, Paukkonen K, Jurvelin J (eds) Joint loading. Biology and health of articular surfaces. Wright, Bristol, p 64–88

Thorstensson A, Arvidson Å 1982 Trunk muscle strength and low back pain. Scandinavian Journal of Rehabilitation Medicine 14: 69–75
Thorstensson A, Nilsson J 1982 Trunk muscle strength during constant velocity movements. Scandinavian Journal of Rehabilitation Medicine 14: 61–68
Trafimow J H, Schipplein O D, Andersson G B J, Andriacchi T P 1989 The effect of quadriceps fatigue on the technique of lifting. The International Society for the Study of the Lumbar Spine, Kyoto, Abstract 22–23
Troup J D G, Chapman A E 1969 The strength of the flexor and extensor muscles of the trunk. Journal of Biomechanics 2: 49–62
Troup J D G, Foreman T K, Baxter C E, Brown D 1987 The perception of back pain and the role of psychophysical tests of lifting capacity. 1987 Volvo Award. Spine 12: 645–657
Waddell G 1987 A new clinical model for the treatment of low-back pain. 1987 Volvo Award. Spine 12: 632–644
Westing S H, Seger J Y, Karlson E, Ekblom B 1988 Eccentric and concentric torque-velocity characteristics of the quadriceps femoris in man. European Journal of Applied Physiology 58: 100–104
Young R J 1979 The effect of regular exercise on cognitive functioning and personality. British Journal of Sports Medicine 13: 110–117
Zeh J, Hansson T, Bigos S, Spengler D, Battié M, Wortley M 1986 Isometric strength testing. Recommendations based on a statistical analysis procedure. Spine 11: 43–46

Annotated bibliography

MUSCLE PERFORMANCE: PRINCIPLES & GENERAL THEORY

Mayhew T P, Rothstein J M 1988 Measurement of muscle performance with instruments. In: Rothstein J M (ed) Measurement in physical therapy, Churchill Livingstone, New York, ch 3, p 57–102
This chapter is an excellent overview of the strengths and weaknesses of commonly used instrumentation for measurement of muscle performance. The authors stress the reliability and validity of each of the instruments presented, as well as addressing the clinical applicability of the instruments and testing protocols. The chapter also includes an extensive reference list on measurement of muscle performance.

Riddle D L, Finucane S D, Rothstein J M, Walkerė M L 1989 Intrasession and intersession reliability of hand-held dynamometer measurements taken on brain-damaged patients. Physical Therapy 69: 182–192
This study is a good example of how a well-defined testing protocol can be used by clinicians to yield consistent testing results in a select group of patients. The authors have written an excellent discussion addressing many of the important testing issues that arise in the clinic and offer concrete suggestions for controlling some of the confounding variables that may negatively influence testing results.

Rose S J, Brooke M H 1982 Muscle biology. Physical Therapy 62: 1751–1830
This special issue of the Physical Therapy Journal contains several excellent articles integrating research findings with clinical applicability. Articles address muscle mutability, length associated changes in muscle, muscle anatomy and physiology and clinical considerations.

St. Pierre D, Gardiner P F 1987 The effect of immobilization and exercise on muscle function: a review. Physiotherapy, Canada 39: 24–35
This article is a 'must read' for those people who wish to learn more about the effects of immobilization on muscle function. The authors have produced a thorough review of the literature and apply the research findings to the practice of physical therapy. There is also an extensive reference list included for those who want more information.

Stauber W 1989 Eccentric action of muscles: physiology, injury and adaptation. Exercise and Sports Science Reviews, American College of Sports Medicine, Williams and Wilkins, 7: 157–185
Dr Stauber's article is a comprehensive discussion about the eccentric action of muscles. He explains clearly the physiology of the stretch shortening cycle of

muscle, the physiologic changes that occur with eccentric exercise and the adaptive responses of muscle to eccentric training. This article is highly recommended for those who are incorporating eccentric exercise training into their treatment programmes.

EVALUATION OF SKELETAL MUSCLE PERFORMANCE

Clarkson P M, Trembly I 1988 Exercise-induced muscle damage, repair, and adaption in humans. American Physio Society 1–6

This is an excellent article reporting the effects of eccentric exercise on human muslce. Although muscle initially responds to eccentric exercise with soreness and pain, recovery takes place with time depending on the exercise stress imposed. However, with repeated bouts of eccentric exercise, the recovery time takes place in a shorter time span, suggesting an adaptive response by the muscle. This article is very interesting for those people who would like to understand more about adaptive responses of muscle to imposed stress and the effects of eccentric exercise.

Davies G 1985 A compendium of isokinetic usage, 2nd edn. S & S Publishers, LaCrosse, Wisconsin

This book is a good reference for those who wish to learn more about the use of isokinetic testing and training with patients. Principles of testing, interpretation of the measures and the rationale for exercise protocols are presented in an understandable style. There are also extensive reference lists included for those people who want more in-depth information.

Jones N L, McCartney N, McComas A J (eds) 1986 Human muscle power. Human Kinetics Publishers, Champlain, Ill, p 1–332.

This extensive textbook on current theories of muscle physiology and human muscle performance was published as a result of a symposium on human muscle power at McMaster University in 1984. This book is highly recommended reading for those who would like more in-depth information about muscle mechanics, morphology, neural influences, energy metabolism, fatigue and adaptation/maladaptation during performance.

Kendall F P, McCreary E 1983 Muscle: Testing and function, 3rd edn. Williams and Wilkins, Baltimore, MD

This book is the best resource on manual muscle testing and applied muscle function. The text is beautifully illustrated which helps the reader to understand common types of muscle weakness patterns. This book is an invaluable resource for all physical therapy clinicians.

Komi P V (ed) 1992 Strength and power in sport. Blackwell Scientific Publications, London

This up to date textbook contains several excellent chapters by well known exercise physiologists integrating current theory with athletic performance. The book is organized into five sections: definitions, biological basis for strength and power, mechanisms of adaption in strength and power training, special problems in strength and power training in sports. Many of the principles discussed in this text are directly applicable to physical therapy practice.

BIOMECHANICS AND EXERCISES

Arborelius U P, Ekholm J 1978 Mechanics of shoulder locomotor system during exercises resisted by weight-and-pulley circuit. Scandinavian Journal of Rehabilitation Medicine 10: 171–177

An investigation of how different ways of using a pulley device influence the mechanics of the shoulder joint and muscles. The resistance effect of various modes of application of the pulley was calculated. It is shown how the resistance load moment is influenced by: i) angle between the horizontal plane and a line between the joint and the pulley (height of pulley); ii) distance between joint and pulley; iii) weight applied to pulley cord; iv) weight of limb.

Ekholm J, Arborelius U P, Németh G, Schüldt K, Harms-Ringdahl K 1982 Biomechanical research methods for analysis of factors influencing load and muscle activation during therapeutic exercise movements. Proceedings, 'Man in Action', IXth International Congress of the World Confederation of Physical Therapy, Stockholm, Sweden. Part I, p 50–57
Methods are described for calculation and measurement of load on muscles, tendons and joints during exercise movements. Relevant elements are presented such as the geometry of movement, distances, angles, gravity forces, ground reaction forces, external forces from device, muscle force, load moment of force about joint axis, and lengths of moment arms. The effects of alterations in the biomechanical factors on the muscular and joint load during some exercise movements of the thigh and shoulder are described, such as the great effect of changes in patient positioning.

Ekholm J, Arborelius U P, Németh G, Harms-Ringdahl K, Schüldt K 1983 On the biomechanics of therapeutic exercises for strength and endurance. Proceedings 'New frontiers that influence disease and rehabilitation'. 4th World Congress of the International Rehabilitation Medicine Association, San Juan, Puerto Rico. p 287–293
The article reviews some studies by the Kinesiology Research Group of the Karolinska Institute, about the load on muscles and tendons of the thigh and shoulder during exercises with, e.g. pulley exerciser and a simple quadriceps training device. The principles related to load quantification during exercise are presented. Basic concepts such as distribution of resistance moment of force over the motion range, relation between load moment of force and maximum muscular moment of force at different joint angles, muscular strength utilization ratio, and level of muscular activity are discussed.

Ericson M O, Bratt Å, Nisell R, Németh G, Ekholm J 1986 Load moment about the hip and knee joints during ergometer cycling. Scandinavian Journal of Rehabilitation Medicine 18: 165–172.
The aim of the study was to calculate the magnitudes of load moments of force acting about the bilateral hip and knee joint axes during ergometer cycling. During cycling at 120 Watts, 60 revolutions per minute with mid-saddle height and anterior foot position, the mean peak resistance flexing and extending knee load moment are 29 Nm and 12 Nm, respectively. For knee load moment levels, work load is important. The resistance flexing knee load moment does not change with changes in pedalling rate. The maximum resistance flexing knee load moment, which the knee extensors counteracts, decreases and the maximum extending load moment, which the flexors counteract, increases with increased saddle height. The authors conclude that the maximum resistance hip and knee joint load moments induced during cycling are small compared with those obtained during other exercises or activities, such as level walking, stair climbing, and lifting.

Harms-Ringdahl K, Arborelius U P, Németh G, Schüldt K, Ekholm J 1982 Biomechanical load and muscle activation during exercise therapy of the

humeroscapular joint. In: World Confederation for Physical Therapy, Proceedings, IXth International Congress, Stockholm. Part I, p 58–65
The aim of the study was to find principles to optimize various ways of exercising humero-scapular rotator muscles. The possibilities for adapting resistance load moment about the longitudinal axis of the humero-scapular joint to maximum muscular moment (strength) were studied for push-ups, exercises with dumbbells and rubber exercise strips. A comparison was made with rotation exercises under resistance from a pulley device. For push-ups, the positioning of the hand in relation to the shoulder is crucial for the resistance load level and load direction, but body position also changes the load. For exercise with dumbells, the body position is of great importance. When rubber strips are used as resistive equipment, the elasticity properties as well as the lengthening and the pretension of the strip can change the curve of the resistance load moment. The load during therapeutic exercises can be varied in many ways by adjustments of the posture and position of the subject.

Harms-Ringdahl K, Arborelius U P, Ekholm J, Németh G, Schüldt K 1985 Shoulder externally rotating exercises with pulley apparatus. Joint load and EMG. Scandinavian Journal of Rehabilitation Medicine 17:129–140
The mechanical load on the gleno-humeral joint and the muscular activity during shoulder external rotation resisted by a pulley device were analyzed using normalized, low-pass filtered EMG recorded from the infraspinatus, deltoid, pectoralis major and trapezius muscles. The effect of subject positioning on the joint load and the muscular activity was studied. The best adaptation between the curves for resistance load moment and maximum muscular moment (strength) is obtained when the subject sits with the pulley located 20° posterior to a frontal plane through the shoulders at a distance of 1.3 m from the joint. Of the four muscles investigated, the infraspinatus was the most active.

Moritz U, Svantesson G G, Haffajee D 1973 A biomechanical study of torque as affected by motor unit activity, length tension relationship and muscle force lever. In: Desmedt J E (ed) New developments in electromyography and clinical neurophysiology. Karger, Basel, 1: 675–682
The relative influence of motor unit activity, muscle force lever and muscle length on knee extensor muscle strength (torque output) was analyzed for subjects seated on a quadriceps table. Muscle activity was recorded using surface electrodes from the vastus medialis and lateralis and the rectus femoris. At maximum voluntary contraction, the average muscle activity level increased as the knee was held in a more flexed position. The maximum strength curve shows a peak in the motion range at 50°–60° with lower values toward 10° and 90° of flexion. In contrast to the shape of the strength curve, the curve for the muscle activity level increases through the whole motion range from 10° to 90°. The authors conclude that there are several, partly interdependent, variables affecting the isometric knee extension torque. Of these, the knee flexion angle may be considered an independent variable affecting all the others.

Németh G, Ekholm J, Arborelius U P, Harms-Ringdahl K and Schüldt K 1983 Influence of knee flexion on isometric hip extensor strength. Scandinavian Journal of Rehabilitation Medicine 15: 97–101
The maximum isometric extensor muscle strength was measured in healthy subjects at different combinations of hip and knee angles. The results revealed that the knee angle does not affect the hip extensor strength. The highest extensor muscular moments occur at 90° hip flexion, decreasing with decreasing hip angle. In prone position, the subjects used 10–24% of the

maximum strength at hip angles 60°–0° to hold the leg, counteracting the induced resistance load due to the weight of body segments.

Nisell R, Ericson M, Németh G, Ekholm J 1989 Tibio-femoral joint forces during isokinetic knee extension. American Journal of Sports Medicine 17: 49–54
A sagittal plane biomechnical model is presented for calculations of tibio-femoral joint compressive and shear forces during isokinetic knee extensions at two different speeds and at two different positions of the resistance pad (proximal and distal). In healthy males, the mean tibio-femoral compressive force and the patellar tendon force reach a maximum of 6300 N, or close to 9 times body weight. The anteriorly directed tibio-femoral shear force reaches a positive magnitude of about 700 N or close to 1 body weight, indicating that high forces arise in the anterior cruciate ligament when the knee is straighter than 60°. The anteriorly directed shear force was considerably lowered by locating the resistance pad proximally on the leg.

Schüldt K, Ekholm J, Németh G, Arborelius U P, Harms-Ringdahl K 1983 Knee load and muscle activity during exercises in rising. In: Recent Advances in Rehabilitation. Medicine Scandinavian Journal of Rehabilitation Medicine Suppl. 9: 174–188
Knee joint and quadriceps muscle load and knee muscle activation during rising exercises in a device with a movable back support were analyzed. The biomechanical methods for such studies are described. Floor-to-foot forces were recorded and the load moment of force about the knee joint axis was calculated. The initial knee load moment with much flexed knees was high and decreased markedly with decreasing knee angle, resulting in no resistance to knee extension at small knee angles. The magnitude in change in knee extension resistance due to adaptive adjustments of the exercise device was mapped.

ECCENTRIC MUSCLE ACTIVITY

Ebbeling C A, Clarkson P M 1989 Exercise induced muscle damage and adaption. Sports Medicine 7: 207–234
This article reviews the current hypotheses for the mechanisms of eccentric induced pain and damage. It pays particular attention to the enzyme efflux from affected muscles and how this is affected by repeated activity.

Jones D A, Round J M 1990 Skeletal muscle in health and disease. University Press, Manchester
This comprehensive book is valuable for all those with an interest in skeletal muscle. Of particular interest to this subject are chapters on the mechanism of force generation, damage, pain, fatigue and training.

Jones D A, Rutherford O M, Parker D F 1989 Physiological changes in skeletal muscle as a result of strength training. Quarterly Journal of Experimental Physiology 74: 233–256
This article reviews the extensive literature on the effects of strength training on peripheral and central factors. It considers the stimuli for hypertrophy, including any possible benefits of eccentric contractions, in addition to specificity and the effect of strength training on power output.

Newham D J 1988 The consequences of eccentric contractions and their relationship to delayed onset muscle pain. European Journal of Applied Physiology 57: 353–359

This is a review article which describes the changes indicative of damage which can follow a bout of eccentric exercise. It considers the temporal relationship between pain and the indications of damage.

Newham D J 1991Skeletal muscle pain and exercise. Physiotherapy 77: 66–70
This article reviews the possible mechanism and aetiology of muscle pain in health and disease. It also discusses the role of physical therapy in treating muscle pain.

Stauber W T 1989 Eccentric action of muscles: physiology, injury and adaptation. In: Pandolf K B (ed) Exercise and Sports Science Reviews, vol 17. American College of Sports Medicine Series. Williams & Wilkinds, Baltimore, p 157–186
This article reviews the physiology of eccentric exercise and its effect on untrained and trained muscle. There is a section on the clinical applications of eccentric exercise.

MUSCLE STRENGTH—MUSCLE LENGTH

Stejskal L 1972 Postural reflexes in theory and motor reeducation, Academia Publishers, Prague. 103 pages

Lewit K 1989 Manipulative therapy, 2nd edn. Butterworths, Edinburgh

Janda V 1983 Muscle function testing. Butterworths, Edinburgh

Skládal J 1976 The human diaphragm in normal and clinical physiology. Academia Publishers, Prague. In Czech, with a long English summary; an excellent book.

MUSCLE STRENGTH TESTING IN CHILDREN AND ADOLESCENTS

Pact V, Sirotkin-Roses M, Beatus J 1984 The muscle testing handbook, ch 8:Pediatric functional assessment, p 124–143
Functional positions and activities are described and pictured to assess muscle strength in young children (ages 2–5) when traditional strength measurement techniques may be difficult.

Espenschade A S, Eckert H M 1980 Motor development, 3rd edn. Charles E. Merrill Publishing, Columbus, OH.
Comprehensive textbook covering the topics of heredity, prenatal maternal influences, differentiation and integration of the sensory-motor system, prenatal development, the neonate, motor behaviour of infants, motor behaviour in early and later childhood, adolescent development, and performance in adulthood and old age.

Muscle and nerve (supplement) 1990 13: S1–S57. Proceedings of a workshop on evaluating muscle strength and function. Sponsored by the Muscular Dystrophy Association
Discussions are provided regarding clinical trials in neuromuscular disease, methodology to measure the strength of spinal muscular atrophy patients, manual muscle testing, biomechanical muscle performance, functional testing, pulmonary function testing, fatigue testing, disease-specific traits, specific tests for polymyositis, statistical considerations, and modelling of time-strength relationships.

McDonald C M, Jaffe K M, Shurtleff D B 1986 Assessment of muscle strength in children with meningomyelocele: accuracy and stability of measurements over time. Archives of Physical Medicine and Rehabilitation 67: 855–861
This is a retrospective study of the accuracy of muscle testing of 825 children with myelodysplasia at different ages, and the stability of the strength measurements on serial examination of these children over time. The predictive validity of strength assessments in this population was also discussed.

Hinderer K A 1988 Reliability of the myometer in muscle testing children and adolescents with myelodysplasia. Master of Science Thesis, Rehabilitation Medicine Department, University of Washington, Seattle
This study examined the reliability of testing the peak isometric strength of individuals with myelodysplasia using the myometer. Procedural, intratrial, test-retest, and interrater reliability coefficients and standard errors of measurement were calculated for measurements obtained from one upper limb and seven lower limb muscle groups on 66 children with myelodysplasia.

Level M B 1986 Spherical grip strength of children. Master's thesis, Rehabilitation Medicine Department, University of Washington, Seattle
This study established pilot grip strength norms of preferred and nonpreferred hands for boys and girls 6 to 9 years old, using the Vigorimeter. Age and sex differences in scores were documented.

MUSCLE STRENGTH AND AGING

Clas-Håkan Nygård 1988 Work and musculoskeletal capacity: A field and laboratory study of 44- to 62-year-old women and men. Kuopion yliopiston julkaisuja, Publications of the University of Kuopio, Lääketiede, Medicine, Alkuperäistutkimukset 17/1988. Original reports
The purpose of the study was to investigate the relationship between work load, musculoskeletal capacity and strain during work among aging employees. One hundred and twenty-nine subjects (mean age 52.0 years) from different municipal occupations participated in the study. Eighty-three of the subjects also participated in the follow-up 3.5 years later. The field methods comprised job analysis and measurement of the cardiorespiratory and perceived strain of the employees at work. The laboratory measurements consisted of maximal muscle strength and mobility tests.

The results indicated that there were significant differences in the musculoskeletal work load of different municipal occupations. The musculoskeletal capacity was systematically lower or on the same level among those in physical work (both women and men) and among those in mixed physical and mental work (men) than in mental work. Furthermore, those subjects with a high musculoskeletal work load had systematically lower maximal muscle strength and muscle endurance than those with a low musculoskeletal load. The 3.5 year follow-up showed a significant decrease in isometric trunk flexion and extension strength (9 and 10%, respectively, among the women and 22 and 16%, respectively, among the men) and an increase in back mobility (9% among the women and 13% among the men).

It was concluded that jobs with mainly physical demands or with a high muscular load do not maintain a high musculoskeletal capacity in elderly employees. Marked changes due to aging also occur in the musculoskeletal capacity of elderly employees in a relatively short time: especially, the loss of trunk muscle strength accelerates. Furthermore, the strain of elderly, employees at work is mainly determined by the work load, and maximal muscle strength has a minor influence on strain.

Vuokko Kovanen, Harri Palokangas, Harri Suominen Effects of aging and physical training on rat skeletal muscle. An experimental study on the properties of collagen, laminin, and fibre types in muscles serving different functions. Department of Health Sciences, University of Jyväskylä, P O Box 35, SF-40351 Jyväskylä, Finland

A series of experiments was designed to investigate the age and training-related changes both in the composition of muscle fibres and in the properties of collagen in rat skeletal muscles serving different functions. Both age and life-long endurance training accelerated the muscle fibre transformation towards more fatigue-resistant fibres with slower contractile properties. The properties of muscle connective tissue seem to be related to the functional demands of skeletal muscles, and these properties are affected both by age and physical training.

Sarianna Sipilä[1], Jukka Viitasalo[2], Pertti Era[1], Harri Suominen[1] 1991 Muscle strength in male athletes aged 70–81 years and a population sample. European Journal of Applied Physiology 63: 399–403

Summary. Muscle strength characteristics of different muscle groups were studied in active male strength-trained (ST, $n = 14$), speed-trained (SP, $n = 16$), and endurance-trained (EN, $n = 67$) athletes aged between 70 and 81 years. A population sample of similar age ($n = 42$) served as a control group. The isometric forces for hand grip, arm flexion, knee extension, trunk extension, and trunk flexion were higher for the athletes than the controls and higher for the ST than EN group. The SP athletes showed higher values in knee extension and trunk flexion than the EN group. When the isometric muscle forces were related to lean body mass, significant differences still existed between the athletes and controls. However, the differences between the ST and EN groups disappeared. The elevation of the body's centre of gravity in the vertical jump was also higher for the athletes than the controls. The SP group performed better in the vertical jump than either the ST or EN group. The results showed that the athletes who trained not only for strength and speed but also for endurance had superior muscle function compared to the average male population of the same age. Although the strength and speed athletes generally showed the highest muscle strength in absolute terms, the endurance athletes also preserved excellent strength characteristics to body mass.

Esko Mälkiä 1983 Muscular performance as a determinant of physical ability in Finnish adult population. Publications of the Social Insurance Institution, Finland, AL:23, Turku

This study is a part of the so-called 'Mini-Finland Health Survey', the aim of which was to evaluate the health situation, need for treatment and restrictions of working capacity and functional ability of a Finnish adult population, and which was carried out between 1977 and 1980. A total of 1100 examinees aged 30–65 years participated in the present study. It was a randomized subsample of the sample of the Mini-Finland Survey. The aim of the study was to measure in cross-section the physical ability of the population by using muscular performance tests, and to evaluate factors related to the level of muscular performance. From the results it is apparent that muscular performance is connected with the subjective physical ability of the examinees. Men, especially, showed a close relationship between muscular performance and ability to manage daily physical tasks. Of the measurements used, the hand grip test and

---

[1] Department of Health Sciences, University of Jyväskylä, P O Box 35, SF-40351 Jyväskylä, Finland

[2] Department of Biology of Physical Activity, University of Jyväskylä, Jyväskylä, Finland

abdominal muscle test gave the best basis for the assessment of physical ability. The muscular performance is best explained by sex and by age. The changes in muscular performance of men across the age groups differ from those of women. The overall muscular performance of men decreases with age quite linearly, while that of women does not decrease until after the age of 40–44 years. The muscular performance of women is about 40–100% of the performance of men depending on the test and on the age group. The anthropometric measurements used in this study do not explain the differences in muscular performance between men and women. Only the physically stressful activities of leisure time, but not of work, correlate with muscular performance.

STRENGTH AND BRAIN LESIONS

1. Knutsson E, Martensson A 1980 Dynamic motor capacity in spastic paresis and its relation to prime mover dysfunction, spastic reflexes and antagonist co-activation. Scandinavian Journal of Rehabilitation Medicine 12: 93–106
The authors examined 18 patients with spastic paraparesis and 6 patients with spastic hemiparesis, using an isokinetic dynamometer and electromyography. Torque was measured during passive movements and maximum voluntary efforts at 30, 90 and 180°/sec. The torque measured during voluntary efforts was less for the patients than for healthy subjects. Torque was reduced more at the faster than at the slower speeds. Spastic resistance to passive movement was generally quite minimal. Spastic restraint reached a notable magnitude only during passive knee flexion at 180°/sec. Antagonist coactivation was shown to be a greater source of restraint than spasticity, particularly at the higher speeds. Therefore the authors concluded that antagonist coactivation 'may constitute a crucial component' of the motor handicap.

2. Sunderland A, Tinson D, Bradley L, Hewer R L 1989 Arm function after stroke. An evaluation of grip strength as a measure of recovery and a prognostic indicator. Journal of Neurology, Neurosurgery and Psychiatry 52: 1267–1272
The function of the paretic upper extremity was examined in 38 recent stroke patients. Used to examine the extremity were a sensitive hand-grip dynamometer, the Motricity Index (an index for motor loss based on manual muscle testing), the Motor Club Assessment, the Nine Hole Peg Test and the Frenchay Arm Test. The patients were examined using each test within three weeks of their stroke, at one month, three months, and six months. Patients demonstrated a fast initial rise in performance at all five test, but only minimal improvement between three and six months. The Motricity Index was the most sensitive test for detecting early recovery. Only at the Nine Hole Peg Test and grip strength tests did a significant proportion of patients improve between each adjacent examination session. Grip strength was correlated significantly with the other test scores, initially ($r \geq 0.71$) and at six months ($r \geq 0.79$). When the Frenchay Arm Test score at six months was used as an outcome measure, both strength measures (hand-grip and Motricity Index) were excellent predictors of outcome. The authors concluded that 'measuring grip over a six month follow up period was a sensitive method of charting intrinsic neurologic recovery' and that the 'presence of voluntary grip at one month indicates that there will be some functional recovery at six months.'

3. Tang A, Rymer W Z 1981 Abnormal force-EMG relations in paretic limbs of hemiparetic human subjects. Journal of Neurology, Neurosurgery and Psychiatry 44: 690–698

Isometric elbow flexion force and electromyographic (EMG) activity of the elbow flexor and extensor muscles were examined while 11 normal and 17 hemiparetic subjects performed elbow flexion efforts using each upper extremity. In the range of forces tested, integrated EMG activity was linearly related to force on the nonparetic and paretic sides of hemiparetic patients. The slope of EMG/force, however, was significantly steeper on the paretic side. The ratio of EMG to force on the paretic side was highly variable between subjects. The authors hypothesized that alterations in the EMG to force ratio may be the consequence of a 'reduction in mean motor unit discharge rate in paretic muscles.'

4. Demeurisse G, Demol O, Robaye E 1980 Motor evaluation in vascular hemiplegia. European Journal of Neurology 19: 382–389
The authors used their result of repeated tests (at 11 days and two, four, and six months since onset) of 100 stroke patients to develop a Motricity Index which is meant to describe motor status in the patients. Initially, 28 tests incorporating the proximal, middle and distal portions of the paretic upper and lower limbs were applied. The scores for the tests were based on manual muscle test grades (0–5). Mathematical analysis was used to reduce the number of tests to one for the proximal, middle, and distal portion of the upper and lower extremities. The tests identified by the analysis were shoulder flexion, elbow flexion, prehension, hip flexion, knee extension and ankle dorsiflexion. Each test score was assigned a weight. The scores multiplied by the weights and summed yielded an index. The authors concluded that the 'Motricity Index is useful to appreciate the severity of the hemiplegia and to follow its evolution in time.'

5. Bohannon R W 1988 Muscle strength changes in hemiparetic stroke patients during inpatient rehabilitation. Journal of Neurologic Rehabilitation 2: 163–166
Thirty-three hemiparetic stroke patients were measured with a hand-held dynamometer during an initial assessment and again prior to discharge. Fourteen muscle groups (seven on each side) were tested. Strength increased in all four extremities (upper, lower, paretic, nonparetic) between initial and final assessment. For seven of the muscle groups, strength increases were expressed as daily percentage increases relative to initial strength. Weaker muscle groups had greater increases in strength, but the increases were significantly greater in only two. The author concluded that 'it is doubtful that higher percentage increases in strength will allow patients with weaker muscles to gain strength to the point that their muscles are as strong as those of patients who were stronger initially.'

6. Riddle D L, Finucane S D, Rothstein J M, Walker M L 1989 Intrasession and intersession reliability of hand-held dynamometer measurements taken on brain damage patients. Physical Therapy 69: 182–189
A hand-held dynamometer was used to obtain repeated measurements within sessions and between sessions (two days apart) of 10 muscle groups of the paretic and nonparetic sides of hemiparetic patients. Intrasession reliability coefficents ranged from 0.88 to 0.98. Intersession reliability coefficients ranged from 0.90 to 0.98 on the paretic side and 0.31 to 0.93 on the nonparetic side. The authors' finding of high reliability on the paretic side contrasts with the opinion of some authorities who claim that muscle strength measurement are unreliable in patients with hemiparesis.

7. Bohannon R W 1989 Selected determinants of ambulatory capacity in patients with hemiplegia. Clinical Rehabilitation 3: 47–53
The strengths of seven lower extremity muscle groups of 33 stroke patients were measured bilaterally, as were four gait variables (speed, cadence, distance,

and independence) and balance. On initial assessment the strength-gait correlations ranged from 0.678 to 0.837 on the paretic side and from 0.343 to 0.600 on the nonparetic side. On final assessment the strength-gait correlations ranged from 0.556 to 0.801 on the paretic side and from 0.310 to 0.662 on the nonparetic side. The author concluded that lower extremity muscle group strength measures appear to provide an indication of gait performance and may be appropriate targets for measurement and therapeutic interventions. Balance, which was also correlated strongly with walking performance (0.864–0.912 on initial assessment and 0.544–0.715 on final assessment), was also recommended as a target.

8. Inaba M, Edberg E, Montgomery J, Gillis M K 1973 Effectiveness of functional training, active exercise, and resistive exercise for patients with hemiplegia. Physical Therapy 53: 28–35
Seventy-seven patients with hemiplegia were randomly assigned to receive: 1) functional training and selective stretching only, 2) active exercise as well as functional training and selective stretching, 3) progressive resistive exercise as well as functional training and selective stretching. Resistance exercise entailed hip-knee extension against one-half maximum and maximum loads while subjects were supine on an Elgin table. The group receiving resistance exercise showed greater increases in strength. Moreover, a larger proportion of patients in the resistance exercise group showed improvement in activities of daily living.

LOW BACK PAIN

Allan D B, Waddell G 1989 An historical perspective on low back pain and disability. Acta Orthopaedica Scandinavica (Suppl.) 60, no. 234
Pain and disability are related, but have to be distinguished. This review of low back pain and sciatica over the last 3500 years puts our present epidemic of low back disability into historical perspective. Backache and sciatica have affected human beings throughout recorded history. What has changed is how these pains have been understood and managed. Since the nineteenth century, backache and sciatica were considered and treated together, and their management was increasingly dominated by the principle of rest. What is new is chronic disability due to simple backache. Disability is ultimately a form of illness behaviour, and it depends on psychological factors just as much as on physical disease. Disability escalated after World War II, and appears to be closely related to the idea that backache is due to serious spinal injury or degeneration and to medical prescription of rest, which is reinforced by the improved social support which makes rest possible.

Friedlander A L, Block J E, Byl N N, Stubbs H A, Sadowsky H S, Genant H K 1991 Isokinetic limb and trunk muscle performance testing: short-term reliability. The Journal of Orthopaedic and Sports Physical Therapy 14: 220–224
The relationship between precision level and minimum difference in muscle performance requires to be statistically significant is discussed. Measurements of knee and trunk flexion/extension (peak torque and best work as a percentage of body weight at different speeds) were made in normal subjects in two sets 24 hours apart. Correlations between first and second measurements were high. Imprecision (reliability) was estimated as the average coefficient of variation (CV) for paired measurements. There was a wide range of CV variables. It was shown that for a sample of this size ($N = 15$), and with a 3% imprecision level, muscle performance changes have to be greater than 8% to be detected with

95% confidence. This estimate increases to about 33% at an imprecision level of 12%.

Kellet K M, Kellet D A, Nordholm L A 1991 Effects of an exercise program on sick leave due to back pain. Physical Therapy 71: 283–293
In a prospective and controlled study persons with a short-term sick leave were randomized between an exercise group and a control group. The persons were allowed to take part in a physical exercise program 1 hour a week for 1½ years during paid working hours, and had to be willing to exercise at least once a week outside working hours for the same period of time. In the exercise group the number of episodes of back pain and the number of sick leave days attributable to back pain decreased by more than 50% in the intervention period, whereas absenteeism attributable to back pain increased in the control group. The paper includes suggestions for physical exercise programmes.

Klingenstierna U 1991 Back schools : a review. Critical Reviews in Physical and Rehabilitation Medicine 3: 155–171
The concept 'back school' was first used by a Swedish physiotherapist, the back school being an educational programme for persons with low-back pain (LBP) aiming at improving the ability to cope with back pain, to improve self-confidence, and to lower the costs to society. The article focuses on controlled studies, and deals with 3 categories depending on the treated population: programmes dealing with acute LBP, chronic LBP and prevention. This critical look at the efficacy of back schools shows considerable variation in programme content, inclusion criteria, number of sessions, amount of time spent, evaluation techniques, compliance and follow-up. To date there is no conclusive evidence that back schools are effective in the treatment of LBP.

Koes B W, Bouter L M, van der Heijden G J M G, Knipschild P G 1991 Physiotherapy exercises and back pain: a blinded review. British Medical Journal 302: 1572–1576
Computer aided search of published papers during 1966–90 was conducted (key-words: backache, musculoskeletal diseases, joint diseases, spinal diseases, physical therapy, evaluation studies, out-come, process assessment). Only randomized clinical trials were considered, only exercise therapy provided by physiotherapists, and not group training. Blinded assessments were performed according to 4 main categories: study population, interventions, measurement of effect, data presentation and analysis. Only 4 studies scored more than 50 points (maximum 100). No conclusion can be drawn about whether exercise therapy is better than other conservative treatments for back pain, or whether a specific type of exercise is more effective. Further trials are needed in which greater attention is paid to methodology of study.

LeBlanc F E (ed) 1987 Scientific approach to the assessment and management of activity-related spinal disorders. A monograph for clinicians. Report of the Quebec task force on spinal disorders. Spine 12: (S1–S59)
This is an abridged version of a consensus conference on spinal disorders, published originally in French. The report gives an overview on the problem, costs, terminology, approaches, magnitude, diagnosis, treatment, management guidelines, and recommendations. It is imperative to develop studies into the sensitivity, specificity and predictability of clinical diagnostic methods. Clinicians should identify, as early as possible, factors likely to lead to chronic distress and chronic functional disability. There is a pressing need to improve the mechanisms by which the various therapeutic modalities should be identified and evaluated. There is no single research priority that deserves

unique and special attention. No particular solution could be expected to rectify the whole problem.

Ljunggren A E, Eldevik O P 1986 Autotraction in lumbar disc herniaton with CT examination before and after treatment, showing no change in appearance of the herniated tissue. Journal of Oslo City Hospital 36: 87–91
Fifteen hospitalized patients who were candidates for lumbar disc surgery, were examined by computed tomography (CT) before and after one week of autotraction therapy. Seven patients had to be operated, whereas complete or considerable reduction of clinical signs and symptoms was registered in 8 patients. CT did not show change in size, shape or position of the prolapse in any patient shortly after the traction or after 3 months in 4 of the unoperated cases. The reason for clinical improvement after traction in some patients is still a matter of conjecture.

Ljunggren A E 1991 Discriminant validity of pain modalities and other sensory phenomena in patients with lumbar herniated intervertebral discs versus lumbar spinal stenosis. Neuro-Orthopedics 11: 91–99
The importance of somato-sensory pain description in the discrimination between two different causes of lumbago-sciatica (herniated intervertebral discs and spinal stenosis) was evaluated. Three groups of pain descriptions have diagnostic potential: localization of pain (bilateral pain in stenosis); quality of pain (in herniation, gluteal punctate pressure, a taut feeling in the back of the thigh and calf and constrictive calf pressure; and in stenosis, aching pain); and the variation in time of both localization and its quality (patients with stenosis gradually develop pain and they can get pain relief when assuming a subjectively suitable position).

Sikorski J M 1985 A rationalized approach to physiotherapy for low-back pain. Spine 10: 571–579
A systematic approach to treatment of low-back pain is presented that relies on classification of patients according to their symptoms: non-spinal, non-mechanical, acute mechanical, chronic anterior element, chronic posterior element, chronic movement-related, chronic unclassified. Rational systems of physiotherapy are proposed for each group, and these have been incorporated into an algorithm. Patients were offered education, exercise, spinal manipulation, back supports and analgesics. The response to treatment was assessed by a postal questionnaire. The most effective treatment was education, followed closely by an exercise programme (benefit claimed by 69 and 64%, respectively). The responses were different in the various subgroups, and a series of flow charts is presented as a basis for further evaluations.

INDEX